CLINICAL DELEGATION SKILLS

A Handbook for Professional Practice

D0484774

CLINICAL DELEGATION SKILLS

A Handbook for Professional Practice

FOURTH EDITION

Ruth I. Hansten, PhD, RN, MBA, FACHE
Principal Consultant
Hansten Healthcare PLLC
Port Ludlow, Washington

Marilynn Jackson, PhD, RN, CCA, CHTP
Intuitive Options
Ontario, Oregon

JONES AND BARTLETT PUBLISHERS
Sudbury, Massachusetts
BOSTON   TORONTO   LONDON   SINGAPORE

World Headquarters
Jones and Bartlett Publishers
40 Tall Pine Drive
Sudbury, MA 01776
978-443-5000
info@jbpub.com
www.jbpub.com

Jones and Bartlett Publishers
Canada
6339 Ormindale Way
Mississauga, Ontario L5V 1J2
Canada

Jones and Bartlett Publishers
International
Barb House, Barb Mews
London W6 7PA
United Kingdom

Jones and Bartlett's books and products are available through most bookstores and online booksellers. To contact Jones and Bartlett Publishers directly, call 800-832-0034, fax 978-443-8000, or visit our website, www.jbpub.com.

Substantial discounts on bulk quantities of Jones and Bartlett's publications are available to corporations, professional associations, and other qualified organizations. For details and specific discount information, contact the special sales department at Jones and Bartlett via the above contact information or send an email to specialsales@jbpub.com.

Copyright © 2009 by Jones and Bartlett Publishers, LLC

All rights reserved. No part of the material protected by this copyright may be reproduced or utilized in any form, electronic or mechanical, including photocopying, recording, or by any information storage and retrieval system, without written permission from the copyright owner.

The authors, editor, and publisher have made every effort to provide accurate information. However, they are not responsible for errors, omissions, or for any outcomes related to the use of the contents of this book and take no responsibility for the use of the products and procedures described. Treatments and side effects described in this book may not be applicable to all people; likewise, some people may require a dose or experience a side effect that is not described herein. Drugs and medical devices are discussed that may have limited availability controlled by the Food and Drug Administration (FDA) for use only in a research study or clinical trial. Research, clinical practice, and government regulations often change the accepted standard in this field. When consideration is being given to use of any drug in the clinical setting, the health care provider or reader is responsible for determining FDA status of the drug, reading the package insert, and reviewing prescribing information for the most up-to-date recommendations on dose, precautions, and contraindications, and determining the appropriate usage for the product. This is especially important in the case of drugs that are new or seldom used.

Production Credits
Publisher: Kevin Sullivan
Acquisitions Editor: Emily Ekle
Acquisitions Editor: Amy Sibley
Associate Editor: Patricia Donnelly
Editorial Assistant: Rachel Shuster
Associate Production Editor: Amanda Clerkin
Associate Marketing Manager: Rebecca Wasley
Manufacturing and Inventory Control Supervisor: Amy Bacus
Text Design and Composition: Shawn Girsberger
Cover Design: Brian Moore
Cover Image Credit: © SSilver/Shutterstock, Inc.
Printing and Binding: Malloy, Inc.
Cover Printing: Malloy, Inc.

Library of Congress Cataloging-in-Publication Data
Hansten, Ruth I.
  Clinical delegation skills : a handbook for professional practice / Ruth I. Hansten and Marilynn Jackson. -- 4th ed.
    p. ; cm.
  Includes bibliographical references and index.
  ISBN-13: 978-0-7637-5579-9 (alk. paper)
  ISBN-10: 0-7637-5579-6 (alk. paper)
  1. Nursing services--Personnel management. 2. Delegation of authority. 3. Differentiated nursing practice. I. Jackson, Marilynn. II. Title.
  [DNLM: 1. Nursing, Supervisory--organization & administration. 2. Decision Making. 3. Nursing Services--organization & administration. 4. Personnel Management. WY 105 H251c 2009]
  RT89.3.H36 2009
  362.17'3068--dc22
                    2008032926

6048

Printed in the United States of America
12 11 10 09 08   10 9 8 7 6 5 4 3 2 1

Contents

About the Authors

We began this journey of delegation and professional development after years of clinical experience in diverse healthcare arenas, from public health and visiting nursing, ICU, CCU, medical surgical, PACU, OR, to educator, and supervisory roles. You might wonder if we could keep a job, but we would reframe this experience with the fact that we were both preparing for our future work as healthcare consultants and educators. Both BSN graduates of the University of Northern Colorado, we pursued different advanced educational courses. Ruth completed her MBA in Health Care Administration in Seattle, while Marilynn received her MA in Organizational Development and Human Behavior at the University of Phoenix. Kennedy Western University provided the venue for doctoral studies, with Ruth completing a PhD in Healthcare Administration, and Marilynn receiving her doctorate in Business Psychology.

As part of our consulting work, we have written numerous articles addressing outcomes-based care, critical thinking, teamwork, and, of course, delegation. Our roles as national consultants, seminar leaders, and speakers provided us with abundant opportunities to work with those who care for others and to continue our efforts to develop both personal and professional excellence with all those we served.

As time has moved on and the fourth edition of the delegation text is written, we both offer consulting services, continuing to emphasize delegation skills training, support of outcomes-based care, improving care delivery systems, and critical thinking. For more information regarding our workshops and consulting options, contact:

Ruth I. Hansten, PhD, RN, MBA, FACHE
Principal Consultant
Hansten Healthcare PLLC
101 Merridith St.
Port Ludlow, WA 98365
Telephone: (360) 437-8060
Fax: (360) 437-8070
www.Hansten.com
www.HanstenRROHC.com
Ruth@hansten.com

Marilynn Jackson, PhD, RN, CCA, CHTP
Intuitive Options: Restoring Balance and Harmony Energetically
Healing Practitioner
855 SW 3rd St.
Ontario, OR 97914
www.intuitiveoptions.com
mj@intuitiveoptions.com

Contributors

Karen Haase-Herrick, MN, RN
Northwest Organization of Nurse Executives
Seattle, Washington
Presently, Consultant, Edmonds, Washington

Karen A. McGrath, RN
Former Associate Executive Director
Washington State Nurses Association
Seattle, Washington

Loretta O'Neill, MN, RN
Director of Nursing
Manorcare Health Services
Lebanon, Pennsylvania

Acknowledgments

We express continued appreciation for the support and involvement of Karen Haase-Herrick, MN, RN, past Executive Director of the Northwest Organization of Nurse Executives and 2004 President of the American Organization of Nurse Executives. Her leadership and vision for nursing has inspired many to continue their commitment to nursing and the health of their communities. We also applaud the continued contribution of Loretta O'Neill, MN, RN, whose expertise with assertive communication and training techniques has been a model for us. The first edition of this handbook, granted the AJN Book of the Year Award in 1994, was developed partially from the combined efforts of a group of creative nurse executives across the state of Washington, including Loretta O'Neill and Karen Haase-Herrick, as we strove to meet the needs of groups of nurses learning for the first time to delegate to unlicensed assistive personnel.

Numerous other individuals have contributed to the book in so many ways! We appreciate so much their generosity and their legacy to nursing! We thank Karen McGrath, RN, for her considerable expertise in the area of collective bargaining and her contribution to Chapter 4; Dennis Burnside, who in the early stages of computerized graphic design, used his creativity, patience, and impressive ability to give life to our ideas—he designed the original key logo; Randall DeJong, MSN, RN, CCRN, another visual talent who shared his pictorial care pathways; Donna Fabian who was helpful in sharing her patient care experiences in updating the text; Virginia Kenyon for her work on the companion edition, *Home Care Nursing Delegation Skills*, and her significant ongoing contribution to patient care; Margaret Conger, RN, EdD, for her work in delegation decision making; Rosalinda Alfaro-LeFevre, MSN, RN, the grand dame of critical thinking in nursing, for continued generosity in sharing her research and the critical thinking indicators, and especially for her practical, down-to-earth approach to realities in nursing; Gayle Garland, RN, C, MSN, CNA, for her tool on assessing nurses' advancement from novice to expert; Pat Auracher for the use of the decision-making model from Columbia Swedish Medical Center in Englewood, Colorado; the Washington State Department of Health and Human Services, and Kay Kramer-Sievers and the State Unit on Aging for discussing the process of developing and revising nurse delegation documentation in community settings; Rosemary Gahl of the National Council of State Boards of Nursing for her immediate timely responses and continued support in keeping us updated; and Anne DeWitt for the opportunity to guide nurses in creating a living philosophy at University of Texas Health Center in Tyler, Texas.

A heartfelt note of gratitude from Marilynn to the numerous friends, family members, and clients who have continued to enrich her journey, adding meaning and possibilities with each encounter. The love and energy shared by everyone is the backbone of this text, setting the highest intentions for the growth and enrichment of a profession based on the intimacy of caring.

And finally, Ruth would like to thank her wonderful family, her husband Phil, her five children and three grandchildren, for their ongoing love and support through challenging times and "growth" adventures. Snakey Boy and Yoda were especially inspirational when they would offer their prey, including dead rodents, as gifts. And most of all, a heartfelt Hurrah! to the nurses and other healthcare professionals who have been involved in Hansten Healthcare's Relationship & Results Oriented Healthcare™ certification program and have offered advice about changes in the book. I appreciate your commitment to making a positive difference in the lives of those you serve with your gift of presence.

The Overall Process of Delegation

Ruth I. Hansten and Marilynn Jackson

CHAPTER SKILLS

+ Define delegation.
+ Review a model for delegation that parallels the nursing process.
+ Describe the purpose of perfecting delegation and supervision skills as an integral part of professional practice.

RECOMMENDED RESOURCES

▶ Visit the National Council of Boards of Nursing Web site and search the keyword "delegation": www.ncsbn.org.
▶ Review the relationship of good teamwork and communication and patient safety by visiting the World Health Organization's Nine Patient Safety Solutions at www.who.int/mediacentre/news/releases/2007/pr22/en/index.html.
▶ Read one of the articles listed in the references to understand the evidence behind excellence in professional practice and delegation.

"All this talk about delegation—we seem to be going in circles. First you're by yourself, then you're in a team trying to do everything with everybody else, then primary nursing came along, now there's another nursing shortage and every plan flies out the window. Nursing assistants come and go depending on what the budget looks like. Why should I bother to learn about delegation? Tomorrow it will be something different anyway."

There's no doubt about it; nursing has tried on many different styles of delivering care and no doubt will continue to do so in the future. But it is apparent to us that we must better understand how to work with other members of the healthcare team to provide the safest and most effective care to our patients. If nurses are to assume their rightful position as coordinators of care, systematically implementing the holistic approach that is the foundation of our profession, then we must be certain of the process necessary for this coordination.

THE DEFINITION

Just as a surgeon establishes anatomical boundaries before he or she operates, we need to establish boundaries, in the form of a definition, when delegating to other personnel. We cite the operational definition adopted by the National Council of State Boards of Nursing beginning in 1990 (1990, p. 1) in their Concept Paper on Delegation and will use this as the basis of our discussion throughout the book: "Transferring to a competent individual the authority to perform a selected nursing task in a selected situation." This definition has stood the test of time, becoming a part of the Concepts and Decision-Making Process National Council Position Paper of 1995–1996. It is currently found on their Web site (www.ncsbn.org) in the practice and discipline section and is the cornerstone of the delegation glossary (National Council of State Boards of Nursing, 1997). It is important to note the generic approach of this definition, which makes it timeless while allowing the practicing nurse a great deal of freedom in selecting the task and the individual to perform that task. As we will note in some detail in future chapters, the primary ingredient of this concept is that the nurse ensures the competency of the individual to whom he or she is delegating. To some, this is an added dimension of responsibility—and one that is not always willingly adopted. The challenges for nurses in this area are apparent because many do not feel they are adequately prepared to teach individuals to perform tasks that have been a part of their own scope of practice. Further, many nurses do not welcome the added responsibility of assessing competency of teammates. This has become a significant issue for our regulatory agencies and will be discussed at length in Chapter 3.

This book will assist in developing that skill by applying a process that is very familiar to all of us: the nursing process. By following the four major steps of the nursing process, we can systematically analyze what is necessary for any practicing professional nurse to know in order to develop a skill that will be a fundamental of practice.

Delegation: "Transferring to a competent individual authority to perform a selected nursing task in a selected situation."

THE MODEL: THE KEY TO DELEGATION

The activities of delegation, like those of the nursing process itself, are cyclical, beginning with a gathering of data, continuing with the utilization of those data as plans are made and carried out, and concluding with the analysis of the activity; the cycle then repeats itself. We have developed a key model that illustrates this process (**Figure 1–1**) and will refer to the sequence of events often to make our point that this is not a singular process. The ongoing cycle of events will be the result of your ability to connect one component with the other until you have an integrated skill that allows you to perform many of the fundamentals concurrently. We will isolate each step for the purpose of our study and allow you to focus your attention on the areas of the process in which you determine you need the most skill building.

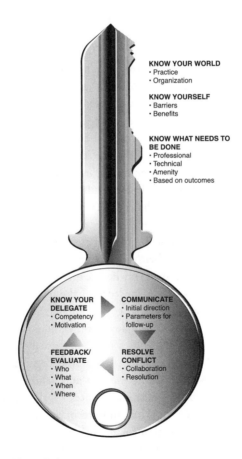

FIGURE 1–1 The Key to Delegation

Assessment

- ✦ Know Your World
- ✦ Know Your Organization
- ✦ Know Your Practice
- ✦ Know Yourself
- ✦ Know Your Delegate

A foundation must be laid upon which to build the decision making that is implied in the concept of delegation. Selecting the right task for the right individual sounds a little like the job of the human resources manager and is foreign to many of us. We must do a certain amount of assessment, as we would in any situation in which we were determining the best course of action for the patient.

Assessment implies knowledge: the interpretation of information to provide an overview of the total picture of factors that affect the current condition. Such a review will help us to understand how best to respond and to plan for the future of health care. To "know your world" in terms of demographics, economics, and social changes will be essential in understanding why we are pursuing a skill that some believe is outside the domain of our profession. Analyzing these factors will help us to prepare for changes ahead and to position nursing as a profession to lead the way instead of following a path determined by others as a reaction to the healthcare reform movements of the last century.

Knowledge of the nurse practice act, including the numerous regulatory changes that are being made as a result of the changes in care delivery systems, cannot be overemphasized. The responses of the individual boards of nursing, as they strive to protect the public by setting up ground rules for the changes in nursing personnel, have been significant. Many nurses feel at risk, voicing their concerns in the heartfelt statement, "I'm not putting my license on the line to work with those people!" Knowledge of the practice act, the statutes and rules that govern nursing practice, and the policies of the employing institution will help the nurse to allay those fears and to practice more professionally.

> Assessment implies knowledge: the interpretation of information to provide an overview of the total picture of factors that are affecting the current condition.

> Many nurses feel at risk, voicing their concerns in the heartfelt statement, "I'm not putting my license on the line!"

The knowledge of the organization in which we work, its mission and values, will help nurses to assess the attributes of their environment in terms of its support of nursing practice. What is the plan for quality? What are the policies for working with other personnel? Is nursing directly involved with the decision making regarding the changes in care delivery systems, whether they occur in a community setting or in the acute care arena? Is this organization on the journey to Magnet status, a national benchmark for nursing excellence? Answers to such questions will prepare the nurse for the decisions to be made regarding how he or she practices and delegates clinically.

> There is no substitute for attitude, which will make all the difference in how successful you are in your practice with others.

Knowledge of our own attitudes and beliefs is an area that each of us must explore if we are to fully develop the skill of delegation; reflection is a basic critical thinking skill. What personal barriers make it difficult for me to work with someone else? What do I do best that makes working with others the most reasonable choice? And what benefits can I get from this whole thing, anyway? Often we find that nurses know the fundamentals of delegation and appreciate the principles, but they just aren't buying it. There is no substitute for attitude, which will make all the difference in how successful you are in your practice with others.

Speaking of others, it is also necessary to assess the delegates. Who are these people that you are being asked to share your practice with? Individuals with gifts and challenges like the rest of us, delegates have their own strengths, weaknesses, preferences, motivations, and cultural backgrounds. Because the basic tenet of safe delegation is the assurance of the competency of the delegate, a careful assessment of this individual is an absolute necessity. We will ask you to refocus your thinking, however, by first emphasizing the strengths of your delegate and optimizing the resources you have available, rather than focusing on all of the tasks she or he cannot do. We will ask you to examine these areas of weakness as potential growth areas and to determine what can be done to overcome an apparent inability to perform a procedure—is more teaching necessary, or is this task truly beyond the scope of the individual?

Having completed an assessment of the external environment, the internal environment (that's you), and the delegates with whom you are asked to work, you are ready to proceed to the next step of the cycle. The foundation of knowledge you have developed in your assessment will allow you to plan the best use of resources and coordinate a high-performance team.

Plan

+ Know What Needs To Be Done

The first step in planning involves gathering the knowledge of what needs to be done. You have some latitude here: As a practicing professional

For many of you, thinking in terms of outcomes will be an uncomfortable experience, and you will seek to return to the comfort of a task list, which quantifies the amount of "work" you have done and certainly gives a sense of accomplishment.

coordinating a plan of care, you are in the position to prioritize which outcomes are the most important to attain. Notice that we are talking about outcomes; we will continue to ask you to focus your attention in this direction. Before you can plan anything or determine who will carry out the plan, you must think in terms of outcomes, the goals that your patient and you want to achieve from this experience.

Often tasks are done for the sake of getting work done and clocking out on time, and very little thought is spent on the analysis of what the performance of these tasks contributes to the patient and family's bottom line or outcomes (and we don't mean budgets!).

In Chapter 6, we will look at a model of nursing that divides our work into three areas of focus: the professional, the technical, and the amenities aspects of nursing care. From this "PTA model" we will be able to determine the emphasis of our care and those parts of our practice that can be performed by others.

Intervene

+ Prioritize and Match the Job to the Delegate
+ Know How To Communicate
+ Know How To Resolve Conflict

Continuing our cycle, we arrive at the point where the majority of delegation takes place. Procedures and tasks can be taught to unlicensed personnel, but the critical components of the remainder of the nursing process rely on the knowledge and experience of a professional licensed nurse. Herein lies one of our greatest challenges, for we are faced with the need to determine which parts of our practice to let go of, and we often find that some of those direct care tasks might be what we have found the most personally satisfying. Once again, according to the operational definition of delegation, the registered nurse (RN) is selecting the tasks and the appropriate situation in which to delegate. Matching the job to the delegate then becomes a decision we can control, and we must continue to make the choice wisely, based on sound judgment. Numerous studies have demonstrated that the nurse spends considerable

Although we might strongly voice our concerns about the quality of care when someone else is performing the task, we must assume control of the decision and make the best choice by mastering the skill of delegation and directing the process.

time performing tasks that can more easily and efficiently be done by someone else. We owe it to ourselves and to our patients to free up this time so that we can do what we were educated to do.

> Knowing when to take the lead and assuming a calm but assertive stance will assist you in clarifying what work is to be done and by whom.

Working successfully with others requires communication. This skill is one we perform quite readily in interactions with our patients; we need to transfer that skill to the directing and supervising of our delegates. Clearly outlining expectations, giving complete and concise directions for implementation, and providing parameters for following up with the nurse are essential ingredients to successful communication. Being able to be assertive without being aggressive when the response is not the eager and willing "yes" that we would like is also part of the skill of effective delegation.

We have implied that the response given by the delegate might not be enthusiastic, and indeed it might be an absolute refusal. Knowing how to resolve conflict when the members of the healthcare team do not agree is fundamental to a successful working relationship. Passivity and a strong desire to avoid conflict will not lead to the desired outcome of a high-performing partnership with your delegates.

Evaluate

- ◆ Know How To Give Feedback
- ◆ Evaluate and Problem Solve

The final step of the process is one to which we are held accountable by law, yet it is the one area that we do not often find time for and that we willingly shift to management. However, the contract of delegation carries with it the legal expectation that you will be supervising the delegate. Once again, an operational definition is provided by the National Council of State Boards of Nursing (1995, p. 2):

> Supervision: "Provision of guidance or direction, evaluation and follow-up by the licensed nurse for accomplishment of a nursing task delegated to unlicensed assistive personnel."

Evaluation and follow-up of the activity means that you oversee the performance (again, you determine the frequency of this observation) and offer feedback to the delegate in terms of an appraisal of his or her performance. This is certainly part of your obligation to ensure the

> Rules and statutes will tell us that the supervising nurse (that's you any time you delegate) will be held accountable for the correction of any error made by the delegate.

competency of the individual, as well as to close the loop by giving the delegate an evaluation of how things are going.

Whether you choose to pass that on to the manager for resolution or take action yourself by directly discussing the situation with the delegate, corrective action must take place.

Feedback and follow-up can be as simple as a thank you for a job well done or as formal as the documentation of an unusual occurrence accompanied by a lengthy investigation. Whatever the situation calls for, you must be prepared to provide it. Just as you provide a thoughtful appraisal of the patient you have just taught to perform his own central line catheter care, you will need to evaluate the progress of the home health aide who is performing range of motion exercises on an elderly patient with impaired mobility.

THE SKILL

You have probably determined by now that the majority of the components of the delegation process are not new to you. In fact, you perform many of them continually as you plan and implement your care for your patients. What will be required, then, is not the development of new knowledge but the transfer of skills that you have already developed. Assessment of the patient is a skill that you have developed and practiced all of your professional life and is no different in technique when you transfer that attention to the new delegate who arrives at your work setting ready and eager to do his or her job. The teaching that you do with each of your patients requires planning, clear communication, and evaluation to complete the process and is similar to the planning, communication, and evaluation you will do with delegates.

Throughout this book we will focus on fundamentals, offering exercises for you to check your knowledge and to apply any new material. There will be repetition (we warn you) because this is a basic principle of learning. Using this book will help open the door to growth in professional nursing.

CHECKPOINT 1-1

Delegation and supervision skills are related to successful professional practice because

a) our team leadership ability is comprised of complex skills of emotional intelligence, communication, and critical thinking, along with knowing the patient/family.

b) nurses need to be able to use an extra set of eyes and ears in any setting, for observation and reporting on clinical changes.

c) we need to be able to match the patient and family's condition and preferred outcomes with excellent team communication skills and the personalities and abilities of our team members.

d) all of the above

See the end of the chapter for the answers.

CHECKPOINT 1-2

List at least three reasons that an RN should be an expert delegator and supervisor.

See the end of the chapter for the answer.

DELEGATION AS INTEGRAL TO PROFESSIONAL PRACTICE

Delegation and supervision skills are fairly complex because we must match the patient and family's condition and outcomes with excellent team communication skills and triple digit emotional intelligence. Our professional practice as nurses requires integrated critical thinking skills, creating synergy with others' personalities and abilities. A few readers are probably wondering, is all this effort worth it, to perfect our leadership skills as nurses? Although we will tackle details of the evidence driving the necessity of developing our delegation and supervision talents in subsequent chapters of this book, we would like to provide sufficient motivation in this first chapter for you to keep reading this entire book.

+ With the current shortfall of nurses in the United States and internationally, nurses will continue to have to provide care by maximizing the use of their knowledge and expertise by employing the skills of others. The shortage of nurses is expected to grow to 340,000 by 2020, and the over age 65 population will nearly triple between 1980 and 2030, further impacting the caregiver crisis (Runy, 2007).

- Medical errors kill more people in the United States per year than AIDS, breast cancer, and motor vehicle accidents combined, an approximate 200,000 per year (IOM, 2001). Healthcare accrediting agencies, as well as the National Patient Safety Foundation and the World Health Organization, cite the need to improve team communications as essential for providing better patient safety (WHO, 2007). If we don't assign, delegate, communicate, and supervise well, we can compound the number of failures to rescue and other care delivery errors.

- Research about optimal methods of providing patient care abounds. There are no "perfect answers" for care delivery, and experts encourage ongoing patient-centered studies that analyze quality and its correlation to nurse staffing, skill mix, and professional autonomy (Currie, Harvey, West, McKenna, & Keeney, 2005). A study that examined errors or lapses in treatment when unlicensed assistive personnel (UAPs) were involved in the care delivery model showed about 61% of patient care concerns within the care team were related to the UAP not following through with requests or normal departmental procedures. However, the role of the RN was crucial for patient safety and clinical outcomes in fulfilling the leadership roles of delegating and follow-up. Nearly 14% of care lapses were due to the RN not providing optimal direction or delegation and nearly 12.5% were due to inadequate supervision of the delegated tasks (Standing, Anthony, & Hertz, 2001). Another study cited by Kopishke attributed a higher infection rate and increased blood borne central venous catheter infection rates when a lower ratio of RNs to UAPs meant difficulty with RNs providing adequate supervision (Kleinman & Saccomano, 2006, p. 165).

- Care providers are not satisfied with their jobs when teamwork fails. For example, when teamwork was based on building relationships within the team and with the patients and their families, including clear roles and communication, work satisfaction improved 14% (Allen & Vitale-Nolen, 2005).

> Nearly 14% of care lapses were due to the RN not providing optimal direction or delegation and nearly 12.5% were due to inadequate supervision of the delegated tasks (Standing, Anthony, & Hertz, 2001).

- Many nurses are not comfortable with delegation and supervision of assistants. Delegation is sometimes done blindly without envisioning a clear match between a role description and the actual capabilities of a worker. New graduates are focused on organizing their own assignments and express discomfort with asking someone else to help them (Kleinman & Saccomano, 2006). A national survey on the elements of nursing education concluded that delegating tasks to other personnel and supervising care delivery were evaluated as lacking in undergraduate education (NCSBN, 2006). Taking the risk of offering honest feedback to a coworker is difficult and therefore rare. Hierarchical relationships (nurses acting like queens or kings to "serf" assistants), over delegation of work, and RNs' unwillingness to do any tasks that are in the nursing assistant (NA) job role seem to be normal problems with teamwork (Kalisch & Begeny, 2005).

Working toward the goal of sustaining world class teams, the most recent science of team success would recommend that the same skills be developed as we are teaching in this book: face-to-face interaction, clear roles, shared goals, effective ongoing communication, the ability to confront and resolve conflicts, and the process of evaluation and feedback as the team "disengages from action" (Kozlowski & Ilgen, 2007, p. 60).

♦ The delegation process we have outlined in this book follows recommendations from the National Council of State Boards of Nursing and other healthcare organizations as well as our own hard-earned nursing practice experience and decades of consulting with hundreds of hospitals. We also applied recent human performance research. Working toward the goal of sustaining world class teams, the most recent science of team success would recommend that the same skills be developed as we are teaching in this book: face-to-face interaction, clear roles, shared goals, effective ongoing communication, the ability to confront and resolve conflicts, and the process of evaluation and feedback as the team "disengages from action" (Kozlowski & Ilgen, 2007, p. 60).

Following the logical conclusion of these statements, delegation and supervision are scarce but essential nursing skills to provide safe, effective health care within our communities in a future with insufficient RNs to meet the growing needs of an aging population. Few are expert at these leadership abilities. Further, the professional practice of delegation and supervision enables healthcare workers to grow together effectively as team members, affecting healthcare outcomes for patients and

Our goal, our planned outcome for you, is to develop your ability to implement the process of clinical delegation with confidence and completeness so that you have the time to do what you do best.

loved ones as well as nurses' joy in their work. Would it be worth it to you to keep reading and apply the principles to achieve better results and happier patients, families, and healthcare professionals despite a challenging future? We think so! We will try to make the journey enjoyable.

ANSWERS TO CHECKPOINTS

1–1.   d, all of the above

1–2.   The current shortfall of nurses means that nurses will continue to provide care by employing the skills of others. Our ability to delegate and supervise effectively means that we could avoid some of the over 200,000 medical errors per year. When registered nurses are unable to supervise effectively, studies show there is a higher infection rate and increased blood borne central venous catheter infection rates. Job dissatisfaction and turnover of staff occur when team members are not working together well. Recent human performance research shows that the science of team success recommends the skills that are developed in this book: face-to-face interaction, clear roles, shared goals, effective ongoing communication, ability to confront and resolve conflicts, and the process of evaluation and feedback.

REFERENCES

Allen, D., & Vitale-Nolen, R. (2005). Patient care delivery model improves nurse satisfaction. *The Journal of Continuing Education in Nursing, 36*(6), 277–282.

Currie, V., Harvey, G., West, E., McKenna, H., & Keeney, S. (2005). Relationship between quality of care, staffing levels, skill mix, and nurse autonomy: Literature review. *Journal of Advanced Nursing, 51*(1), 73–82.

Institute of Medicine. (2001). *Crossing the quality chasm: A new health system for the 21st century.* Washington, DC: Author.

Kalisch, B., & Begeny, S. (2005). Improving nursing teamwork. *JONA, 35*(12), 550–556.

Kleinman, C., & Saccomano, S. (2006). Registered nurses and unlicensed assistive personnel: An uneasy alliance. *The Journal of Continuing Education in Nursing, 37*(4), 162–170.

Kozlowski, S., & Ilgen, D. (2007, June/July). The science of team success. *Scientific American Mind,* 54–61.

National Council of State Boards of Nursing. (1990). *Concept paper on delegation.* Chicago: Author.

National Council of State Boards of Nursing. (1995, December). *Delegation: Concepts and decision-making process.* Retrieved October 23, 2007, from https://www.ncsbn.org/323.htm

National Council of State Boards of Nursing. (1997). *Glossary–delegation termi-nology.* Retrieved April 14, 2008, from https://www.ncsbn.org/glossary.pdf

National Council of State Boards of Nursing. (2006, July). *NCSBN research brief, executive summary, a national survey on elements of nursing education—Fall 2004,* (24).

Runy, L. (2007). Nurses' satisfaction not guaranteed. *Hospital and Health Networks,* 6(71), 76.

Standing, T., Anthony, M., & Hertz, J. (2001). Nurses' narratives of outcomes after delegation to unlicensed assistive personnel. *Outcomes Management for Nursing Practice,* 5(1), 18–23.

World Health Organization. (2007). *Nine patient safety solutions.* Retrieved July 12, 2007, from http://www.who.int/mediacentre/news/releases/2007/pr22/en/index.html

Know Your World

CHAPTER SKILLS

+ Link together social, economic, cultural, and environmental factors that are driving changes in health care and your nursing practice.
+ Describe the evolution of care delivery models throughout the continuum of health care.
+ Integrate the tools of clinical pathways, case management, and disease management in your professional practice.

RECOMMENDED RESOURCES

▶ Join a reading group at the local library or bookstore.
▶ Read the daily newspaper.
▶ Attend one national/international nursing conference this year.
▶ Discover results obtained from new care delivery models by visiting www.IHI.org (the Institute for Healthcare Improvement) and click on your specialty, or review outcomes at www. hansten. com/rrohc/success.html.

The ancient redwood trees, huge as they are, have a very shallow root system. Yet, they cannot be blown over by the strongest wind. The secret of their stability is the interweaving of each tree's roots with those that stand by it. Thus a vast network of support is formed just beneath the surface. In the wildest of storms these trees hold each other up. (Dawna Markova, PhD)

What in the World Is Going On?
Karen Haase-Herrick

The past three decades have seen unprecedented change in the work world for the registered nurse (RN). Critical pathways; ever-shortening lengths of stay; and terms like disease and demand management, continuum of care, case management, telenursing, and outcomes have become mainstays of conversation. Alternative care providers have "come of age" with the public. Consequently, RNs need to develop their roles in relation to naturopathic therapies, aroma therapy, massage therapy, music therapy, and acupuncture. More and more nursing care is being delivered outside the traditional acute-care hospital. Nurses are becoming more involved in public policy discussions, as evidenced by the increasing numbers running for public office and participating in the processes of local, state, and federal governments.

Perhaps the biggest area of change affecting your RN practice involves the giving of care through others: the delegation of some traditional nursing tasks to others (Blegen, et al., 1992; Porter-O'Grady, 2003a). You are switching from a model of nursing care delivery in which the RN provides all the care to a model in which you delegate to others many of the tasks involved in the care of patients. You are being asked to work on teams or in partnership with another person. You are sometimes being asked to work with caregivers about whom you know nothing and in whom you have little or no trust.

More changes are on the way. The nursing shortage of the early 21st century, along with technology changes, is driving this. Later on in this book, you'll be asked to explore your own personal barriers to the use of clinical delegation skills. To get to a point where you are ready to explore the why and how of clinical delegation for the management of patient care, however, you must first know the world in which you are working and understand the driving forces behind this change. The purpose of this chapter is not to provide you with new information so much as to bring to the forefront of your thinking those environmental factors that are influencing the world in which you work or are about to work. You know that all of these things are happening. What you might not have done up to this point is to link all of them together into an assessment of why you are now in such a period of change in your work life.

> Perhaps the biggest area of change affecting each of you as an RN involves the giving of care through others—the delegation of some traditional nursing tasks to others.

Consider your environment at large. Take a few minutes to think about things that are going on around you. What do you hear in the news? What articles in nursing journals have you read recently about changes in patient care delivery? What programs and systems has your facility initiated over the last five years? How many businesses in your area have laid off employees in the last five years and might now be either rehiring or laying off even more? What is happening to your own healthcare costs? What are you seeing with respect to the length of time patients remain in an acute care facility? What types of patients are you now caring for in the home or in residential long-term care facilities that you did not see 5 or 10 years ago? What about the age of your patients? What about the knowledge level of your patients? What have you and your coworkers said about your workloads over the past 5 years? How many times have you been able to do all the necessary patient and family education prior to discharge, especially when the discharge is from an acute care facility?

Now list at least five things that you think are shaping these changes, things around you in your community, your state, and the country.

1. _____
2. _____
3. _____
4. _____
5. _____

Your list of five things will most likely fit into one or more of the following six categories:

1. influence and memories of past nursing shortages
2. evolution of healthcare payment systems
3. demographic trends
4. healthcare delivery trends
5. changing nature of work
6. evolution of the art and science of nursing practice

INFLUENCE OF NURSE SHORTAGES

In the past, vacancy rates for nursing personnel were cyclical; periods of high vacancy rates were followed by RN layoffs and oversupply. In the

1980s, hospitals across the country reported persistent vacancies; nursing school enrollments dropped. A devastating nursing shortage developed very quickly. Positions were going unfilled for over a year in many rural facilities. And yet patients were in hospitals and needed care. Home care agencies had growing caseloads. Long-term care facilities were full and needed RNs. Public health agencies, schools, and prisons all needed RNs, and schools of nursing had vacant faculty positions. States across the country set up commissions to study the nursing shortage and identify ways to address and resolve the issue.

The American Medical Association proposed the creation of a new job category: the registered care technologist or RCT, a suggestion that sent shock waves through the nursing profession because the RCT was not truly part of the nursing care delivery team.

Otis R. Bowen, secretary of the U.S. Department of Health & Human Services, established the Secretary's Commission on Nursing in December 1987. The commission, which became known as the Bowen Commission, delivered its final report with recommendations in 1988. The Bowen Commission held hearings across the country to hear first-hand from RNs what issues were contributing to the current shortage. The conclusion reached was that the nursing shortage was primarily the result of rapidly escalating demand for RNs. The final report of the Bowen Commission contained 16 specific recommendations that were grouped according to the following issues:

1. Utilization of nursing resources
2. Nurse compensation
3. Healthcare financing
4. Nurse decision making
5. Development of nursing resources
6. Maintenance of nursing resources

Recommendations in the "utilization of nursing resources" category called on employers of nurses to develop innovative models of care delivery that would use scarce RN resources efficiently and effectively (U.S. Department of Health & Human Services, 1988). Meanwhile, back at the site of care delivery, especially for acute care patients, nursing leaders had already begun to develop innovative ways to provide the needed care with the resources available. Nurse managers and staff nurses began talking about new ways to get the job done. Out of this evolved the increased use of clinical delegation. However, the evolution of these innovative care delivery models was shaped by other environmental influences as well.

After months of study, the Pew Health Professions Commission released two reports in 1995 that set the healthcare industry abuzz: "Reforming Health Care Workforce Regulation: Policy Considerations for the 21st Century" and "Critical Challenges: Revitalizing the Health Professions for the Twenty-First Century." The first of these reports recommended broad changes in the regulatory environment for all health professions to increase consumer involvement and create a type of "shared governance" among the state licensing boards of all healthcare professionals (Pew Health Professions Commission, 1995b). This report has stimulated many state governments to look at their regulatory environments and seek ways to better align the licensing processes across all healthcare professions. States have increased consumer membership on licensing boards, and in response to telemedicine and other interstate care modalities, the National Council of State Boards of Nursing issued the report of a task force on interstate licensure that provided the groundwork for a true "interstate license" and formed the basis for a mutual recognition model via an interstate compact agreement. While many states have passed the needed legislation to join the compact, others continue to consider it. In 2001, the model was expanded to include advanced-practice RNs.

The second report focused more on the future of the reformed healthcare system and what needed to be done for future survival in this evolving system. Integrated training across professions, where feasible, was viewed as a key recommendation for all professions, encouraging an interdisciplinary team approach to care. Recommendations specific to nursing related to the need to decrease the numbers of nurses educated at the associate degree or diploma level and increase the numbers of nurses trained at the master's level and above. Central to the concepts that were discussed in this book was this recommendation: "Recover the clinical management role of nursing and recognize it as an increasingly important strength of training and professional practice at all levels" (Pew Health Professions Commission, 1995a, p. vi).

By 1994, the nursing shortage had eased. The advent of healthcare reform discussions in 1993, the growth of multiple cost management strategies by the government and insurers, and the drop in occupancy rates brought on by shortened lengths of stay for patients in acute care facilities triggered staff nurse layoffs. Then,

> The Pew Commission reports recommended review of state regulations for healthcare professionals, integrated training across professions, an increase in the number of nurses prepared at a master's degree or higher, and recovery of the clinical management role of the RN.

as early as 1998, some western states began reporting a growing nursing shortage once again. By 2000, most states reported severe shortages, especially in specialty practice areas and in nursing education faculty.

This shortage is considered to be far more serious and definitely not cyclical because various factors converge in what some have called "the perfect storm" (Buerhaus, Staiger, & Auerbach, 2000a, 2000b, 2000c; Auerbach, Buerhaus, & Staiger, 2000; Staiger, Auerbach, & Buerhaus, 2000). Current forecasts predict a shortage from 340,000 to 400,000 RNs in 2020 (Health Resources and Services Administration, 2002).

EVOLUTION OF HEALTHCARE PAYMENT SYSTEMS

Public debate over health care has resurfaced with the growth in healthcare insurance premiums, the rise in dollars spent on medications, and an economic downturn. The number of uninsured people in the United States has increased from an estimated 34 million in 1993 to an estimated 47 million in 2008, and the uninsured are more likely to have advanced diseases when diagnosed (Dunham, 2008). Although national healthcare reform failed in the early 1990s, the passage of the Kennedy–Kassebaum bill in 1996 and the Children's Initiative in 1997 implemented steps at the national level to address financial access to care for defined, limited populations. Healthcare professionals in all disciplines have been talking for decades about healthcare reform as a means to ensure access to care for all. Business leaders have returned to the discussions since the economic slump began in 2000 with the bursting of the "technology bubble." As health insurance premiums for businesses again began to rise faster than the cost of living in the early 2000s, employers also renewed their search for means to reduce that cost of doing business. Pressure for changes in healthcare reimbursement, including state insurance for all children and plans for national health insurance, have been building.

For a long time, many Americans had thought very little about the cost of health care. They were covered through their place of employment by insurance, paid out of pocket for what little care they could afford, or sought care only in emergencies. In the 1960s, when Medicare was passed, government became a major purchaser of healthcare services for one segment of the American people: the elderly. As this group grew in size, the amount of money paid out by the government for health care increased. At the same time, federal and state governments were paying for additional healthcare services for the poor through the Medicaid program. The number of people served by Medicare continues to grow. In 1970, there were 20.4 million beneficiaries; in 2000, there were 39.9 million. By 2020, that number is expected to increase to 61.5 million (De Lew, 2000). In an effort to hold down the amount of federal money spent for Medicare, prospective payment in the form of diagnosis-related groups (DRGs) was introduced in the early 1980s. Medicaid budgets were also tightened. Consequently, the amount of money the government reimbursed to providers for Medicare and Medicaid patients ceased being equal to the amount the care cost. That reimbursement figure has run from 60 cents for every dollar of costs in 1993 to much lower amounts depending on the organization's case mix, costs, quality, and overhead. (Prospective Payment Assessment Commission, 1993). Following the lead of states such as Minnesota and California and the National Quality Forum, as of October 2008, CMS (Centers for Medicare and Medicaid Services) will not reimburse at all for "never events" such as pressure ulcer, air embolism, blood incompatibility, objects left in the patient after surgery, catheter-associated urinary tract and Staphylococcus aureus septicemia, patient falls with disabling consequences, when death or disability are due to clearly preventable errors (O'Reilly, 2008).

> CMS (Centers for Medicare and Medicaid Services) will not reimburse at all for "never events" such as pressure ulcer, air embolism, blood incompatibility, objects left in the patient after surgery, catheter-associated urinary tract and Staphylococcus aureus septicemia, patient falls with disabling consequences, when death or disability are due to clearly preventable errors (O'Reilly, 2008).

CHECKPOINT 2-1

1. Private insurance and CMS reimbursement is becoming more limited. What are the implications for your practice as an RN?

2. "Never events" are those conditions that are related to healthcare acquired mistakes or inadequate care, and hospitals will not be reimbursed for care when some of these occur. What are the implications for my practice, care delivery models, and delegation skills?

See the end of the chapter for the answers.

The costs of providing the care—salaries, buildings, equipment, and expanding technology—did not go down. All contributed to skyrocketing healthcare costs. Providers had to secure additional revenue to continue to operate. Cost shifting to payers other than the government

Clearly, financial access to health care will remain a public policy concern well into the 21st century.

became the means. The payer other than the government was most often a healthcare insurance plan. Insurance premiums had to rise to cover these increased costs.

Insurance companies have developed innovative ways to curb the growth of premium increases. Managed care, securing discounts from providers, and narrowing the scope of coverage have been tried with varying success. Experimental procedures are seldom covered. There is limited coverage for alternative therapies, although providers still deliver these services, and the cost of delivering the services continues to escalate. In the mid-1990s, healthcare costs to individuals and corporations leveled off. The rate of increase stayed at or below the level of inflation through 1996; however, double digit premium increases averaging 15% to 17% have been the continuing trend for the past decade (Aon, 2007). Employers who provide healthcare insurance for their employees once again see their costs increasing annually, increasing the cost of their products or services. The options for businesses are to hold down the cost of the healthcare insurance benefit, discontinue the benefit, increase the price of their products or services, or allow profits to decline.

In addition, many people over age 50 find themselves caught in a gap. They lose their healthcare coverage when they are laid off or when their spouse dies. They cannot secure new coverage, cannot afford coverage on their own, and are too young for Medicare (Perkins, 1997). The trend in employer-sponsored health insurance is downward. In 1990, 77.7% of American workers were covered; as of 1995, 83.7% were covered. In 1997, 76% of employees in businesses with over 100 employees were covered, and in 2006, 17.0% of people under age 65 (43.3 million) were without health insurance (NCHS, 2007). Clearly, financial access to health care will remain a public policy concern well into the 21st century.

CHECKPOINT 2–2

List the two demographic trends that are influencing the changes in patient care delivery models.

1. _____

2. _____

See the end of the chapter for the answers.

DEMOGRAPHIC TRENDS

The preceding discussion of the driving forces for healthcare payment mentioned several demographic changes that are influencing how we deliver health and wellness care to the American people.

Age

In 1970, 9.5% of our population was over 65 years of age. This percentage increased slowly over three decades so that in 2000, 12% were over 65. However, the forecast for 2020 is that 15.8% of the U.S. population will be over 65 years of age (De Lew, 2000). Put another way, there is a baby boomer turning 50 years old every 7 seconds (Wolf, 2007)! This trend means there will be more people with chronic and debilitating conditions who require more care than ever before. This increased demand for services means increases not only in total healthcare expenditures but in every category: more long-term care, more home care, more support services, more community-based wellness services, more health education services, more alternative therapies, and more training for family members to provide care. In addition, as the baby boomers move into the role of caretaker for frail elderly and aged parents, they are demanding expanded wellness-oriented services for their parents. Continuous care retirement communities, including services for cognitively impaired seniors as well as simple and complex assisted living arrangements, are increasing in numbers, and the need for RNs is increasing with that growth. Moreover, the size of the baby boomer generation far outstrips the size of the next two generations, so, as boomers retire, a nationwide overall worker shortage is highly likely.

Poverty

Anyone who reads a newspaper or listens to national news coverage hears that the number of poor people in this country continues to increase, as has been the case since the so-called Decade of Greed, the 1980s. It is not as necessary to delineate why this is happening as to look at what it means for health care. The poor tend to wait longer to seek healthcare services and are thus sicker when they do come for care, so they end up utilizing more services. They tend to suffer more violent crime, so they end up utilizing more services. They tend to have more children born to mothers with substance abuse problems, so they end up utilizing more services. They tend to avoid engaging in preventive health activities because they don't have the money to pay for such care, they don't know about such measures, and

As in every other facet of their lives, the majority of Americans are becoming more involved in their health status.

they don't have the time to engage in such measures, so they end up utilizing more services. Community-based services jointly developed by community people and healthcare professionals are increasing in an effort to create healthier communities.

Consumer Involvement

Americans are engaging in healthier behaviors with regard to smoking, eating, exercise, and stress management. They are also exploring the use of alternative medicine with increasing zeal. Congress, in 1992, passed benchmark legislation that directed the National Institutes of Health to study the effectiveness of alternative medicine therapies. As consumers increase their involvement in healthcare decisions, they become more involved in the way healthcare services are provided in their communities. They also demand more information about health care so they can make informed decisions, as evidenced by the growing numbers of resources on medical conditions and treatments available on the Internet. All of this increased consumer involvement is driving a need for more health teaching and advocacy services from the healthcare discipline that claims accountability for delivering this aspect of wellness care: professional nursing. Thus the need for services from a relatively stable pool of nurses is increasing.

Value Orientation of the Consumer

The American consumer switched horses in midstream, so to speak, in the early 1990s. Business and news magazines as well as news broadcasts highlight this change quite often. Rather than buy the most expensive item, consumers now want value for the dollar. This doesn't mean they won't spend money for something, but they will spend only to the level necessary to get the value they want. They are demanding that providers of goods and services deliver increasing value at less, or at least at stable, cost. Healthcare providers are facing this consumer demand as much as Rubbermaid, IBM, or any of the auto makers.

Trends in RN Supply

As previously discussed, we are in the midst of a new and different nursing shortage. The average age of RNs is increasing (Buerhaus, 1998). In 1996, the average age of an RN was 44.3; in 2000, it was 45.2 (Spratley, Johnson, Sochalski, Fritz, & Spencer, 2000). Not only are there more older nurses in the workforce, but the average age at graduation from the basic nursing education program is also increasing, which means that the aging of the workforce will not abate in the near future (Spratley, et al., 2000). It also means they will retire from the RN workforce sooner (Buerhaus, et al., 2000a, 2000b).

> The current nurse shortage does not have easy solutions, and it further threatens the economic viability of provider organizations that lack strategic improvements to the workplace environment of health professionals.

Over 80% of the RN population is employed in nursing (Risher & Applebaum, 2002; Spratley, et al., 2000). This is good news. However, it does mean that an effort to bring those who are not currently working back into the workforce is not the answer to the shortage.

Nursing schools, after several years of declining enrollments, have seen their enrollments increase in a trend that continues. AACN (2004) reported that enrollment in entry-level baccalaureate programs increased 10.4% in 2004, although more than 25,000 applications were denied. Schools in the Pacific Northwest, for example, report having two to four times as many qualified applicants as funded student slots. State budgets are so strapped that increased funding for schools of nursing to accommodate the number of applicants is not likely to occur. Consequently, providers are entering into creative agreements with schools of nursing at community colleges and universities to fund additional training slots. In 2004, an AACN survey determined that 32,797 qualified applications to baccalaureate, master's, and doctoral programs were not accepted, and an insufficient number of faculty was cited by 47.8% of responding schools as the major reason for not accepting all qualified applicants (Berlin, Wilsey, & Bednash in AACN, 2005).

Faculty shortages also affect the ability of schools to maintain or increase enrollments. The median age of faculty, 51.2 years in 2002, is even higher than that of the entire RN workforce (Nurses for a Healthier Tomorrow, 2007). In addition, faculty salaries lag behind those in the provider settings, making faculty recruitment very difficult.

Work environments for nurses are stressful and are a source of legislative maneuverings against mandatory overtime and for mandated staffing ratios. Nurses who intended to leave the profession within a year cited 11 factors that influenced their decisions, with the top three including working conditions, salary, and company policies/administration (Borkowski, Amann, Song, & Weiss, 2007). With the coming overall workforce shortage due to baby boomer retirements, we will need to develop new care models that use fewer workers to deliver more services. This means leveraging technology, skill levels, consumer involvement, and family systems support to provide care in the future. That care will be managed overall by RNs. Clearly, this means that professional nurses must continue to develop and refine efficient and effective patient care delivery models that appropriately use all available skill levels of other staff to the extent of their education and critical contributions to the care team.

HEALTHCARE DELIVERY TRENDS

To continue to deliver increasing healthcare services while raising prices as little as possible, providers have been forced to find ever more efficient ways to do so, which leads us to a discussion of environmental factors with which you are intimately familiar. Even without healthcare reform legislation at the federal level, healthcare providers and insurers have created reforms of their own in an effort to deliver services at much lower rates of price increase, at the same cost, or with fewer workers due to shortages across the healthcare workforce. Providers knew that the economy of the United States simply could not sustain the spiraling healthcare costs of the last century.

More and more businesses are offering employees cafeteria options of health maintenance organizations (HMOs), managed care/preferred provider plans, or medical savings accounts for their healthcare insurance coverage, and workers are covering more of their own healthcare expenses as premiums rise. In the managed settings, the need to deliver services at a lower cost than previously thought possible is forcing many providers, especially hospitals, to rethink how they deliver care. Hospitals often must accept significant discounting on their costs to be included in the insurance plans offered by a major employer in a given area. But to be competitive in the eyes of the consumer, providers also must find a way to deliver value. The good news about this is the inclusion of staff personnel in the planning and discussion of how to deliver the same quality care for a lower or stable cost.

Another key trend is the change in the length of stay in acute care facilities. New technologies have enabled the ambulatory care setting and short-stay or niche hospitals to provide more and more services that were previously only available in a hospital. This same growth in technology means that many patients are spared invasive procedures that are usually done in the hospital and are able to go home faster. In addition, management of the costs of care has led to shorter and shorter stays for those patients who still require hospitalization. Clinical roles of both the physician and nurse must change as the patient assumes the locus of control and therapies advance, which require less hospitalization and only a minor disruption of the patient's normal routines (Porter-O'Grady & Malloch, 2007).

Patients still require nonacute care after these shorter stays, and this means that home health care, long-term care, hospice care, and other community-based care will continue to grow. As our population ages, more preventive and community-based services for the elderly will be needed.

> Nurses are learning to work in different ways as case managers—through others and as part of multidisciplinary teams—to provide continuity of care (Sherer, Anderson, & Lumsdon, 1993). The growth in nursing jobs will come not in acute care but in community-based nursing, case management, and advanced practice nursing.

CHANGING NATURE OF WORK

This chapter started with a picture of rapid change in the work environment in the world today. Now it is time to put it in the context of your work world in health care. The 1990 to 1991 recession with its cuts in defense spending brought about an increase in unemployment across the country. Then, with the bursting of the technology bubble in 2000, an economic downturn again hit the United States. Job growth is at a standstill. Managers and professionals are losing jobs at a rate that has alarmed even the most previously secure healthcare professionals. Job security now seems to be a thing of the past in all sectors of the economy in America. This bad news comes as companies and organizations flatten their structures in an attempt to get rid of the hierarchy. At the same time, mergers and acquisitions are occurring across all industries, even health care.

Specific changes are also occurring in health care that are dramatically altering the work world of the nurse. Lengths of stay in acute care hospitals are alarmingly short. One very frustrating consequence of this change is that nursing personnel have less time to get to know their patients. Teaching, discharge planning, and individualizing care are all affected by this shortened time with patients. More procedures are moving to the outpatient setting, and with this shift comes the movement of RN jobs to the outpatient site as well. Tim Porter-O'Grady describes this complex of changes and highlights the meaning for professional nursing

> The traditional boundaries and structures of organizations are being radically altered, and nurses are being challenged daily to use their holistic, systems-focused knowledge base to create the continually changing environment in which they work to provide care for individuals as well as communities.

practice by calling it a switch from an institutional model of work to a mobility model (Porter-O'Grady, 2003a; Porter-O'Grady & Malloch, 2007). Mergers and acquisitions mean that RNs must learn new organizational cultures as well as procedures and structures. Also, many hospitals are closing their doors with consequent loss of jobs, perhaps necessitating a move to a new community in search of a nursing job or a change in type of job within the same community.

All of these changes have strengthened the expectation that all workers will play a more active role in decision making in the organization. (That's the good news!) We call this empowerment, and it might strike fear in the hearts of some who feel ill prepared to make the decisions they are now called upon to make. As early as the eighties, the trend toward empowering staff evidenced itself in nursing departments through shared governance, implementation of quality programs, and the movement toward self-managed units (Wake, 1990).

SAFETY AND BALANCED ASSESSMENTS

Two Institute of Medicine publications, *To Err is Human: Building a Safer Health System* (1999) and *Crossing the Quality Chasm* (2001), began a trend to focus healthcare delivery on patient safety as well as the system needs within health care. Scores of subsequent reports, such as the 2006 report on emergency medicine "Hospital-Based Emergency Care: At the Breaking Point" (IOM, June 2006), continue to highlight healthcare disparities and crises as they emerge, nationally and globally.

CHECKPOINT 2-3

Consider what's good about the trends we have discussed so far in terms of nursing as a profession. Describe two current issues that could have a positive impact on nurses or the future of health care.

1. _____

2. _____

See the end of the chapter for the answers.

The renewed public concern about patient safety stimulated the emergence of The Leapfrog Group (www.leapfroggroup.org) as a critical driver in the quest for enhanced safety in patient care in acute care facilities. The

National Patient Safety Foundation (www.NPSF.org) and consumer-directed care and patient/family advocacy groups have been promoting research and use of technology to avoid errors. Nurses everywhere are involved in their organizations' work to identify system improvements that lead to safe environments not only for patients but also for staff. Technology enhancements for medication administration, patient transport and lifting, and communication are being adopted at rapid rates to achieve these safer environments. Technological advances in equipment, such as patient beds, are in development. These advances will change much of the work of patient care and redefine the tasks nurses do that align with the critical and unique essence of care delivered by RNs.

The gaps in care in the healthcare system highlighted in *Crossing the Quality Chasm* have changed the content of discussions of what the healthcare system should look like in the future. That publication is also helping provider organizations look at themselves with a more systematic view. Balanced scorecard assessments help administration and governing boards look at the organization as a whole system. Out of this has grown an intentional measuring not only of fiscal performance but also of patient and staff satisfaction.

Critical assessments of the drivers of the shortage of personnel in health care, especially the shortage of nurses, have resulted in a renewed interest in creating positive, healthy work environments. There are many measurement tools for work environment appraisals, but the American Nurses Credentialing Center (ANCC) Magnet Recognition Program has captured the attention of many nurses. This interest in positive, healthy work environments has opened doors for staff nurse involvement in shaping the nature of their work world now and into the future.

EVOLUTION OF THE ART AND SCIENCE OF NURSING PRACTICE

This involvement of nurses in creating their new world of work has led to another environmental trend that actually bridges all the other trends: the increased focus on clinical delegation skills for the management of patient care. It has brought about an evolution of the art and science of nursing practice that incorporates and revels in new technologies and ways of delivering care.

Different foci and different environmental factors have influenced this evolutionary development. During the mid-1970s, the focus of nursing was on establishing an identity as a profession. The profession was greatly

Nursing has discovered it is not a lone profession caring for patients while at the same time fine-tuning its understanding of what exactly professional practice means to nurses. The profession is learning respect for the values and perspectives of other professions and for others who might help perform those tasks that constitute the "doing" part of nursing.

influenced by the need for a truly scientific research basis for practice. Primary nursing, interpreted by many to mean that the RN did everything for a patient, was perfect for this phase of development. The search for a unique body of nursing knowledge and the quest for autonomy of practice coalesced in a struggle for identity (Rodgers, 1981).

Now the profession has moved to evidence-based practice. Nursing has a set of values and readily tests them out in the real world. Nurses have come to realize that doing tasks is not the essence of nursing. The nursing process, which requires thinking as well as doing, is part of the profession's set of values, as are holism and systems thinking. The profession is entering another phase of evolution. It is learning to work with others, with new technologies, and in new settings in new ways. In this learning, nursing is growing in understanding its exquisite role in sustaining and supporting the health of individuals and populations. It is increasingly certain of its unique contribution to quality outcomes (Aiken, Clarke, Sloane, Sochalski, & Silber, 2002) and the health of the communities.

In discussing her concept of primary nursing, Marie Manthey stated, "The all-RN staff became very popular. That was never part of the original work nor was that ever a requirement" (Villaire, 1993, p. 102). RNs are able to work with other disciplines and other workers on quality teams and task forces and develop new ways to shape their world of work. They embrace new technology with vigor and in the process redefine what "caring" and "nursing care" will mean in our future world of work.

As the profession evolves further, who knows what changes in practice will develop or what professional practice will come to mean? The vibrancy of the nursing profession's art and science allows it to continue learning and shapes the understanding it will bring to this learning in years to come. All of this means that more change is yet to come in your work world—change that will be shaped by you as professional nurses, based on the needs of patients and communities. Who knows where virtual reality, robotics, and genomic therapy will take nursing? That is your world to know and to create!

CHECKPOINT 2-4

List major trends that are shaping the world in which you work.

1. _____

2. _____

3. _____

4. _____

5. _____

6. _____

See the end of the chapter for the answers.

Nursing's Responses to the Changes
Ruth I. Hansten and Marilynn Jackson

Having discussed many of the factors affecting our practice, we now have a clearer understanding of the challenges facing the profession. Many of us will embrace this time as an opportunity for growth, looking forward to changes with excitement and anticipation. Others of us will approach the demands of the future with trepidation and reluctance, longing for "the good old days" of hospital nursing and job security. The sense that "we're not in Kansas anymore" can be a cause for celebration or sadness, depending on our perspective.

As nurses, we have historically risen to the challenges facing us, from the halls of Florence Nightingale's Scutari filled with wounded soldiers to the streets of New York City lined with homeless to the newly emergent global communicable diseases and the hazards of terrorism. The nurses of today will again rise to meet the realities of the present and future to do what we do best: protect and promote the health of our communities. We have implemented many innovative and creative ideas, realizing the importance of our role in shaping the delivery of care to our patients.

> As nurses, we have always risen to the challenges facing us, and we will continue to do so if we keep in touch with our successes and fight the tendency to succumb to victim behavior.

CHECKPOINT 2-5

List four changes you have observed that nursing has implemented in response to the dynamic environment of health care.

1. _____

2. _____

3. _____

4. _____

See the end of the chapter for the answers.

It's important that we get in touch with our successes, keeping a focus on the positive control that we do have over the direction of our practice. Many of us must fight the tendency to succumb to victim behavior, adopting a "poor me" attitude as organizations, physicians, and government regulations vie to regulate and control nursing practice. Joseph Califano (1993, p. 10), former secretary of Health and Human Services, reminds us of our control:

> But few of us have a greater responsibility or opportunity than the American nurse. Revolutions, like nations, do not drift in a vacuum. They move in a direction. And in the coming years, the opportunity for nurses to help shape the direction of America's healthcare revolution is enormous.

While this statement was written more than a decade ago, we believe that nursing's role in shaping health care is continually evolving. There is no time like now to be involved in the growth of the profession!

Keeping our focus on the positive, your list of the changes nursing has made in response to the dynamic forces (Checkpoint 2-5) might have included some of the following accomplishments that have been implemented by nursing:

+ early discharge planning in acute care settings
+ implementation of clinical pathways and care mapping
+ evaluation of technology
+ health maintenance education
+ increase in home care management and community connections
+ redesign of care delivery systems, including rapid response teams in acute care settings

✦ integration of alternative therapies and a focus on welcoming, healthy physical environments for care

CONTINUAL PLANNING FOR TRANSFER AND DISCHARGE

The previous focus on discharge planning in the acute care setting has shifted to a continual emphasis on planning for the next phase of care throughout the continuum of care. The luxury of time that nurses had in acute care settings in past decades is gone. Gone are the days of lengthy hospitalizations; DRGs and other factors have created a demand for streamlined care. Nurses responded early on by realizing that plans for discharge must begin on the day of admission to any care setting or sooner, when the preadmission data are obtained. New positions have been created in acute and community-based settings, where it is not uncommon to find at least one "discharge planner" on staff, along with many case or care managers, typically RNs.

IMPLEMENTATION OF CLINICAL PATHWAYS

Clinical pathways, or critical paths, came into use in the mid-1980s as an interdisciplinary version of standardized medical orders combined with a tracking tool. These project management aids are based on multidisciplinary input regarding a particular DRG and are used as road maps or guidelines for effective planning and monitoring of patients' progress. The literature reveals numerous reports of studies that demonstrate the effectiveness of these plans in terms of reducing lengths of stay in acute care settings and achieving desired outcomes in a more cost-effective manner (Walter, et al., 2007). These benefits are being sought in other settings as well, and the term "extended-care pathway" is now an integral part of the process. Clinical pathways are also the backbone of case management, a care delivery design that will be discussed later in this chapter. As nursing continues to move the planning process outside the walls of acute care and foster the "seamless approach" to continuous care, we will continue to see clinical pathways adapted to all settings. Managed care networks have developed care management plans that do just that: track a patient in any environment—from home to the primary care provider's office to subacute care, rehabilitation, and back home again. Critical or clinical pathways are an interdisciplinary progress plan based on physician's orders and standardized care, allowing for effective planning and tracking

Critical or clinical pathways are an interdisciplinary progress plan based on physician's orders and standardized care, allowing for effective planning and tracking of the patient's progress.

of the patient's progress. (See Disease Management later in this chapter.) Examples of two versions of clinical pathways, in written and pictorial pathway form, are shown in **Exhibits 2–1 and 2–2**.

There are several important points to remember when using critical paths for patient care planning. The most obvious is that not all patients will fit neatly into a critical path diagnosis, a medical patient with multi-system failure being the first that comes to mind. RNs must always assess the patient as an individual, clearly identifying those nursing diagnoses that fit for that patient, recognizing and dealing with those needs that do not fall into a standard critical path, all the while working in partnership with the patient and his or her family for true family-centered care based on their preferred outcomes. Recall that critical paths were first applied in engineering and construction to assist in project guidance and control and, as they were introduced into health care, were "simple direct timelines that focus on an episode of illness. They are not standards of care nor care plans . . . [but] are at a glance reminders of the predictive (routine) care for a condition or situation" (Carpentino, 1996, p. 6). When a nurse looks only at the critical path as a guide to tasks to be done—without full assessment of the individual patient, planning preferred outcomes with the patient and family and continuing the process by evaluation of the patient's responses to the care—the focus remains on tasks that will get the job done. The patient then becomes a cog in the wheel of his or her progress out the door of the hospital, and the valuable assistance of a critical path becomes a stumbling block to comprehensive, integrated patient care for that patient in all settings.

When critical paths are used in close collaboration with the patient and his or her interdisciplinary care team with the RN providing for individualization of the total plan of care, assessment, and evaluation of the patient's progress toward preferred outcomes, the results are exciting. Improved quality, shorter hospitalization, better pain control and comfort, and better functional ability are some of the documented results (Ireson, 1997; Renholm, Leino-Kilpi, & Suominen, 2002). The message is clear: Use critical paths as guides, but don't substitute them for what nurses do best—assessment, nursing diagnosis, planning, evaluation of the results of interventions—coming full circle to redesigning the plan.

Clinical paths have the following characteristics. They:

+ are a critical guide to track progress and streamline processes in patients whose diagnoses and care can be fairly standardized

EXHIBIT 2–1 Clinical Pathway, Written Form

	Day 1	O	C	Day 2	O	C	Day 3	O	C	Day 4	O	C
Consults	Cardiologist if indicated			Cardiac rehab ————— ^ Nutritional consult ————— ^ Physical therapy consult (if indicated)			Physical therapy consult ————— ^ (if appropriate)					
Tests	EKG ————————— ^ CXR ————————— ^ CBC ————————— ^ SMAC ———————— ^ Mg level U/A PT, PTT (if indicated) Special tests if indicated Cardiac enzymes/ISOs			Echo ———————— ^ MUGA ———————— ^ Mg level—repeat as ^ needed						EKG prn		
Medications	Review medications prior ————— ^ to admission			————————————— ^			Review current meds— give appropriate drug ^ monograph			Review monographs		
Treatment	O₂ (if indicated) ———— ^ Saline plug Monitor Daily weights (fasting) Strict I&O ——————— ^ VS q 4 hours ————— ^			————————————— ^ Daily weights ————— ^ VS q 8 hours ————— ^			————————————— ^ Evaluate monitor as ^ needed ——————— ^ ————————————— ^			————————————— ^ ————————————— ^ ————————————— ^		
Nutrition	Diet (as indicated) Fluid restriction as indicated ^			————————————— ^			Reevaluate diet accord- ^ ing to D/C plan ——— ^			Reinforce D/C diet plan ^		
Activity	Bedrest			Bedrest if indicated Up in chair ————— ^ Bathroom privileges			Ambulate in room Increased activity if ^ appropriate ———— ^			————————————— ^		
Teaching	Orient to unit and routine			CHF teaching initiates			Evaluate specific patient ^ needs ——————— ^			————————————— ^		
Discharge Planning	Case Management/ Social Services/Home Health			Assess and implement discharge planning needs			Evaluate discharge needs					
Variance												

EXHIBIT 2-1 Clinical Pathway, Written Form (continued)

	Day 5	O	C	Day 6	O	C	Day 7	O	C	
Consults										
Tests	EKG prn									
Medications	Reinforce medication teaching			Reevaluate discharge medication plans Appropriate monograph Complete appropriate wallet cards			Review medication plans			
Treatment	VS q 8 hours O₂ as indicated Daily weight (?) D/C monitor (if indicated)			Evaluate O₂ as needed						
Nutrition	Reinforce D/C diet plan			Evaluate and reinforce discharge diet						
Activity	Increased activity									
Teaching	Evaluate specific patient needs			Review all discharge plans						
Discharge Planning	Referral to community resources									
Variance										

EXPECTED OUTCOMES
1. The patient can expect to _____ date   O = Ordered
2. The patient can expect to _____ date   C = Completed
3. The patient can expect to _____ date

Courtesy of Harbor Hospital Center, Baltimore, Maryland.

Source: Courtesy of Harbor Hospital Center, Baltimore, Maryland.

EXHIBIT 2-2 Clinical Pathways Pictorial Form

Total Knee Joint	Preadmission Visit Date:___	ADMISSION Date:___	DAY #2 Date:___	DAY #3 Date:___	DAY #4 Date:___	DAY #5 Date:___	DAY #6 Date:___
NUTRITION		Nothing					
ACTIVITY	Walking	Exercises Dangling	Chair 5-25'	25-75'	100+'	100+'	100-400'
EQUIPMENT	—	CATHETER DRAIN IMMOBILIZER PASSIVE MOTION	CATHETER DRAIN IMMOBILIZER PASSIVE MOTION	IMMOBILIZER PASSIVE MOTION	IMMOBILIZER PASSIVE MOTION		
PAIN CONTROL & OTHER MEDS	Discussed	IV	IV to Pills	Pills			
DISCHARGE PLAN	Order Equipment	Discharge plan discussed	Discharge plan finalized				

Adapted from Randall DeJong. © 1993, Providence Hospital, Everett, Washington.

+ tend to decrease length of stay and improve resource utilization
+ tend to improve patient and family understanding of the patient's illness and allow for greater patient participation
+ are a useful tool to improve communication among the healthcare team members and the patient and his or her family

Critical paths are not:

+ a substitute for individualized nursing care plans dealing with all the patient's nursing diagnoses and critical problems
+ useful for all patients with many diagnoses and complex care
+ necessary for all patients

Critical Paths for the Caregivers

Care paths for the caregivers have also been developed for nurses and their colleagues during times of stress to remind themselves of the need for self-care. Individualized, specific goals and the steps to achieve the goals include the following:

+ Improve one health habit each week by using stairs instead of an elevator, taking scheduled breaks, and drinking 6–8 glasses of water daily.
+ Restore intershift and interdisciplinary communication by greeting others or listening actively to someone from another discipline or shift.
+ Develop career paths by reading a professional journal or joining a committee or task force.
+ Learn one new stress management technique per week.
+ Develop a new self-image by introducing yourself and articulating your role to patients and families.
+ Support peers by writing a note to someone who did a great job or practicing outcomes-based communication techniques (see Chapter 8).

Care paths transfer skills from quality management processes while using the nursing (scientific) process and are a tool that can be used in personal growth and family life as well as patient care.

TECHNOLOGY EVALUATION

Modernization can be either a blessing or a curse in that we often see new technological breakthroughs result in increased costs and questionable impact on the outcome of patient care. Nurses are positioning themselves on new product committees, evaluating the need for "new and improved" supplies, and participating in the decisions about updating and purchasing equipment. As frontline providers, we are continually evaluating the effectiveness of treatment and monitoring the usage of technology with a watchful eye. Computers at the bedside and handheld data centers are a supportive adjunct to care professionals only when patients are still treated as human beings with unique needs.

We have been at the forefront of the ethical and moral dilemmas created by advanced technology; often it is a nurse who initiates the discussion regarding the plans for the comatose patient on a respirator or the premature infant with irreversible brain damage.

Utilization review nursing has become another specialty for many of us. As we consider how to make health care available to all while we grow our technology in a positive direction, costs and benefits of new technology are being weighed and evaluated more completely than in the days when fee-for-service healthcare plans were common and new gadgets were easily purchased.

Nurses who are approaching retirement share their enthusiasm for new technology such as assistive lifts and other devices to make their work less physically demanding. As healthcare systems strive to coordinate electronic medical records with ambulatory care and all sites across the system so that care is truly seamless, nurses and other professionals can benefit from computerized decision support systems, careful drug interaction screening, and other advances. Computerized physician order entry, scanning of patient identification and name bands for medication administration, use of handheld computers, and other methods of streamlining care and recording of data have been noted to be of benefit for patient safety. Nurses have become "telenurses," and some provide advice, counsel, and triage over the telephone or Internet.

CLIENT ACCOUNTABILITY FOR CARE: HEALTH EDUCATION

Nursing has traditionally focused on the holistic approach to patient care needs, realizing that education is an integral part of patients' abilities to maintain their optimum level of health. As Sister M. Olivia Gowan once wrote:

> Nursing in its broadest sense is an art and a science which involves the whole patient—body, mind, and spirit: promotes his spiritual, mental and physical health, by teaching and by example; stresses

health education and health preservation as well as ministration to the sick (Hansten & Washburn, 1990, p. 11).

Recent changes in the economy of healthcare delivery are now supporting this position as insurance groups reimburse for preventive treatment and the system shifts from the traditional episodic, crisis-driven medical model to a continuum of wellness supported by preventive education. As patients and their families arrive for an appointment with their care provider waving a sheaf of information gleaned from their Internet searches, we have evidence of the advent of patient and family participation in their diagnosis and care.

Relationship- and Family-Centered Care

From the inception of nursing, nurses themselves have understood that the gift of their presence has had a unique impact on healing. Whether it is called patient-focused care, relationship-centered care, or a healing environment, and whether or not the model and vision of treatment includes the family and significant others, these holistic approaches allow nurses to give credence to their need to know the patient and his individual idiosyncrasies. Partnering with the patient within his social structure and environment is nothing new but is certainly fundamental to successful care. What nurses have known instinctively has now been proven by research: An interdisciplinary, holistic approach to healing, with nurses and other care providers being present and in relationship with the patient, involving all those persons who are important in the patient's life, brings better clinical outcomes and ensures greater job satisfaction for those who provide the care.

The Institute for Family-Centered Care's Web site (www.familycenteredcare.org) gives evidence of the following positive results from family-centered care.

+ Patients' physical and emotional health improved, along with better patient satisfaction, better adherence to treatment plans, more appropriate medical decisions, and better health outcomes.
+ One-year studies of former NICU infants and their families show that when the child has developmental delays, family-centered care results in increased satisfaction, decreased maternal depression and stress, and improvement in mother–child feeding interactions.
+ Combined intervention (interdisciplinary care) rather than just pharmaceutical care showed lower levels of distress during invasive procedures.

+ Family-centered care for collaborative rounds with adult cardiac surgery patients, cut the death rate by more than half (4.8% to 2.1%) (Concord Hospital, Concord, New Hampshire).
+ In pediatric emergency rooms using family-centered care, staff members have more positive feelings about their work and exhibit improved job performance, and there is less staff turnover and a reduction in the cost of care.
+ There is evidence of better use of resources, decreased costs, shorter length of stay, and better use of preventive care.
+ With the Newborn Individualized Developmental Care and Assessment Program, NICU patients spent fewer days receiving ventilator support and O2, nipple fed more quickly, and were discharged sooner, with savings of $90,000 to $129,000 (Children's Hospital, Boston).
+ With labor support from a doula, mothers had 56% fewer C sections, 85% less use of epidural anesthesia, and 25% shorter labor than those who did not receive this support.
+ From a risk management standpoint, patients and families do not tend to initiate lawsuits, even when mistakes are made, when there are open and positive relationships.
+ From an error prevention viewpoint, the research shows that patients who are more involved in their care get better clinical results (Institute for Family-Centered Care, 2002).

The Agency for Healthcare Research and Quality refers to preventing worker detachment from the process of error-free patient care (therefore knowledge of, and connection with, the patient) as a component of mistake-proofing patient care (Grout, 2007).

We also know from our research into emotional intelligence, neurobiology, and the impact of our emotions on others that the gift of being truly present and connected with a patient can have such effects as were noted in a recent ICU study. When a comforting person was in attendance, the patient's blood pressure was lowered to a more normotensive reading, and there was a diminished secretion of fatty acids that block arteries. The actual emotions of the nurses affect patient care as well. Cardiac units where the nurses' general mood was depressed had a death rate four times higher than comparable units (Goleman, Boyatzis, & McKee, 2002). As nurses, we will continue to hold tightly to the ability to know and relate to our patients and their community so that care will not only be the most effective and healing for them but also more energizing for us as care providers.

GROWTH OF HOME CARE

When Lillian Wald began the Henry Street Settlement in 1893, she organized a system of delivering nursing care that had been in existence for centuries. Did she realize the distance we would travel in hospital development before returning home? As we complete the circle, we are now seeing an increased trend in home health and community nursing, settings where nursing has always been the predominant provider.

The growth in this area is so significant that overall employment of home health aides (including nursing aides and psychiatric assistants) will grow faster than ever before through 2014, and home health aides are expected to be one of the fastest growing employment categories overall (Bureau of Labor Statistics, 2006–2007). Home care is truly nursing's arena, and as the trend increases, nurses will continue to identify this as a successful response to the patient's changing needs.

REDESIGN OF CARE DELIVERY SYSTEMS

We have repeatedly stated that nursing is responding to the demands of the environment by redesigning or reengineering delivery systems. Let's take a look at the progression of the more predominant systems to better understand where we are today in terms of the organized structure of nursing. Our discussion will begin with the acute care setting and continue through extended care and the community-based network of the future. We encourage you to read the success stories of some organizations who reengineered, restructured, or redesigned in our *Toolbook for Health Care Redesign* (Hansten & Washburn, 1997). We also encourage you to read the extensive in-depth analysis of both traditional and nontraditional models of care published by nursing professors (Lookinland, Tiedeman, & Crosson, 2005; Tiedeman & Lookinland, 2004).

As part of the growing body of evidence regarding nursing's contribution to patient outcomes, researcher Linda Aiken has reported significant findings:

> Mortality rates are 44% lower in hospitals with good working environments, 1:4 nurse/patient ratios and where 60% of nurses have degrees, compared to hospitals with poor environments, 1:8 nurse/patient ratios and where just 20% of nurses have degrees (Analysis, 2005).

The important message here is that no matter what model of care delivery is being used, the factors of work environment, patient ratios, and nursing education have a considerable impact on the outcomes of care. A review of available data has led to the conclusion that three important elements should be considered when looking to future care redesigns: 1) there is evidence that RNs positively affect patient outcomes; 2) assistive personnel can be beneficial in providing care; and 3) outcome success is dependent upon coordination of care over time and clearly established accountabilities (Wolf, 2007).

Team Nursing

Team nursing began as early as the post-World War II period, when the nursing shortage in hospitals called for the creation of licensed practical nurses (LPNs), nurse's aides, and other auxiliary nurses to meet the increased demand for health care. The attempt to organize these workers into cooperative work groups was the beginning of the team nursing concept that was to last throughout the early 1970s. In this model, the RN functioned as the team leader and led a group of LPNs and nursing assistants who cared for a given group of patients. Tasks were differentiated according to skill level, and the work was divided among the team members based on the assignments made by the RN leader. A series of studies commissioned by the American Nurses Association during the 1950s revealed the following conclusions regarding the differentiation of these tasks among a variety of workers (Hughes, et al., 1958, p. 150):

> The practical nurse and the nurse's aide, often spoken of as temporary, are certainly permanent members of the hospital team. The occupational standard of living, if one may call it that, of the professional nurse has risen so much that she is unlikely to wish to have back all her old tasks. Hence, when, if ever, the division of labor in hospital nursing is stabilized, we can be sure it will recognize a variety of ranks of nurse.

TEAM NURSING STRUCTURE

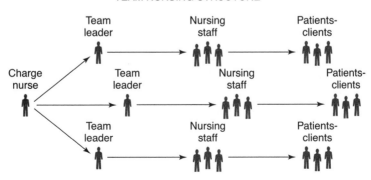

Some form of team nursing has been the norm for decades and continues to be the basis for many of the nontraditional models of care that have been developed in recent years. The configuration of the teams and the scope of practice of the personnel that make up the teams change depending on the qualifications and supply of employees in that geographic area, especially during a patient–care personnel shortage. The benefits of team nursing can be numerous and measurable. One Emergency Department (ED) administrator of an Illinois hospital reports that employee satisfaction increased over 37% after team nursing was implemented. DiMarco attributes the correct skill mix of nurse, technician, unit clerk, and physician, and partnering new nurses with more seasoned ones, as key ingredients in a team's success (DiMarco, 2004).

Functional Nursing

Modifications to the coordinated work groups of team nursing began as adaptations that were needed to meet the various needs of patients. The functional model involves a leader in the form of a charge nurse, with the workload grouped according to the type of tasks to be done. In this system, a medication (med) nurse, a treatment nurse, and nursing assistants provide care according to their functions for the entire population of patients. The med nurse (either an RN or an LPN) is responsible for the administration of medications to all patients within the setting (unit, floor, or section of the facility). The treatment nurse, similar to the med nurse, provides treatments for the entire patient population. The patients are seen throughout their day by a number of care providers, and the care received is segmented.

FUNCTIONAL NURSING STRUCTURE

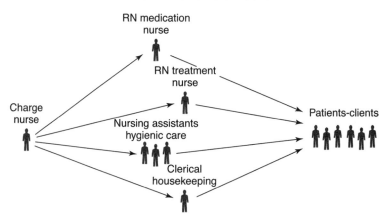

CHECKPOINT 2-6

Have you ever practiced nursing in a team model? If so, what were the similarities to the model described here? Can you identify advantages and disadvantages to this system?

See the end of the chapter for the answers.

This type of system lends itself to areas where patient turnover is less frequent and the patient population is more stable, as in an extended care facility or rehabilitation unit. Unfortunately, care can become segmented. No one focuses on the total picture of the patient except the charge nurse, whose workload generally precludes the attention necessary for coordinating individual care.

TOTAL CARE NURSING STRUCTURE

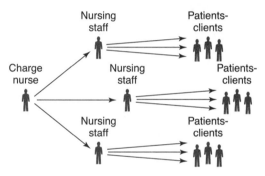

Total Patient Care

Another modification to the team concept developed in the 1970s when many of us had been accustomed to working in teams and had recognized the benefits of nursing assistants. These nursing assistants (and LPNs) were removed from the staff, or at least limited, as many hospitals sought a short-lived benchmark of quality, the all-RN staff. With a charge nurse to lead the way, a staff of only RNs was assigned to provide all of the care needed by a given group of assigned patients. Care was no longer segmented, and the advantages to this system were thought to be that the highest level of worker was always available to the patient—a worker who knew the entire spectrum of needs for that particular patient. The following argument was made:

> In contrast to team nursing and the assignment of less skilled tasks to cheaper categories of wage labor, primary nursing employs labor

power that although more expensive, may also be more productive in that RNs can be assigned to perform a broader range of nursing and nursing-related tasks with little supervision (Chernomas & Chernomas, 1989, p. 642).

This model remains popular in specialty settings such as intensive care units, trauma and emergency care, neonatal care, postanesthesia care, and select ambulatory care settings. Some acute care organizations in the mid- to late 1990s returned to this model and found cost savings due to decreased turnover of assistive personnel and smaller training budgets, with positive results in patient satisfaction surveys. Other organizations have added assistive personnel who are specially trained to work in those areas, such as intensive care aides and emergency medical technicians.

CHECKPOINT 2-7

1. In what ways is functional nursing different from team nursing?

2. If you have had experience working in either system, can you recall:

   a) Who was responsible for documentation of care?

   b) Who interfaced with the other disciplines, such as physicians, physical therapy, and pharmacy?

   c) How the reporting process occurred and by whom?

See the end of the chapter for the answers.

Primary Care

Primary care nursing must be distinguished from "total patient care." The RN is accountable for the patient's care planning throughout the hospitalization but does not have to be the individual who performs all the required tasks.

When Marie Manthey introduced her model of care in 1970, she set out to change the organization of nursing's work. Similar to total patient care, and often confused with it, the original concept of primary nursing "simply means one nurse accepting responsibility for managing the care of a small number of patients" (Villaire, 1993, p. 100). As in the total patient care model, the RN is responsible for meeting all of the needs of the patient, but the responsibility extends beyond the limits of a traditional shift because it is expected that the "primary nurse" will coordinate the plan of care for the entire 24-hour period throughout the entire hospitalization. The patient is able to identify one nurse as his or her "own," thereby limiting confusion and providing a sense of continuity. Many variants of primary nursing sprang up all over the country as nursing units embraced the philosophy and the innovative idea of coordinated care.

There are many arguments to support the value of the primary nursing concept and just as many to refute it. Those of you who have worked in some type of primary care system can well understand both the drawbacks and the advantages. One of the unintentional by-products, we believe, was the unfortunate separation of nursing in yet another arena. The title of associate nurse was created to describe the caregivers who were not the patient's primary nurse, and this title led to some feelings of inferiority and separation that are still present today. Also, the model implied that a nurse should be able to meet or at least plan for all the needs of his or her patients. The idea of being all things to all people became an unreasonable expectation fostered by nursing curricula and management, and it led to reality shock for new graduates and burnout for veteran staffers. Organizational systems, in many instances, could not or would not provide the time and resources needed for this model to work as originally envisioned, and frustration ran high. However, the essence of this model, as described by Manthey, has truly shaped the latest and most responsive care delivery system, case management.

PRIMARY NURSING STRUCTURE

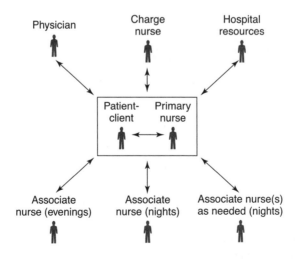

Case Management

The concept of case management involves the determination of what care is needed, when, and by what provider so that patient outcomes can be achieved with the most effective use of time and other resources. Using critical pathways as a guide, the case manager coordinates the services of a multidisciplinary team and may or may not provide direct patient care personally. The impact of this model in acute care settings has been significant: The literature abounds with survey results that demonstrate dramatic decreases in lengths of stay, reduction in utilization of resources, and increased quality of care. The model is still evolving as nursing leaders and other healthcare providers adapt the process in all settings of health care.

CASE MANAGEMENT MODEL

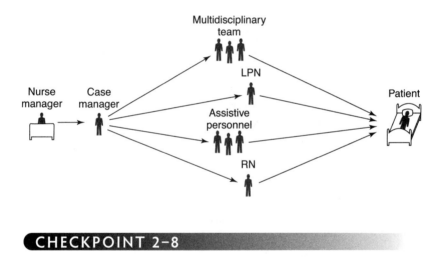

CHECKPOINT 2-8

Describe the major differences between total patient care and primary nursing.

See the end of the chapter for the answers.

One of the most recent models to reflect the evolution of case management into the community, crossing the boundaries of acute care and establishing a more effective "care network" approach, is that of Holy Rosary Medical Center in Oregon. **Figure 2-1** illustrates their approach in a rural environment that is supported by the large corporate structure of Catholic Health Initiatives.

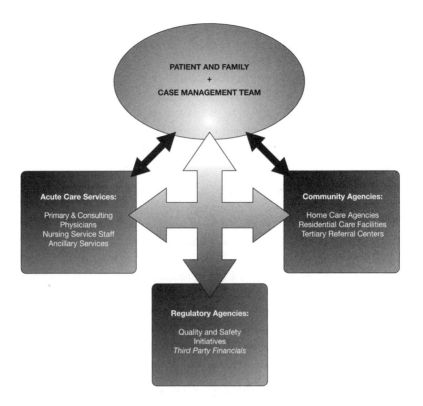

FIGURE 2-1 Holy Rosary Medical Center. Integrated Case Management Network Model. A collaborative team of professional nurses and social workers partnering with patients/families to work with primary/consulting physicians, unit based nursing staff, ancillary service providers (PT, OT, Speech, Pharmacy, Dietary) and community agencies to maximize individualized patient outcomes and create seamless patient transitions into and out of hospital based services, while facilitating compliance with all regulatory, quality and reimbursement standards. Reprinted with permission from Holy Rosary Medical Center, Ontario, OR.

CHECKPOINT 2–9

Which of the following are true descriptions of the case manager role?

a) Coordinates an interdisciplinary approach

b) May or may not provide direct patient care

c) Utilizes clinical pathways to organize care

d) Effectively manages resources

e) All of the above

See the end of the chapter for the answers.

Disease Management

> "Nursing makes a major contribution to clinical outcomes through powerful interventions based on a diagnostic reasoning process, and by making the system work for the physicians and the patients." (Zander, 1988, p. 28).

Blending the strengths of case management and critical pathways with recognition of the managed care requirements for cost-effective care, discrete populations of patients with special needs are managed with improved efficiency and results in disease management. As Karen Zander (1997, p. 85) so aptly describes it:

Disease management employs the concepts of critical pathways and care planning to "conceptually and operationally organize care, essentially care of chronically ill people, to achieve lower costs yet optimal clinical outcomes. Disease management is actually case management on the continuum level, with emphasis on prevention and reduction of the risk of exacerbation, hospitalization, and further functional decline/disability." In all cases, current healthcare leaders are striving to use evidence-based practice to clarify the impact of interventions within specific disease groups, consulting ongoing research results and applying them to care in a timely fashion.

> The emphasis in disease management is on using scientific data and a systems approach, including evaluation of patient clinical outcomes, a holistic picture of the patient's total care, and prevention of avoidable symptoms and debilitation. This begs for nursing involvement.

In the late 1990s, disease management became a potential savior for managed care providers and has been embraced by others as a way to deal effectively with the chronic outliers who consume so much of our healthcare resources. Instead of evaluating a specific hospitalization, disease management looks at the continuum of care for a patient with a given diagnosis in all settings, then it uses the disease as such to measure cost, from diagnosis of the illness to its end stages, which allows for interesting and helpful studies of how best to treat patients for optimal function, satisfaction, and decreased costs. What a natural place for nurses to take leadership!

Care Delivery Systems in Nonacute Settings

As we struggle for meaningful healthcare reform, there have been changes in care delivery systems in virtually every organization along the healthcare continuum. Whereas acute care providers, such as community hospitals, once seemed to set the pace for changes in the care of the ill, now extended care within the home and community has taken a proactive lead in holistic health care of the public. To be able to care, with fewer dollars, for the ever-growing population with temporary or chronic disabilities, these organizations have adapted the actual methods of providing care in creative ways.

Long-Term Care

Many skilled nursing facilities have used a modified functional nursing structure, with an RN leading in care planning and supervision, an LPN or LVN (licensed vocational nurse) giving medications and some treatments, and nursing assistants performing hygienic and activities-of-daily-living tasks. With a new emphasis on rehabilitation of their changing and ever more acutely ill client population, they have developed new roles for the nursing assistants. One such role is that of the restorative aide. These individuals receive additional supervision and training related to range of motion, transfers, and other activities and can work in a team with physical and occupational therapists.

In some states, nursing assistants in long-term care or residential facilities receive additional training to administer oral medications under the supervision of an RN, who evaluates the medication regimen and determines whether the medications should be administered as planned. This function is carefully regulated. Conversations with state board of nursing officials in several states reveal that this practice has been quite effective to date and reflects a trend (see Chapter 3).

Some extended care facilities that use many nursing assistants have developed the role of team leader. These experienced, skilled assistants have exhibited additional leadership potential and are able to help the RN train, mentor, and evaluate the tasks completed by orientees. Because this group of assistants often exhibits a fair amount of turnover, the creation of this position has also become a means to develop and recognize highly competent, tenured employees.

Some facilities have developed a care triad: an RN, LPN (LVN), and certified nursing assistant. This team is assigned a group of patients, and work is divided among them based on their licensure, job descriptions, and their special strengths. In some settings, personnel who were once thought to be "outside" the care team are considered to be valuable members of the treatment team. Consider an Alzheimer's residential

Working together in pairs or larger groups has been very effective in providing care for patients in these facilities. "Bath teams" are able to turn debilitated or frail patients with a minimum of potential for employee back injury. The staff who work together enjoy the teamwork and find that time is saved through working together systematically.

facility and how important it might be for the housekeeper, who often spends a fair amount of time interacting with the patients, to understand current methods of answering questions and directing or helping the residents to their rooms. In other facilities, combining the skills of former environmental services personnel with those of the certified nursing assistant has created a job description for a cross-trained worker who is able to respond to many possible needs. In theory and often in fact, cross training provides the worker with additional job growth and added potential for individual job mobility and provides the manager with more productive workers.

RN-led case management has also been used as a very effective method of providing the highest quality care, using all members of the team, within extended care organizations. Just as acute care must focus on discharge planning and effective use of resources, the RN case manager coordinates the care given in the long-term care facility as he or she organizes the discharge plan and aftercare with the interdisciplinary team from the present care site to the community. Many acute care organizations have established linkages with subacute, ambulatory, home care, and extended care facilities so that one RN case manager oversees the care of a particular patient throughout the continuum.

Assisted Living

Assisted living and various gradations of care provided to the elderly and those with chronic diseases or disabilities, from independent living to skilled nursing facilities and adult family homes, have grown in popularity as our population ages and requires cost-effective care provided in a shielded environment. Considerable variations of models are being developed, and states are responding to the marketplace by developing rules about nurse delegation, definitions of assisted living, and reimbursements for care (Monroe, 2003). Delegation, supervision, and administration of medications in assisted living settings is expected to continue to change dynamically on a state-by-state basis over the next decades as regulatory agencies respond to the glut of baby boomers who require assistance in their activities of daily living.

Home Care

Home care enjoyed a rebirth of interest in the 1980s as hospitals dealt with the realities of the prospective reimbursement system (DRGs: diagnosis-related groups or "Da Revenue's Gone") and began to discharge patients as quickly as possible. The acuity of patients within the home increased along with the number of elderly and acutely or chronically disabled people. This trend fostered the need to intensify the coordination of care that originated in public health programs at the turn of the century. Driven by increasing acuities and diminishing resources, case management has become more sophisticated in the setting where it had its beginnings.

Home health continues to use a multidisciplinary approach to illness care within the home, employing physical, occupational, speech, and respiratory therapists; social service workers; and nutritionists. Psychiatric care is provided by RNs or other mental health therapists. Chores and activities of daily living are provided by homemakers or home health aides. These assistive personnel also can provide transportation, shopping, and other important living maintenance tasks that do not require licensed health professionals. Supervision of unlicensed healthcare assistants has been a long-term reality for home healthcare RNs.

In some states, notably Oregon and Washington, specific regulations have been written to guide RNs in supervision of unlicensed assistive personnel in such settings as adult family homes or homes for the developmentally disabled. In Washington, a study was commissioned to evaluate the safety and effectiveness of trained, unlicensed assistive personnel in these settings who perform such tasks as insertion of rectal suppositories; administration of oral and topical medications and nose, ear, and eye drops; dressing changes; catheterization using clean technique; blood glucose monitoring; and gastrostomy feedings (Washington State, 1995). From the results of the study, state rules were developed to guide RN practice in delegation and supervision of assistive personnel in those settings. Task lists were eliminated in 2002, encouraging the use of nursing judgment for specific situations, and in 2003 nurse delegation was authorized for private home settings (Washington State Code Reviser's Office, 2003). What an excellent example of meeting the needs of the community using research and evidence to build the necessary structures!

As we reform our system and community-based organizations scramble to adapt to the changing configuration of health care, home health providers continue to use the concept of case management and multiskilled, unlicensed assistive workers to provide care.

CHECKPOINT 2-10

Long-term care organizations, such as skilled nursing facilities, step-down units, subacute care, swing beds, nursing homes, or adult residential care homes, have responded to healthcare trends by developing innovative methods of delivering care. Ambulatory and home healthcare providers have also adapted their systems. What similarities are evident?

See the end of the chapter for the answers.

Ambulatory Care

In ambulatory care arenas, such as physicians' offices, outpatient clinics, adult day care centers, short-stay surgery centers, and mental health clinics, assistive personnel are employed much as they are in acute and long-term care settings. Positions and job descriptions are created to adapt to the needs of the organization. Surgical technicians, medical assistants, mental health technicians, and rehabilitation aides are trained and perform according to the specific state's practice codes and organizational job descriptions. Experiments with new types of team approaches and combinations of workers to fulfill specific needs are being conducted throughout the country to adapt to healthcare trends and contingencies.

WHERE DO WE GO FROM HERE?

We have heard many nurses respond to the need for clinical delegation skills with the opinion that this is a passing phase and that when reform is implemented, assistive personnel will vanish, leaving RNs to provide all the care once again. We think not. Nor will we return to the nursing of 30 years ago, to become generalists who assign tasks to other personnel, utilizing the principles of the work teams of the postwar era. There are distinct differences between the team concept of the past and the current systems we see emerging. We are responding to a shortage of nurses and to a shortage of professional nursing care. Prescott (1989) describes this shortage of professional nursing care as occurring when nurses are too busy performing tasks that do not require their knowledge and skill base. Personnel with the minimal base of knowledge to perform tasks will be utilized to perform task assignments, not patient assignments.

Whether you practice in an acute care setting or in the community, you will always be involved in working with other people. Not practicing in a vacuum, you will be called upon to use your skill and expertise to delegate wisely to the multidisciplinary

> There is no doubt about it, some form of team process will always be part of the care delivery system of the future. Whether as "practice partners," case managers, or coordinators of patient-focused care, nurses will be part of a group of providers that spans the disciplines.

members of the team, maximizing your resources for the most beneficial outcomes for your patient. As Connie Curran sums it up,

> We can look at our history and realize that being in nursing is being in the patient care business, and being part of the largest group of care givers in this country. That would produce a redefinition of nursing based on the ethics that underlie the profession, some basic competencies, patient advocacy, clinical outcomes, and coordination of other healthcare workers in a variety of settings (Friedman, 1990, p. 3120).

As healthcare professionals we are charged with meeting our commitment to the public—despite the ever mounting challenges we face in terms of lack of human and financial resources and environmental and social ills—to continue to care and provide healing services. We know we are up to meeting the test of creativity.

AN INVITATION

We invite you to respond to an international invitation that exemplifies nursing's creative leadership role in global health: The Nightingale Declaration for Our Healthy World (www.nightingaledeclaration.net). Numerous strategies are outlined in preparation for the Decade for a Healthy World, 2011–2020, as led by the United Nations. An important strategic initiative for nurses includes the proposal to the 2008 UN General Assembly that seeks a resolution to make 2010 The International Year of the Nurse, a century after the death of Florence Nightingale. You can go to the Web site listed above to sign the The Nightingale Declaration for Our Healthy World statement, joining signatories from over 85 countries:

> "We, the nurses and concerned citizens of the global community, hereby dedicate ourselves to the accomplishment of a healthy world by the year 2020.
> We declare our willingness to unite in a program of action, sharing information and solutions to resolve problems and improve conditions—locally, nationally and globally—in order to achieve health for all humanity.
> We further resolve to adopt personal practices and to implement public policies in our communities and nations, making this goal for the year 2020 achievable and inevitable, beginning today in our own lives, in the life of our nations and in the world at large." (Reprinted with permission from B. Dossey, 2007.)

ANSWERS TO CHECKPOINTS

2–1.   1.

- Be cognizant of the material and human resources used on a daily basis (i.e., supplies, time, and people).

- Be aware of public healthcare funding and my social responsibilities in communicating healthcare effects to those who do not understand the system (here we are talking about members of a parent teacher organization or your church but not telling patients "we are too short today because of healthcare reimbursement.")!

- Consider involvement in professional and patient/family advocacy or political organizations.

- Communicate with policy-makers regarding my best guess at methods to improve health care.

- Participating in research that would support best use of healthcare resources.

- Other answers may be supplied on an individual basis.

2.

- The quality of care that nurses are able to provide is linked to healthcare reimbursement and the financial viability of our employing organizations. Nurses and nursing care can be viewed as essential quality and economic assets!

- Careful assessment of current care delivery models and how nurses delegate care is essential for preventing catheter induced urinary tract infections, skincare, turning, and nutrition/hydration tasks that nurses may delegate.

- Avoiding patient falls is a nursing intervention: Assistive personnel are often involved in fall prevention interventions and ongoing monitoring of fall risk patients.

- OR nurses must clearly lead and coordinate preoperative time outs (for correct site and patient surgical interventions) and postoperative sponge and equipment review (to avoid left-behind objects).

> • Nurses can review current research about best practices to encourage the highest quality health outcomes—not just because we believe in the highest ethics and standards, but because we care about the health of our communities and nation.

2–2. Increase in the number of elderly people; increase in the number of poor people.

2–3.

> 1. Mobility and empowerment allow nurses to flourish in their ability to make decisions about their work and the ways they care for their patients.
>
> 2. Public emphasis on safety and consumer satisfaction supports the nurses' advocacy role and could potentially provide reinforcement for promotion of health care or workplace safety.
>
> 3. Public focus on the nursing shortage might spur legislation to support nursing education and other programs to encourage students to enter nursing.
>
> 4. Nursing compensation might increase in a nursing shortage period.
>
> 5. As the baby boomer generation ages, there will certainly be a variety of available jobs in health care.

2–4. Influence of nursing shortages; evolution of health care; demographic trends; healthcare delivery trends; changing nature of work; payment systems; evolution of nursing practice.

2–5. Some of the changes nursing has implemented include:

> 1. Multi-state licensure
>
> 2. Advanced and expanded roles of practice
>
> 3. Progressive education programs that include LPN to BSN and RN to MSN
>
> 4. Degree opportunities
>
> 5. Online continuing education programs that provide immediate professional support

2–6.   Possible advantages to this system include flexibility in adapting to changing patient needs with varying levels of caregivers, decreased personnel costs with fewer RN salaries than in total RN patient care systems, teamwork divides the burden, more personnel are involved with patients so that amenity needs are met. You might have experienced other advantages. Possible disadvantages are that the RN must be able to supervise the care given by others. More personnel can contribute to confusion and communication problems if care is not well organized. If roles are also unclear, conflict can occur and the quality of care can suffer.

2–7.

1.   Instead of focusing on patients as a whole, it divides up by function the tasks that must be completed for each client. This system can also use many different categories of caregivers in addition to the RN.

2.

a)   Documentation of care is often completed by each person as he or she completes a function.

b)   The RN generally interfaces and coordinates the care with other disciplines, although in many long-term care facilities, LPNs can complete some of this communication.

c)   Reporting by all persons involved with the patient must be completed in such a manner that the RN is able to coordinate the total nursing process for the patient.

2–8.

1.   The span of accountability for primary nursing is 24 hours a day throughout the patient's hospitalization, whereas total patient care is limited to the time on duty.

2.   Total patient care implies that one nurse will provide all services; primary nursing coordinates services that are provided by a number of personnel.

2–9.   e)   All of the above

2–10.   Use of creative multiskilled job descriptions, case management, varying team configurations, use of all healthcare workers and disciplines in the delivery of care, linkages throughout the healthcare continuum, and an ever-present need for the RN to lead, coordinate, and supervise.

REFERENCES

AACN. (2004). *Enrollment increases at U.S. nursing schools are moderating while thousands of qualified students are turned away* [Press Release]. Retrieved May 1, 2008, from http://www.aacn.nche.edu/Media/NewsReleases/2004/enrl04.htm

AACN. (2005). *Faculty shortages in baccalaureate and graduate nursing programs.* Retrieved May 1, 2008, from http://www.aacn.nche.edu/Publications/White-Papers/FacultyShortages.htm

Aiken, L., Clarke, S., Sloane, D., Sochalski, J., & Silber, J. (2002). Hospital nurse staffing and patient mortality, nurse burnout, and job dissatisfaction. *JAMA, 288*(16), 1987–1993.

Analysis. (2005). Degree-level nurses lead to fewer deaths. *Nursing Standard, 20*(11), 15.

Aon Corporation. (2007, Spring). *Health care trend survey.* Retrieved November 16, 2007, from http://www.aon.com/us/busi/hc_consulting/employee_benefits_cons/health_welfare/healthcare_trend_survey_spring07.pdf

Auerbach, D., Buerhaus, P., & Staiger, D. (2000, July/August). Associate degree graduates and the rapidly aging RN workforce. *Nursing Economic$, 18*(4), 178–184.

Blegen, M. A., et al. (1992). Who helps you with your work? *American Journal of Nursing, 92*(1), 26–31.

Borkowski, N., Amann, R., Song, S., & Weiss, C. (2007). Nurses intent to leave the profession: Issues related to gender, ethnicity and educational level. *Health Care Management Review, 32*(2), 160–167.

Buerhaus, P. I. (1998, May/June). Is another RN shortage looming? *Nursing Outlook, 46*, 103–108.

Buerhaus, P. I., Staiger, D., & Auerbach, D. (2000a). Implications of an aging registered nurse workforce. *JAMA, 283*(22), 2948–2954.

Buerhaus, P. I., Staiger, D., & Auerbach, D. (2000b, November/December). Policy responses to an aging registered nurse workforce. *Nursing Economic$, 18*(6), 278–284.

Buerhaus, P. I., Staiger, D., & Auerbach, D. (2000c, May/June). Why are shortages of hospital RNs concentrated in specialty care units? *Nursing Economic$, 18*(3), 1–6.

Bureau of Labor Statistics, U.S. Department of Labor. (2006/2007). *Occupational outlook handbook, 2006–2007 edition. Nursing, psychiatric, and home health aides.* Retrieved November 15, 2007, from http://www.bls.gov/oco/ocos165.htm#outlook

Califano, J. A., Jr. (1993). The nurse as a revolutionary. *Missouri Nurse, 62*(2), 10.

Carpentino, L. J. (1996, January/March). Critical pathways: A wolf in sheep's clothing? *Nursing Forum, 31*, 3–6.

Chernomas, R., & Chernomas, W. (1989). Escalation of the nurse-physician conflict. *International Journal of Health Services, 19*(4), 641–643.

Claxton, G., Gable, J., Gil, I., Pickreign, J., Whitmore, H., Finder, B., et al. (2006). Health benefits in 2006: Premium increases moderate, enrollment in consumer-directed health plans remains modest. *Health Affairs, 25*(6), w476–w485.

De Lew, N. (2000, Fall). Medicare: 35 years of service. *Health Care Financing Review, 22*(1), 75–103.

DiMarco, L. (2004). Team nursing improves staff morale, patient care, teamwork improves employee retention. *Rehab Continuum Report.*

Dunham, W. (2008). *More advanced cancer seen in uninsured Americans.* Retrieved April 14, 2008, from http://www.reuters.com/article/domesticNews/idUSN1521748820080218

Friedman, E. (1990). Nursing: Breaking the bonds? *JAMA, 264*(24), 3117–3122.

Goleman, D., Boyatzis, R., & McKee, A. (2002). *Primal leadership: Realizing the power of emotional intelligence.* Boston: Harvard Business School Press.

Grout, J. (2007, May). *Mistake-proofing the design of health care processes* [AHRQ Publication No. 07-P0020]. Retrieved May 1, 2008, from http://www.ahrq.gov/qual/mistakeproof/mistakeproofing.pdf

Hansten, R., & Washburn, M. (1990). *I light the lamp.* Vancouver, WA: Applied Therapeutics.

Hansten, R., & Washburn, M. (1997). *Toolbook for health care redesign.* Gaithersburg, MD: Aspen.

Health Resources and Services Administration. (2002, July). *Projected supply, demand, and shortages of registered nurses: 2000–2020.* Retrieved May 1, 2008, from http://www.ahcancal.org/research_data/staffing/Documents/Registered_Nurse_Supply_Demand.pdf

Hughes, E.C., et al. (1958). *Twenty thousand nurses tell their story: A report on studies of nursing functions sponsored by the American Nurses Association.* Philadelphia: J.B. Lippincott.

Institute for Family-Centered Care. (2002). *Family-centered care in the US and Canada: The rationale, 2002.* Retrieved July 29, 2003, from www.familycentered-care.org

Institute of Medicine. (1999). *To err is human: Building a safer health system.* Washington, DC: National Academies Press.

Institute of Medicine. (2001). *Crossing the quality chasm.* Washington, DC: National Academies Press.

Institute of Medicine (2006). *Hospital-based emergency care: At the breaking point.* Washington DC. National Academies Press.

Ireson, C. (1997). Critical pathways: Effectiveness in achieving patient outcomes. *Journal of Nursing Administration, 27*(6), 16–23.

Lookinland, S., Tiedeman, M., & Crosson, A. (2005). Nontraditional models of care delivery: Have they solved the problems? *Journal of Nursing Administration, 35*(2), 74–80.

Monroe, D. (2003). Assisted living issues for nursing practice. *Geriatric Nursing, 24*(2), 100–105.

National Center for Health Statistics (NCHS). (2007). *Faststats A to Z: Health insurance coverage.* Retrieved May 2, 2008, from http://www.cdc.gov/nchs/fastats/hinsure.htm

Nurses for a Healthier Tomorrow. (2007). *Nursing faculty shortage facts and figures.* Retrieved November 16, 2007, from http://www.nursesource.org/04FacultyShortage

O'Reilly, K. B. (2008, January 7). No pay for "never event" errors becoming standard. *Amednews.com.* Retrieved May 2, 2008 from http://www.ama-assn.org/amednews/2008/01/07/prsc0107.htm

Perkins, K. (1997, May 3). Caught in the post-50 insurance gap. *Sacramento Bee*, pp. A1, A18.

Pew Health Professions Commission. (1995a). *Critical challenges: Revitalizing the health professions for the twenty-first century.* San Francisco: UCSF Center for the Health Professions.

Pew Health Professions Commission. (1995b). *Reforming health care workforce regulation: Policy considerations for the 21st century.* San Francisco: UCSF Center for the Health Professions.

Porter-O'Grady, T. (2003a, February). A different age for leadership, part 1. *Journal of Nursing Administration, 33*(2), 105–110.

Porter-O'Grady, T. (2003b, March–April). Of hubris and hope: Transforming nursing for a new age. *Nursing Economic$, 21*(2), 59–64.

Porter-O'Grady, T., & Malloch, K. (2007). *Quantum leadership: A resource for health care innovation* (2nd ed.). Sudbury, MA: Jones and Bartlett.

Prescott, P. (1989). Shortage of professional nursing practice: A reframing of the shortage problem. *Heart and Lung, 18*(5), 436–443.

Prospective Payment Assessment Commission. (1993). *Medicare and the American healthcare system: Report to the Congress.* Washington, DC: Author.

Renholm, M., Leino-Kilpi, H., & Suominen, T. (2002). Critical pathways: A systematic review. *Journal of Nursing Administration, 32*(4), 196–202.

Risher, P., & Applebaum, S. (2002). *NurseWeek/AONE national survey of registered nurses.* Minnetonka, MN: Harris Interactive, Inc.

Rodgers, J. (1981). Toward professional adulthood. *Nursing Outlook, 29*(8), 478–481.

Sherer, J. L., Anderson, H. J., & Lumsdon, K. (1993). Patients first: Hospitals work to define patient centered care. *Hospitals, 67*, 14–24.

Spratley, E., Johnson, A., Sochalski, J., Fritz, M., & Spencer, W. (2000). *The registered nurse population: Findings from the National Sample Survey of Registered Nurses.* Rockville, MD: U.S. Department of Health and Human Services.

Staiger, D., Auerbach, D., & Buerhaus, P. (2000, September–October). Expanding career opportunities for women and the declining interest in nursing as a career. *Nursing Economic$, 18*(5), 230–236.

Tiedeman, M., & Lookinland, S. (2004). Traditional models of care delivery: What have we learned? *Journal of Nursing Administration, 34*(6), 291–297.

U.S. Department of Health & Human Services. (1988). *Secretary's commission on nursing final report.* Washington, DC: Author.

Villaire, M. (1993, December). Marie Manthey on the evolution of primary nursing. *Critical Care Nurse, 13*(6), 100–107.

Wake, M.M. (1990). Nursing care delivery systems: Status and vision. *Journal of Nursing Administration, 20*(5), 47–51.

Walter, F., et al. (2007, April). Success of clinical pathways for total joint arthroplasty in a community hospital. *Clinical Orthopedics and Related Research, 457,* 133–137.

Washington State. (1995). *House bill report E2SHB 1908.* Retrieved April 14, 2008, from http://www.leg.wa.gov/pub/billinfo/1995-96/Pdf/Bill%20Reports/House/-908-S2.HBR.pdf

Washington State Code Reviser's Office. (2003). *Emergency rules.* Retrieved April 14, 2008, from http://apps.leg.wa.gov/documents/Laws/WSR/2003/22/03-22 -084.htm

Wolf, G. (2007). Blueprint for design: Creating models that direct change. *Journal of Nursing Administration, 37*(9), 381–387.

Zander, K. (1997, June). Classic nursing management skills and disease management: Something old, something new. *Seminars for Nurse Managers, 5*(2), 85–90.

Zander, K. (1988). Nursing case management: Strategic management of cost and quality outcomes. *Journal of Nursing Administration, 18*(5), 28.

Know Your Practice: Is My License on the Line?

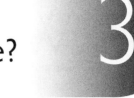

Ruth I. Hansten and Marilynn Jackson

CHAPTER SKILLS

+ Compare the role of the state boards of nursing with the role of a professional nurses' association.
+ Describe the major components of a nurse practice act.
+ Clarify RN accountabilities in the process of delegation.
+ Identify the three aspects of the nursing process that cannot be delegated.

RECOMMENDED RESOURCES

▶ Download or send for a copy of your state nurse practice act.
▶ Attend a state board of nursing meeting or volunteer for one of their committees.
▶ Check out your state board of nursing Web site for the latest issues and news.
▶ Subscribe to a professional journal (e.g., AJN, Nursing Outlook, or RN).
▶ Join a professional nursing organization.

"I am so tired of those nurses whining about their licenses being on the line! Every time we make any changes around here, someone says something about her license being on the line. I hate that phrase! I don't care what you have to do, but get them some information so they know what the law says about their license status, for goodness sakes!" (Hospital administrator who contracted our services)

W e, too, have heard this phrase on numerous occasions, and we share some of the same concerns as the administrator quoted above. However, we recognize the plea for what it is, a cry for help and a sincere statement of concern and fear that the licensure status that allows you to practice as a professional nurse is in danger of being jeopardized by some change in the working conditions or whatever new plan administration has created for you. The resolution of this situation lies in Adelaide Nutting's statement, "Knowledge is our only working power" (Hansten & Washburn, 1990, p. 66). Nurses must have a fundamental knowledge of the practice act, both the statute and the rules, that governs the practice of nursing in each state. Armed with that knowledge, nursing can better evaluate new care delivery systems and requests from administrators who are focused on effectiveness and efficiency and not necessarily the standard of nursing practice.

CHECKPOINT 3-1

It is important to know about my nurse practice act because:

a) This information will help me to do a better job clinically.

b) It's not important to me; the board of nursing is paid to tell me when something is not legal, so I don't have to worry about it.

c) This law directs my practice and is the legal foundation for what I do as a professional nurse. An understanding of the law and the rules will help me to evaluate the safety and legality of actions I am requested to take by my employer and any other member of the healthcare team.

d) As long as I pay my fees and keep my license current, that's all I need to know.

See the end of the chapter for the answers.

The statement, "My license is on the line," has been overused by nurses and in many cases is a "fighting phrase" that triggers a very negative response from many members of the management team. If you are justifiably concerned about the legality of the changes in your practice (and you might very well be!), we cannot emphasize enough that you must support that concern with knowledge of the law that governs nursing practice. Unfortunately, most nurses have received

"Knowledge is our only working power."
—ADELAIDE NUTTING

very little education about the practice act, and educational reforms are seeing nursing trends classes and professional issues classes deleted from many nursing curricula. In addition, practicing nurses of today have not kept themselves informed regarding the current status of the laws that define their individual practice. If you have not had the opportunity to receive some information regarding the law of nursing, all is not lost. This chapter will focus solely on the topic of the nurse practice act (NPA) specifically as it addresses the issue of delegation, and it will provide you with many resources that are readily available to you. Read on!

CHECKPOINT 3-2

The primary purpose of the board of nursing is to:

a) advocate for nurses who are accused of unsafe practice

b) approve schools of nursing and grant or revoke licenses

c) regulate the practice of nursing

d) protect the public from unsafe practice of nursing

See the end of the chapter for the answers.

THE STATE BOARD OF NURSING

Every state in the nation is replete with governing bodies that overlook various professions, occupations, and pastimes. From the board of pharmacy to the board of game and fish, we have a significant number of agencies devoted to monitoring our personal and professional behaviors. The board of nursing is one such regulatory agency created by the state government, but most nurses have contact with it on only an annual or biannual basis as licenses are renewed and fees are paid. What does the board of nursing do the rest of the year, when they are not collecting fees?

Many nurses are confused about the purpose of the board of nursing and might find out the hard way that this particular agency is not in existence to advocate for them. Just as the game and fish department writes rules to protect the public from unsafe habits of hunters and other sportsmen, the board of nursing is primarily interested in the safety of the public you serve as a nurse. If you are looking for support and the advancement of nursing practice on a professional level, try one of the professional associations, such as the state nurses association. The role of the state nurses association is often confused with the role of the board, when in reality the two are very different. **Table 3–1** clarifies some of the basic differences.

For further information about membership in various professional organizations, you can contact the American Nurses Association (http://www.ana.org) or the American Organization of Nurse Executives (http://www.aone.org). The nurses association in your state will also be a good resource for the various specialty organizations. Let's take a look at each of the answers in Checkpoint 3–2 to clarify some common misperceptions.

TABLE 3–1　Roles of Boards of Nursing and Professional Organizations

	Board of Nursing	**Professional Organization**
Membership	Appointed by the governor to regulate practice of nurses in a given state	Based on criteria such as credentials, specialty, geographical location
Membership Fees	None	Membership fees as required by the group, usually annually
Purpose	To protect the safety of the public	Varies with the organization, from networking opportunities for nurses with the same interest, promotion and advancement of the profession, collective bargaining representation, research specific to the specialty
Meetings	Open to the public except for executive sessions, matter of public record, required by law	Can be restricted to members or potential members or by invitation only
Communication	Periodic newsletter sent to all registered nurses licensed in the state	Newsletters, faxes, district forums, workshops for education, and networking

a) **advocate for nurses who are accused of unsafe practice:** If you are ever involved in a board investigation as the result of a complaint made regarding your professional practice, you might find that the approach taken by the board is adversarial and not supportive. Remember, this agency is there to protect the public, not you. If there is reason to believe that you are practicing in a manner that is unsafe to the public, it is the board's responsibility to take corrective action and to ensure that the public is protected. Thus, they often do not come across as being on your side—indeed, they might not be! Here again, a working knowledge of how the board functions, particularly their disciplinary process, will give you a better understanding of the legal side of your practice.

b) **approve schools of nursing and grant or revoke licenses:** These are certainly duties of any board of nursing and are methods by which it governs the practice of nursing to ensure public safety. It is important to remember a little history here: Nursing as a profession in the United States did not have licensure until 1903. The first licensing law for nurses was actually passed in Cape Colony, South Africa, in 1891 (Donahue, 1985). After many years of struggle, British nurses and American nurses began to make progress, and lawmakers began to recognize the need to protect the public from inconsistent standards and questionable practices. Prior to this time, a "nurse" could receive education through the mail, attend any one of a growing number of nursing schools with a great variety of curricula, or train on the job. Sophia Palmer spoke of poorly qualified schools and nursing impostors in her editorial in the *American Journal of Nursing* in 1903: "How long will nurses permit such conditions to exist when only a strong, concerted action is needed to improve the educational standard, to protect the public and nurses themselves against impostors, and to give trained nursing a place among the honorable professions!" (Donahue, 1985, p. 375). Shortly after this publication, several states adopted nurse practice acts providing for the standardization of education and the regulation of practice through licensure.

Today it is the duty of the board of nursing in each state to establish criteria and approve schools of nursing that meet those criteria, thus upholding a standard of education. Through licensure and the disciplinary process for revoking or suspending licenses, the board also supports its prime directive to protect public safety. Such regulation of licensure eliminates the risk of impostors and ensures that anyone practicing nursing will have acquired a specific standard of education.

The primary responsibility of any regulatory board, whether the board of nursing or the board of cosmetology, is to protect the public safety.

c) **regulate the practice of nursing:** The process by which each board of nursing regulates nursing practice varies from state to state. Generally, each board is empowered by law to adopt rules or issue advisory opinions concerning the authority of nurses to perform certain acts. Criteria, in the form of standards of conduct, are established by each board and regulated through the investigative process. Powers of regulation extend to schools of nursing and to individual licensees but not generally to institutions or agencies that employ nurses. These groups are generally regulated in other sections of the law. It is not the duty of the board to regulate practice by overseeing what policies an employing agency or institution creates for the employment of a nursing staff. State licensing laws for hospitals and other healthcare facilities, The Joint Commission, and the Health Care Financing Administration (HCFA) are examples of institution-regulating agencies.

d) **protect the public from unsafe practice of nursing:** The board of nursing is empowered to implement a disciplinary process that ensures the safety of practice. Although the actual system might vary from state to state, the outcome is the same: Nurses found to be practicing in an unsafe manner will be disciplined. Generally there are paid staff members working for the board of nursing who function in the roles of consultants and investigators. In addition to administering the process of licensure, these staff members receive complaints made by the public or by nursing personnel themselves and begin an investigation. The results of their investigations are then presented to the board members for review and action. Hearings can be involved; the individual nurse can have representation by an attorney (the attorney general's office will represent the board), and the case can be presented to the board in this very formal manner. The board members are empowered to rule on the outcome of the hearing or investigation and to take disciplinary action, usually in the form of: 1) issuance of a letter of concern; 2) allowance of practice with limitations; 3) suspension; or 4) revocation of the license.

Lawsuits versus Discipline

There is often confusion regarding the potential action that can be taken against a nurse if there should be a negative outcome to a patient's care. Many times we hear the statement, "I might get sued," and we suspect you have heard it too. But you might not be clear about what happens if a nurse is sued. Disciplinary action taken by a board of nursing occurs when a complaint has been made regarding someone's nursing practice and an investigation reveals that the practitioner was indeed at fault. The steps available to the board are as noted in the preceding paragraph, and they involve measures that will directly affect the nurse's practice in terms of where, when, and with what limitations or restrictions he or she can work or, indeed, whether the nurse would be allowed to continue to practice at all. Although the board is represented by the attorney general's office and the nurse might also have legal representation during the hearing, this is not a civil case or a lawsuit. It is indeed possible to be disciplined by the state board and not be sued by the patient. Likewise, it is possible to be sued by an unhappy patient and/or family and not have the board of nursing involved at all. The fear of legal reprisal is intensified when you delegate tasks to others, and it can become a significant barrier to effective delegation because many nurses believe they are accountable for the delegate's actions as well. We will explore this in detail after you take the test later in the chapter (Exhibit 3–1).

Composition of the Board

Now that we have established the significant power of this group of individuals, it is important to know who they are. The composition of the board is defined in statute, with a law specifying the number of members appointed to serve on the board and the area of expertise that each individual will represent. This ensures that major areas of practice, from management to education, are represented. It is not unusual for the state to require representation from a member of the public as well to represent the public perspective on nursing practice. Other stipulations regarding geographical location of each member might also be specified, again to guarantee broad representation of the profession. In addition to the qualifications of each member, the terms of service are also defined, usually ranging from a two-year to a five-year appointment. The appointment of board members is a political decision, typically from the governor's office, and board members are not paid.

CHECKPOINT 3–3

Powers and duties of the board of nursing include:

a) approving schools of nursing

b) granting or revoking licenses

c)　regulating practice of the profession

d)　all of the above

See the end of the chapter for the answers.

———————————————————————————————

Appointed members, who are defined by law and serve unpaid terms, make up the board of nursing in each state. The board will employ staff members to fulfill the administrative, clerical, and investigative needs of the board. These individuals are hired by the board and do not participate in the decision-making process of the board regarding licensure or other matters. The leader of the personnel will most likely be the executive director or executive secretary. This individual oversees the staff and is present at all board meetings for assistance and administrative support. The executive leader and the president of the board represent each state at the National Council of State Boards of Nursing (NCSBN), a source authority to which we will refer often in this book. Collectively this group strives for standardization among the states and issues position papers and advisory opinions, commissioning studies and investigations of current practice trends from a national perspective.

Meetings

The board convenes on a regular basis, from as frequently as monthly to as infrequently as quarterly. Meetings are open to the public, and agendas and locations for meetings are easily available from your board office. Attending one of these meetings can be very educational and will quickly familiarize you with the process of the functioning of the board. Some boards offer an "open mike" time when nurses can come forward and address specific practice questions for the board's advice and consideration. This is an excellent time to get to know the members of the board and to establish a very important professional relationship.

Resources

Several resources are at your disposal to help you to build your knowledge about the board and the nurse practice act.

The Nurse Practice Act

With the advent of the Internet and the move toward paperwork reduction and cost containment, most nurse practice acts are now available on the Web site for the respective state. If your state makes hard copies available, thus saving you the download, you might want to contact them directly and find out the fee and process for obtaining your own copy. Whether online or in hand, the important issue is to have access to the practice act itself. It is also important to be aware that the majority of healthcare practitioners (physical therapists, pharmacists, respiratory therapists, nursing assistants [NAs], etc.) will also have regulatory documents to govern their practice. If you delegate to an interdisciplinary team, you will want to have an awareness of the framework of regulation and discipline for each of these roles.

> The statute relating to nursing is typically very general in terms, allowing for broad interpretation and application over an extended period of time.

Board Consultants

Members of the staff might be called consultants or investigators or advisors, and they have specific areas of expertise. There might be individuals on staff who advise regarding scope-of-practice issues, impaired nurse programs, nursing school criteria, and so on. These individuals are excellent resources for questions you might have regarding the safety of your working environment and the use of assistive personnel, and they might be of valuable assistance in answering that question that led you to believe your license might be on the line. Consultants or other staff members, including the executive director, often make themselves available to visit schools of nursing, professional association meetings, or healthcare facilities. They are usually very willing to provide an overview of the law and the duties of the board and to advise on specific questions. They might not issue black-and-white answers, but they will be able to direct you in the process of evaluating your particular situation.

Advisory Opinions

Often the law is written in very generic terms and requires some interpretation. It is usually not possible or practical to write law that speaks to every unique situation that a nurse might encounter. In this case, the board can issue an advisory opinion that further clarifies the law and addresses practice in a more specific manner. In recent years, as the use of assistive personnel has increased, several state boards

> If you do not have a copy of your state's practice act, we highly recommend that you call the board office and request a copy. Make certain that there is one where you work, as well as one for your own personal reference. Be certain to request the statute and the administrative code so that you have all of the legal documents regarding your practice.

have issued advisory opinions to offer assistance to the practicing nurse in interpreting the expectations of the law. Since that time, many state practice acts have been changed, and the requirements of the delegating nurse have been more clearly delineated. You can request a copy of any advisory opinion written by the board and are encouraged to do so if you are uncertain about any practice issue. Subjects of advisory opinions can include abandonment, mandatory reporting, acceptance of assignments, and delegating to unlicensed personnel.

Committee Involvement

Within the working structure of any board of nursing is the creation of committees for overseeing specific areas of practice. These committees are chaired by a board member and staffed by one of the investigators or consultants who are employed by the board. Committee members are professional nurses who have an interest in the work of the committee and have expertise in that area. For example, a board might appoint a committee to look at scope-of-practice issues for the advanced practitioner or might create a committee to look into the legal and legislative interests of nurses in the state. These committees might review a particular part of the rules that is confusing or controversial and can draft an advisory opinion (see the previous section) that is then presented to the board for approval. Prior to legislation (a lengthy process), many advisory opinions were issued on the subject of delegation.

Committee meetings are open to the public and are another source of information regarding what is happening on a state level in terms of nursing practice. Your membership on one of these committees might be an opportunity for you to share your expertise and to develop your leadership and professional skills.

THE NATIONAL COUNCIL OF STATE BOARDS OF NURSING

We have referred to the National Council of State Boards of Nursing (NCSBN) often in citing the basic definitions of delegation and supervision. A little background regarding this organization will be helpful in understanding the framework of regulations from a national perspective. As noted previously, this organization has a Web site, which will provide you with an abundance of important information regarding the profession of nursing.

Contact the National Council of State Boards of Nursing at its Web site: http://www.ncsbn.org.

The NCSBN is just that, a national representative group of 59 members made up of two representatives from each state's board of nursing, including the District of Columbia and five U.S. territories (Guam, Virgin Islands, American Samoa, Puerto Rico, and the Northern Mariana Islands). Four states, California, Louisiana, Georgia, and West Virginia, have separate boards of nursing for RNs and LPNs.

"The National Council of State Boards of Nursing (NCSBN), composed of member boards, provides leadership to advance regulatory excellence for public protection" (https://www.ncsbn.org/182.htm, accessed November 12, 2007). In their continued approach to excellence, the NCSBN adopted eight Guiding Principles of Nursing Regulation at their 2007 Delegate Assembly, among which are the recognition of nursing involvement in regulation, strategic collaboration, responsiveness to the marketplace, and the use of evidence-based practice standards in developing regulatory language (for the complete list of principles see https://www.ncsbn.org/Guiding_Principles.pdf, accessed November 12, 2007). Major functions of the NCSBN include the development of the NCLEX exams for RNs and LPNs (NCSBN, 2007), the competency evaluation for nursing assistants, policy analysis, networking information, and ensuring uniformity in regulation of practice on a state-to-state basis. The council also performs research, monitors issues and trends in public policy, and, most important, serves as the communication clearinghouse on nursing regulation.

Mutual Recognition

With the increasing mobility of our practice, nurses often find themselves working across state lines and moving from state to state in a network health system. What laws then govern this multistate practice? Does a nurse need licensure in all states? To respond to these questions, the NCSBN convened a task force in 1996 to gather data and to issue a recommendation regarding further action. In December 1997, the delegates at a special session approved the proposed language for an interstate compact in support of a standard approach to a mutual recognition model for nursing regulation. As of this edition, 22 states have enacted mutual recognition legislation. These states are Arizona, Arkansas, Colorado, Delaware, Idaho, Indiana, Iowa, Kentucky, Maine, Maryland, Mississippi, Nebraska, New Jersey, New Mexico, North Carolina, North Dakota, South Dakota, Tennessee, Texas, Utah, Virginia, and Wisconsin. (See **Figure 3–1**.) If you are a resident of any one of these states and hold a nursing license in that state, you will be able to practice nursing in all Nurse Licensure Compact (NLC) member states. There are many other factors to consider when practicing as a member of the NLC,

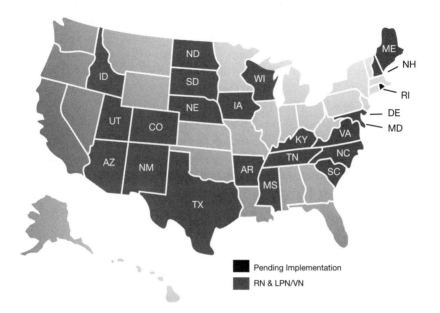

FIGURE 3–1   **Mutual Recognition Legislation.** Reproduced from the NCSBN Web site (www.ncsbn.org) and used with permission from the National Council of State Boards of Nursing (NCSBN), Chicago, IL, Copyright 2007. Note: No states have passed the APRN Compact rules as of this printing, but updated information is available on the NCSBN Web site.

which are expertly answered in the NCSBN publication "Frequently Asked Questions Regarding the National Council of State Boards of Nursing (NCSBN) Nurse Licensure Compact (NLC)," available at https://www.ncsbn.org/NurseLicensureCompactFAQ.pdf. Nevertheless, you are held to the laws of the state in which you are practicing, so it is always wise to know that particular nurse practice act!

We are one giant step closer to a standardized model of practice, reducing the variations that currently exist from state to state and eliminating the need for expensive licensure in multiple states. Significant steps have been taken to begin a national standard of licensure.

> Boards of nursing have agreed to support "an interstate compact, under which nurses would hold a license in one state and be able to practice in any state, provided they follow the laws and regulations of the state in which they are practicing."

THE NURSE PRACTICE ACT

With the advent of multistate recognition, it becomes even more important to have a solid knowledge of the nurse practice act for the state in which you are

ADVANTAGES OF THE NURSE LICENSURE COMPACT (NLC)

- Ease of access to nurses for employers
- Increased mobility of nurses
- Elimination of costly and duplicative licensure
- Improved access to nurses in times of natural disaster or national crisis
- Clarification of nursing authority when practicing telenursing or in inter-state settings
- Improved information sharing and discipline among member states

(NCSBN, FAQs Regarding the NCSBN Nurse Licensure Compact, April, 2004)

licensed. Because there are numerous references to this document, we believe it warrants more than a word or two of explanation. Let's start with the basics: The nurse practice act is the general term applied to the law or statutes written in each state to regulate the practice of nursing. In fact, it has different names in different states: Wisconsin Statutes Relating to the Practice of Nursing, the Law Relating to Registered Nurses, the Revised Code of Washington, the Texas Administrative Code, and so forth. Whatever the title, this document is the legal framework of practice. It is written through the legislative process, meaning that any changes in the language must be initiated in the form of a bill passed by both the state house and senate and signed into law by the governor of the state. For this reason, the statute relating to nursing is typically very general in terms, allowing for broad interpretation and application over an extended period of time. Changes in law might require several years to enact, depending on the nature of the change and the amount of support or controversy it engenders.

Basic components of the practice act will include:

- the creation of a board of nursing, defining membership and qualifications
- the listing of the powers and duties of the board, including meetings
- the licensure process, including qualifications, fees, renewal, permits, reciprocity
- definition of nursing
- approval process for nursing schools
- authority to adopt rules and regulations

RULES AND REGULATIONS

The law is like a skeleton, providing the framework for the muscle and flesh of the rules. Only rules that have support by statute can be written, but they can be much more specific in nature.

Because of the durability of the law, specific areas, such as staffing ratios, acceptability of assignments, complete listings of the procedures allowable for nurses to perform, detailed definitions of such concepts as supervision and delegation, and so forth are not usually addressed in law. However, the statute (law) enables the board to adopt rules and regulations that serve to clarify and amplify the intent of the law. If you are confused, consider the following anatomical analogy: The law is like a skeleton, providing the framework for the muscle and flesh of the rules. Only rules that have support by statute can be written, but they can be much more specific in nature.

CHECKPOINT 3–4

Check the following statements that apply to you:

O I have looked up my state's board of nursing Web site and am familiar with the resources available there.

O I have a copy of the nurse practice act for my state.

O I know who the members of the board of nursing are.

O I have attended at least one board meeting.

O I have served on a committee for the board.

O I have spoken with one of the staff or members of the board regarding a question I had.

If you checked two or more, congratulations! You are well on your way to having a solid foundation of knowledge about your practice. If you checked fewer than two, oops! Call your board of nursing now, and start getting informed.

CHECKPOINT 3–5

The following is one of the major differences between a rule and the law:

a) There are no differences because nurses are disciplined according to the law and the rules.

b) Law is more specific in nature because it must go through the legislative process for approval.

c) Rules are more detailed in nature than the law and must be based on and supported by law.

d) Rules can be written by anyone, and laws must be written by legislators.

See the end of the chapter for the answers.

Members of the board of nursing can write rules and will often use committee input to create them. When written, rules undergo a similar yet simpler process of promulgation to become official. Many issues that cause concern about whether your license is on the line are addressed in the more detailed rules and regulations. For example, the increased use of assistive personnel has caused most states to clarify the reporting relationship of these individuals and to be more specific in the definition of supervision as it pertains to the process of delegation. This topic will be explored in greater detail in the rest of this chapter.

THE TEST

We have now spent considerable time building your foundation of knowledge about the state board of nursing, the NCSBN, and the nurse practice act. It's time to put that information to the test and ask you some key questions that will be major determinants of whether your practice with assistive personnel puts you at risk. Please answer the questions given in **Exhibit 3–1** as true or false, according to your knowledge of the practice act in your state. Ready?

EXHIBIT 3–1　Test on the Nurse Practice Act

Please answer the following questions as true or false.

_____ 1. When I delegate a task to an unlicensed healthcare worker, I am no longer accountable for what happens.

_____ 2. My state's nurse practice act specifically allows me to delegate nursing care activities.

_____ 3. My state's nurse practice act specifies that I must know the competencies and abilities of the person to whom I delegate.

_____ 4. My state's nurse practice act states that I might be in violation of the standards of conduct if I delegate tasks to those I have reason to know lack the ability or responsibility to perform the function.

_____ 5. If I fail to supervise those to whom nursing tasks have been delegated, I might be disciplined by the state board.

_____ 6. If a nursing assistant makes a mistake during a task I have delegated, it would mean I could lose my license.

_____ 7. Employer policies or directives can relieve me of my responsibility for making judgments about the delegation of nursing activities.

Source: Reprinted with permission from Loretta O'Neil, Ruth Hansten, Marilynn Jackson, and the Washington Organization of Nurse Executives, 1990.

How did you do? Using statements of the NCSBN and a representative sampling of state practice acts, let's review the answers. Please note that some of the referenced laws will be several years old, again recognizing the durability of law and the protracted amount of time it takes to change laws.

Question 1: FALSE
This brings us to the definition of delegation, a fundamental that will be emphasized many times because it forms the basis of the legal expectations of your role. Dictionary definitions of the term "delegation" include to assign, entrust, or transfer. The NCSBN (1995, p. 2) has issued the following definition of delegation as it specifically applies to nursing:

> Delegation: "transferring to a competent individual the authority to perform a selected nursing task in a selected situation. The nurse retains the accountability for the delegation."

Note the general nature of this definition. Those individuals who are looking for a black-and-white list of what may and may not be delegated will be a little concerned at the apparent ambiguity of this defined process. Take heart! The definition, as with statute, is intentionally generalized to allow you, as the RN, to practice the art of nursing. No authority can begin to cover every unique and specific practice issue that might arise. This definition considers your expertise and knowledge to be guiding factors in your decision of which selected tasks and in which selected situations you deem it appropriate to delegate care. Unlike the process of assigning, which the NCSBN distinguishes as "when a nurse directs an individual to do something the individual is already authorized to do," delegation involves that direction to an individual to perform a task she may not normally do (ANA & NCSBN, 2006). Therefore, your primary legal obligation is to ensure the competency of the individual you are working with, and we will explore that issue in detail.

> Your primary legal obligation is to ensure the competency of the individual you are working with.

To answer the first test question, when you delegate a task to an unlicensed assistant, you remain accountable for the delegation, according to the definition just given. What causes concern for many is the concept of accountability and the feeling that "If I am accountable, why delegate in the first place?" The term "accountability" has been applied to the nursing profession liberally and with minimal clarification of the meaning of the term. It is often linked with responsibility, authority, and autonomy, other broadly defined terms that translate to being the one who shoulders the blame if something goes wrong. This is not necessarily the case. Being accountable means being answerable for what one has done (in this case, the decision to delegate the task) and standing behind that decision and/or action. For example, the NA to whom you delegated the task of obtaining vital signs made an error in the procedure of taking the blood pressure. The NA is responsible for his or her performance, and you are accountable to the patient for the decision you made to delegate the task and for taking action and correcting the error. As we continue through the remaining test questions, it will become clear just what you are accountable for in terms of patient care.

Delegation versus Professional Activity

The Connecticut State Board of Examiners for Nursing has tackled the issue of medication administration by child care providers. As a result of interviews, public hearings, legal consultants, research, and analysis of public documents and the role of the Department of Health, it was determined that training a child care provider to administer medications appropriately (a skill) could be differentiated from delegation of a nursing task. Similar to a teacher–student relationship, the nurse would not transfer a specific task but rather teach medication administration skills. This view limits the nurse's liability to the quality of the education she provides rather than assuming accountability for the care of that individual child. A 17-year process of analysis of professional nursing activities, regulation, and practicality clarified a thorny issue for the health of Connecticut nurses and children. Day care

> Being accountable means being answerable for what one has done (in this case, the decision to delegate the task) and standing behind that decision and/or action.

centers are required to have a health consultant RN, with weekly visits by those who care for children under 3 years of age (Heschel, Crowley, & Cohen, 2005). This case supports the use of research in determining the best, safest practices for determining public policy.

Question 2: TRUE

Within the statutes or rules of all nurse practice acts is the definition of nursing. According to NCSBN research:

> Forty-eight (48) boards have some reference to delegation in either the nurse practice act or rules; of these, 35 boards references appear in nurse practice acts and 43 boards references appear in the rules. Forty-four (44) boards included a definition of delegation in either the practice act or rules. Thirty-nine (39) boards authorized delegation by RNs; 23 boards authorized delegation by LPN/VNs. (NCSBN, 2005a, p. 6)

Many of these definitions clearly address the function of delegation; others imply the process, as in the following examples. According to the Arizona Nurse Practice Act (revised August 2002), 32-1601, Definitions: 13, "professional nursing" includes the following:

(a) Diagnosing and treating human responses to actual or potential health problems.

(b) Assisting individuals and groups to maintain or attain optimal health by implementing a strategy of care to accomplish defined goals and evaluating responses to care and treatment.

(c) Assessing the health status of individuals and groups.

(d) Establishing a nursing diagnosis.

(e) Establishing goals to meet identified healthcare needs.

(f) Prescribing nursing interventions to implement a strategy of care.

(g) Delegating nursing interventions to others who are qualified to do so. (http://www.azleg.state.az.us/ars/32/01601.htm, accessed November 12, 2007)

The Idaho Nurse Practice Act, 54-1402, Definitions, provides a more indirect approach, using the word "authorizing" as stated in the following definition:

(4) "Licensed professional nurse" means a person who practices nursing by:

(g) Authorizing nursing interventions that may be performed by others and that do not conflict with this act;

(h) Maintaining safe and effective nursing care rendered directly or indirectly (http://www3.state.id.us/cgi-bin/newidst?sctid=540140002.K, accessed November 12, 2007)

Question 3: TRUE

Many state practice acts have adopted language from the NCSBN and specifically address the legal requirement that nurses know the competencies of the delegate. In its paper, "Delegation: Concepts and Decision-Making Process," the NCSBN (1995, p. 1) says, "Boards of nursing should articulate clear principles for delegation, augmented by clearly defined guidelines for delegation decisions." We anticipate that all states are in the process of promulgating rules that specifically address this area. Colorado's (2003) nurse practice act is only one example of language that addresses the competency of the delegate; so do numerous other states. Chapter XIII Rules and Regulations Regarding the Delegation of Nursing Tasks 5.2 says:

> The delegator shall: A. Explain delegation and that the delegated task is limited to the identified client within the identified time frame; B. As appropriate, either instruct the delegatee in the delegated task and verify the delegatee's competency to perform the delegated nursing task, or verify the delegatee's competence to perform the delegated nursing task. (http://www.dora.state.co.us/nursing/rules/ChapterXIII.pdf, accessed March 7, 2008)

Question 4: TRUE

Knowing that the delegate is not competent or prepared educationally and proceeding to delegate the task anyway will certainly be a violation of the standard of practice in any state. All nurse practice acts list specific acts that are in violation of the standard; indeed, this is where you will find the highest degree of clarity! It's quite easy to identify what will get you in trouble. South Carolina's Code of Regulations, Chapter 91 (2006), specifies the following:

(3) Unprofessional conduct which includes, but is not limited to the following:

o. assigning unqualified persons to perform nursing care functions, tasks or responsibilities and/or failing to effectively supervise persons to whom nursing functions are delegated or assigned. (http://www.scstatehouse.net/coderegs/c091.htm, accessed November 13, 2007)

For example, as an RN in a rehab center, you assign a rehab aide the task of feeding a resident who has dysphagia. You know the aide has had difficulty in the past and in fact can recall one instance when the aide almost caused the resident to aspirate part of a tomato. But you are extremely short staffed today, and it's in the aide's job description, so you guess he'll just have to learn with practice. WRONG! Don't put your license in jeopardy by making this kind of decision. You will be responsible for the correctness of this delegation, and in this case, the task should not be delegated to this individual. Your choices might include working with the aide, assigning another aide (whom you know to be competent) to feed the patient, or doing it yourself.

Question 5: TRUE

This question addresses two of the five rights outlined in **Figure 3-2**, right direction and right supervision. Among the terms commonly defined in every practice act is supervision. The NCSBN (1995, p. 2) defines the term as follows: "The provision of *guidance or direction, evaluation* and *follow-up* by the licensed nurse for accomplishment of a nursing task delegated to unlicensed personnel." Note that the italics identify the important components of supervision.

1. **Guidance or direction**—The instructions you provide when first delegating the task. For example, "Please check the blood pressure on Mrs. Jones and report it to me immediately," or "Bathe Mr. Hawley three times this week, on Monday, Wednesday, and Friday during your visit. Use the bath oil Mrs. Hawley has gotten from the doctor. I'll be in on Friday to assess his skin and see how you are doing."

2. **Evaluation**—The decision you make regarding the frequency of checking back with the delegate is based on your judgment of the current situation. It is a defined expectation that you will provide supervision in the form of follow-up with the delegate. In the previous example, the home health nurse is "evaluating" the home health aide on Friday. He or she might be doing this weekly, or as infrequently as monthly, depending on the circumstances.

3. **Follow-up**—You need to communicate your evaluation findings to those who are in a position to do something about the situation. For example, if you note in your evaluation that the home health aide is not using the bath oil as directed, and Mr. Hawley's skin condition is worsening, you will need to discuss this directly with the aide. Florida Administrative Code (2007), 64B9-14.002 (3), clearly delineates this expectation:

1) **Right Task:** Is this a task that can be delegated? One that is fairly routine, with predictable outcomes, minimal risk, does not require the use of nursing judgment, including assessment, planning and evaluation, and is within the scope of skills of the NAP would be a "right task."

2) **Right Person:** Is this delegate competent to perform this task—how do you know?

3) **Right Circumstance:** Does the complexity of the task match the competency of the delegate and the availability of supervision?

4) **Right Direction/Communication:** Is your direction clear, concise, correct and complete, and does it identify the specific task, timeline, and outcome you would like?

5) **Right Supervision:** How are you monitoring performance? Make sure that after initial direction you are available for follow-up, to intervene if necessary, and to ultimately give feedback to the delegate based on the outcome of the task. Be sure to document your findings.

FIGURE 3–2 The Five Rights of Delegation: A Checklist for Safe/Effective Delegation. Adapted from "The Five Rights of Delegation," NCSBN, 1997. (https://www.ncsbn.org/fiverights. pdf, accessed November 13, 2007)

The delegation process shall include communication to the UAP which identifies the task or activity, the expected or desired outcome, the limits of authority, the time frame of the delegation, the nature of the supervision required, verification of the delegate's understanding of assignment, and verification of monitoring and supervision. (http://www.doh.state.fl.us/mqa/nursing/info_Practice Act.pdf, accessed November 12, 2007)

Failure to provide either the initial direction or evaluation and follow-up will be interpreted as a failure to adequately supervise the delegate and will be the basis for disciplinary action of the RN, as noted in the New Hampshire Nursing Regulations, Chapter NUR 402.04 (c)(2) Disciplinary Sanctions: "(2) Failure of licensee to supervise individuals or groups required to practice nursing or provide nursing-related activities under supervision." (http://gencourt.state.nh.us/rules/nur100-800.html, accessed November 12, 2007)

Supervision: "The provision of guidance or direction, evaluation and follow-up by the licensed nurse for accomplishment of a nursing task delegated to unlicensed personnel."

Supervision can be direct and on-site, with the RN immediately available, as in the acute care setting. It can also be indirect, with the RN still accountable for the supervision of the individual but not physically present at the site of care. Home health practice, community settings, and some long-term care facilities are areas where the supervision by the RN is indirect. In their Joint Statement on Delegation (2006), both the ANA and the NCSBN consider supervision from direct, on-site and indirect, off-site perspectives, recognizing that guidance and oversight can be communicated both verbally and in written communications. Chapter 5, Section 1 (1996) of the Maine Nursing Regulations clarifies this well:

> Supervision may require direct, continuing presence of the registered professional nurse to observe, guide and direct the nursing assistant; intermittent observation and direction by the registered professional nurse who may only occasionally be physically present; or development of a plan of care, in advance, by the registered professional nurse. In the latter situation, the registered professional nurse must be available for supervision, in person, in the event circumstances arise that cause the registered professional nurse to believe such supervision is necessary. (ftp://ftp.state.me.us/pub/sos/cec/rcn/apa/02/380/380c005.doc, accessed November 12, 2007)

Just as supervision can be direct or indirect, there are varying levels of supervision on which you will base your decision regarding the frequency of periodic inspection.

1. **Never delegated**—Certain acts, including the assessment, evaluation, and nursing judgment, are never delegated. In addition, some states specify certain procedures that are never to be delegated but can be performed only by the RN. A detailed discussion about this will follow later in the chapter.

2. **Unsupervised**—When an RN is working with another RN in a collegial relationship, he or she is not in the position of supervising the other RN unless the delivery model identifies the relationship through a charge nurse or other designated capacity. For example, when three RNs are working on one unit, they are not supervising one another and are not accountable for the fundamentals of super-

vision unless one of the three is working in the capacity of a charge nurse, resource nurse, or team leader as defined by the facility.

3. **Initial direction/periodic inspection**—The RN supervises an individual, either licensed or unlicensed, whom the RN knows in terms of competency and has developed a working relationship with over time. An RN working in a dialysis center with a dialysis technician might be comfortable in giving an initial report and direction and then following up two or three times during the shift. A home health nurse in the field might have worked with a home health aide for the past year and be confident in meeting with the aide on a biweekly basis for evaluation of the assigned cases.

4. **Continuous supervision**—When the working relationship is new or the RN has reason to believe that the delegate will need very frequent to continual support and assistance, the highest level of supervision is required. A new graduate nurse who is being oriented on the skilled care unit will need to have someone assigned as a preceptor to provide continuous supervision until the new nurse has demonstrated a level of expertise that the supervising RN is comfortable with. A new graduate should not be placed on the night shift of an extended care unit, where the supervision by another RN is indirect, through the director of nursing at home! A nursing assistant who has just completed the nurses' aide training course will need continual supervision throughout orientation until the RN is satisfied with the new assistant's demonstrated level of skill.

It is important to remember that the RN, in assessing the appropriateness of delegation, also determines whether the level of supervision needed to ensure safe practice is indeed available. We cite Massachusetts Regulations, General Criteria for Delegation, Regulation 244 CMR 3.05:

The degree of supervision required shall be determined by the qualified licensed nurse after an evaluation of appropriate factors involved, including but not limited to, the following: a) the stability of the condition of the patient/client, b) the training and capability of the unlicensed person to whom the nursing task is delegated, c) the nature of the nursing task being delegated, d) the proximity and availability of the nurse. (http://www.mass.gov/Eeohhs2/docs/dph/quality/boards/nursing_faculty/delegate_supervise.rtf, accessed November 13, 2007)

CHECKPOINT 3-6

Determine the level of supervision that is appropriate in each of the following situations:

1. A student nurse who is assigned to your orthopedic unit to care for two patients. Her instructor is in the facility but also has eight other students assigned to her.

2. A fellow RN who is working with you and Marge, the charge nurse.

3. A school health aide who has been assigned to work with you at the junior high school—this is her first day.

4. A mental health assistant who offers to give the IM medications because he "was a medic in the Army."

See the end of the chapter for the answers.

Question 6: TRUE, but only if you delegate inappropriately

This is the question that often stumps nurses we work with and is often the basis for their concern about professional responsibility and "their licenses being on the line." In the eyes of the law, you will be evaluated according to the manner in which you delegate a task and the supervision you provide to the delegate. Delegates are responsible for their individual performance of the task they are trained to perform. You cannot assume (and are not expected to assume) responsibility for the personal performance of all individuals on the healthcare team. Again, we reference the NCSBN (1995, p. 3): "The delegate is accountable for accepting the delegation and for his/her own actions in carrying out the act."

Due to the controversy and concern voiced by nurses across the country, states are responding by adopting rules that more clearly state the nurse's responsibility in working with other personnel. One of the barriers to effective delegation is the fear that the delegating nurse has regarding his or her accountability for the results of a task performed by another individual. Being clear on where that line of responsibility is drawn will help to remove that barrier and allow the nurse to function at the level of his or her professional education, providing optimum care to

> One of the barriers to effective delegation is the fear that the delegating nurse has regarding his or her accountability for the results of a task performed by another individual.

the individual. A legal case review was conducted in 2004 with findings reported by NCSBN: "A case law search found no cases holding a nurse accountable for actions performed by a UAP whether or not the activity was delegable according to the state statutes" (2005a, p. 35).

Knowing what conditions must exist for that line of responsibility to be drawn is also very helpful when making decisions to delegate. According to Colleen Person from Creative Nursing Management:

> Professional nurses who negligently delegate or supervise unlicensed personnel may be subject to a civil liability if a patient is injured, provided the patient can show that:
> * the professional nurse had a duty
> * she or he breached that duty by failing to act as a reasonably prudent nurse would have
> * the professional nurse's conduct caused the harm, or subject of the complaint
> * and the nurse's conduct was the proximate cause of the harm (Person, 1997, p. 12)

Let's discuss the case presented in **Exhibit 3–2**. What is the RN accountable for in this situation? According to our discussion of the legalities of nursing practice, we know the RN is accountable for assessing the situation and the decision to delegate. She is also accountable for supervising the delegate by providing initial guidance and direction, evaluation, and follow-up. According to the scenario described, all of these things were done by the RN.

EXHIBIT 3–2   A Delegation Case Study

An RN on a med/surg unit in City Hospital is working with a nursing assistant (NA) whom she has known and worked with for the past six months. Today she delegates the task of taking vital signs on all patients on the unit, giving particular instruction about Mrs. Avery, a fresh post-op with a new AV fistula in her right arm. Mary, the NA, is instructed to take Mrs. Avery's blood pressure on the left arm, as noted in the Kardex and on a sign above the patient's bed. Mary nods in understanding and begins her assignment. Making her rounds later, the RN finds Mrs. Avery in bed, the blood pressure cuff firmly in place over the new AV fistula in her right arm! The cuff is inflated, and Mary is nowhere to be found!

What is the RN accountable for in this example?

Did she delegate correctly?

Is her license on the line for working with an incompetent aide?

What is Mary (the NA) responsible for?

Did the RN delegate properly? Recalling the regulatory requirements of delegation, you know that the RN delegated properly if she knew the competencies of the NA. Knowing they had worked together for several months, one assumes that she had opportunities to assess job performance and knew that this NA could competently take vital signs.

Is her license in jeopardy? Not at this time. The RN assessed the situation, made a reasonable assignment, and provided initial direction. In the performance of periodic inspection, she has discovered a potentially harmful circumstance. The action she takes now will determine whether she completes the legal expectation of a delegator, that of taking corrective action. The RN must assess the patient's condition, checking the patency of the new fistula, notifying the physician if necessary, and following up with Mary to make certain this does not happen again. (For more on the feedback process, see Chapter 10.)

What is Mary responsible for? According to our legal guidelines, the delegate is responsible for accepting the delegation and for her own actions in carrying out the act. If the patient has been harmed as a result of the improperly placed cuff, Mary is responsible for the damage.

Working with other individuals always poses some risk, but no one individual can provide all of the care that a patient needs. The RN who must rely on the LPN to pass the medications correctly knows that the LPN is responsible for the accuracy of the medication administration and is personally responsible for any error that might be made in performing that act. The physician (the primary delegator on the healthcare team!) who delegates the administration of the chemotherapy to the oncology nurse knows that the oncology nurse is responsible for performing that act correctly. Understanding our legal boundaries helps us to minimize risks and to function at the highest level of our scope of practice.

Question 7: FALSE
The NCSBN (1995, p. 2) clearly states its position:

It is inappropriate for employers or others to require nurses to delegate when, in the nurse's professional judgment, delegation is unsafe and not in the patient's best interest. In those instances, the nurse should act as the patient's advocate and take appropriate action to ensure the provision of safe nursing care. If the nurse determines that delegation may not appropriately take place, but nevertheless delegates as directed, he/she may be disciplined by the Board of Nursing.

> The practice act is the ultimate authority by which your performance will be judged.

Employee policies cannot override the law and rules of nursing and will not protect the nurse who is following policy but acting outside of the practice act. It is clear that the practice act is the ultimate authority by which your performance will be judged. Conflict with an employer may be difficult and unwanted, but as a practicing professional, you will find that it is in your best interests to discuss the differences with the employer. No healthcare facility can stay in business long by breaking the law or asking its employees to do so. (Refer to Chapter 4 for further discussion of the employer relationship.)

A classic example of employer policy differences from years ago involved a research center and their intent to allow UAPs to draw blood, creating a policy to support this. Nurses felt this was unsafe delegation. The employer in this instance had developed a policy allowing NAP (nursing assistive personnel) to be delegated the task of drawing blood. Nurses felt this was an unsafe delegation, citing the following concerns: 1) drawing blood involved the administration of heparin; 2) the procedure is a complex nursing task that requires professional judgment, particularly in the Clinical Research Center where there are frequent blood extractions and the use of long-term indwelling lines; and 3) the RNs were not involved with the NAP or knowledgeable about their skills, training, and qualifications. This conflict posed risks to the RNs: They could face charges of abandonment for refusing to follow the policy, or they could be disciplined by the board of nursing for supervising NAP in an undelegatable task. Fortunately, the RNs were willing to be involved in the resolution, and, using the assistance of the Illinois Board of Nursing, they were able to successfully change the employer policy. NAP at this medical center are now delegated "technical" tasks, and nursing is involved in the decision-making process.

THE LPN ROLE

Very little has been said up to this point regarding the role of the LPN. Rules and statutes that have been cited speak to unlicensed personnel in some instances and to both licensed and unlicensed personnel in other instances. In recent years, the role of the LPN has been altered a great deal in response to closer scrutiny and further clarification of the various roles of nursing. It is not unusual to see the LPN role diminished in many areas as functions previously allowed through employer policy have been eliminated or restricted. We have received letters of concern from LPNs who are struggling to understand the "new" restrictions placed upon them, and we feel it is essential for the RN to understand the legal scope of this delegate as well as that of the unlicensed person.

Roles became blurred as employers responded to shortages, and it was not unusual to find an LPN taking an assignment on a hospital unit similar to that of the RN.

The role of the LPN was created in response to the increased demands for nursing personnel during World War II. Because all of the needs could not be filled with RNs, a new level of caregiver was created: a position that required less education and allowed faster training. Due to the limitations of training, the role of the LPN was defined as being under the supervision of either an RN or a licensed physician, with the understanding that this individual would not have autonomy of practice. During the nursing shortage of the 1970s and then again in the 1980s, there were many instances in which employers expanded the role of the LPN, allowing LPNs to perform functions not clearly outlined within their scope of practice. Assessments, IV medications, tracheal suctioning, and insertion of nasogastric tubes are examples of the procedures that were not originally within the LPN scope of practice. Roles have become blurred as employers respond to labor shortages, and it is not unusual to find an LPN taking an assignment on a hospital unit similar to that of the RN. Little attention has been paid in the past to the differentiation of the roles, and indeed, many RNs still have difficulty articulating the differences! The results of two studies conducted in 2003 demonstrate that this role confusion continues:

> Respondents to each of these studies were asked to comment on the working relationships of RNs and LPN/VNs in their settings. Of those respondents writing comments about RN and LPN/VN working roles, 39% of employers, 52% of LPN/VNs and 62% of RNs wrote that RNs and LPN/VNs in their settings held the same role and performed the same work or that their roles were the same except for specific activities that the RN performed for the clients of the LPN/VNs, such as admitting assessments or IV medications. (Smith & Crawford, 2002 as cited in NCSBN, 2005b, p. 8)

Continuing our discussion of the changing LPN/LVN role, it is important to note some key practice aspects that affect the manner in which an LPN functions. According to the most recent data (2006 LPN/VN Practice Analysis), newly graduated and working practical nurses are most likely to be female, average age of 34, with 54% reporting for work in long-term care settings and only 23.5% in hospitals. Twenty percent report being enrolled in an RN degree program, while 48% work the day shift and report working in an administrative capacity as either a team leader or charge nurse. Task-related issues are still widely variable based on location, with 88% reporting taking verbal/phone orders, 43% performing IV medication administration, 45% completing venipuncture for blood analysis or starting a peripheral line, and 85% organizing and prioritizing care for a group of clients. Fifty-three percent of those responding also reported receiving additional certification, either in basic life support (29.8%), intravenous therapy (21.4%), or phlebotomy (7.5%).

> The difference in the roles of the RN and the LPN should be reflected in policies, job descriptions, assignment methods, and documentation, no matter what the setting.

An LPN is still limited in scope of practice, and whether the practice act and the governing board are separate or combined with the RN boards, the limit is still the same. LPN practice is "recognizing and meeting the basic needs of the client, gives nursing care under the direction and supervision of the registered nurse or licensed physician to clients in routine nursing situations" (WAC 308-117-020, Washington).

Facing yet another significant shortage of nursing personnel, employers might be tempted to again advance the role of the LPN. However, we have learned from past experience, and the majority of NPAs (Nurse Practice Acts) are specific regarding the tasks and activities that can be included in the LPN scope of practice.

In several states (for example, Colorado and Texas) the LPN is prohibited by law from delegating nursing tasks, and this function is allowed only to the RN. The definition of supervision as described earlier is applicable to RNs working with LPNs, and the need for initial guidance and direction, evaluation, and follow-up of these members of the team must be demonstrated. The difference in the roles of the RN and the LPN should be reflected in policies, job descriptions, assignment methods, and documentation, no matter what the setting.

DELEGATION AND THE NURSING PROCESS

Although the operational definition of delegation is purposefully general, there are some guidelines for the RN to use when evaluating the decision

While nursing tasks can be delegated, the licensed nurse's generalist knowledge of patient care indicates that the practice-pervasive functions of assessment, evaluation, and nursing judgment must not be delegated.

of whether to delegate. In fact, as some of you will be delighted to know, there are some very specific statements regarding what may not be delegated under any circumstance. For example, according to the NCSBN (1995, p. 2), "8. While nursing tasks may be delegated, the licensed nurse's generalist knowledge of patient care indicates that the practice-pervasive functions of assessment, evaluation, and nursing judgment must not be delegated."

CHECKPOINT 3–7

1. In my state, the LPN (may/may not) delegate selected nursing tasks.

2. At the facility where I work, there (is/is not) a difference in the role of the RN and the role of the LPN according to policy.

3. I (know/do not know) what the limitations of the LPN are in this state.

See the end of the chapter for the answers.

The part of the nursing process most readily delegated involves the component of intervention. Tasks, procedures, technical duties, and so forth all fall into this category and are part of the patient's care that can be readily performed by another individual besides the RN. However, as a professional registered nurse the decision is yours to make and is one we hope that you base on each specific situation, considering carefully the patient's response and the outcome you desire. In one setting, you might choose to delegate the task of a clean dressing change to the NA, knowing that the wound is healing and that the patient has been taught what to observe in the process. In another setting, you might elect to do the dressing change yourself, wanting to assess the skin and teach a family member to look for signs of infection.

Specific limits to interventions that may not be delegated to unlicensed personnel are outlined in each state and vary according to state law. The more common restrictions are similar to those found in the Massachusetts Nursing Regulation 244CMR 3.05:

(5) Nursing Activities That May Not Be Delegated. By way of example, and not in limitation, the following are nursing activities that are not within the scope of sound nursing judgment to delegate:

(a) Nursing activities which require nursing assessment and judgment during implementation

(b) Physical, psychological, and social assessment which requires nursing judgment, intervention, referral or follow-up

(c) Formulation of the plan of nursing care and evaluation of the patient's/client's response to the care provided

(d) Administration of medications except as permitted by MGL Chapter 94C

(e) Patient/client Health Teaching and Health Counseling. (http://www.mass.gov/Eeohhs2/docs/dph/regs/244cmr 003.pdf, accessed November 13, 2007)

Delegation and the Nursing Process

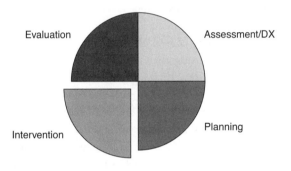

Item (a) in the preceding list is one criterion that is listed in the majority of nurse practice acts and reinforced by the NCSBN, the limiting factors being any task that requires nursing "judgment" and "assessment." The Montana Nursing Regulations (Rule 8.32.1703, Sept. 1996) states that judgment "means the intellectual process that a nurse exercises in forming an opinion and reaching a clinical decision based upon analysis of the evidence or data."

Judgment: "The intellectual process that a nurse exercises in forming an opinion and reaching a clinical decision based upon analysis of the evidence or data."

We would add as a point of clarification that assessment goes beyond the collection of physical data and is really "the initial phase of the Nursing Process which involves the interpretation of the significance of the available subjective and objective data regarding a specific patient situation, performed in order to formulate an individualized plan of care" (Hansten & Washburn, 1995, p. i).

"Assessment is the initial phase of the Nursing Process which involves the interpretation of the significance of the available subjective and objective data regarding a specific patient situation, performed in order to formulate an individualized plan of care."

Many states strictly prohibit the delegation of the administration of medication, but several states are recognizing that this is appropriate in some settings. Group homes for the developmentally or mentally disabled, community settings for the physically handicapped, group homes for the elderly, and long-term care facilities are all examples of areas where assistive personnel may be allowed to administer medication. The Practice and Professional Issues Survey (Smith & Crawford, 2002) conducted by the NCSBN listed eight categories of activities that were delegated to assistive personnel. While basic care tasks were listed more frequently, medication administration was one of the more complex tasks also identified as routinely assigned. LPN/LVNs were more than twice as likely to delegate medication administration. Over 30 states now utilize medication assistants (MAs), and many have certification programs for this type of worker, using the title MA-C. While there is growth in this area, there is still controversy regarding the potential erosion of nursing if this trend is to continue and nurses relinquish the task of medication administration. Support for the use of MAs is largely anecdotal, with comments expressing the increased efficiency and reduction of errors when nurses no longer attempt to administer medications in the midst of numerous other demands. The Arkansas Board of Nursing is only one such state that developed a certification exam, which was available in mid-2007. Citing anecdotal research, they included comments from local nursing home directors who commented on the increased time nurses have to spend assessing residents and complete charting while MAs are more cautiously and attentively passing medications (Murphree, 2007). Wyoming is not as enthusiastic about the use of MAs and references a research study conducted at UC Davis that demonstrated an increase in medication errors after the use of MAs. The medication bill did not pass in this state (Behrens, 2007). Recognizing the continued growth in the use of MAs, the NCSBN conducted an MA Job Analysis in 2006, revealing that most MAs work in long-term care settings (58%), assisted living (32%), and rehab facilities (11%).

The growth of assisted living centers for the elderly or disabled has raised questions about regulation of medication administration in those settings. A University of Virginia study reviewed the status of this emerging practice setting and how state rules differ. They cite a Washington state study with no evidence of harm to residents who are administered medications by nonnurses. California, Connecticut, and Delaware prohibited delegation of medications. Eighteen states allowed the residents to be "reminded" of self-medication by assistive personnel. However, boards voiced concern about whether or not assistive personnel were really administering the medications in assisted living settings without adequate training (Reinhard, Young, Kane, & Quinn, 2006). This area of practice appears to be in a state of flux, and we recommend that readers who work in assisted living care centers contact their state regulatory agency to clarify their state's current policy.

CHECKPOINT 3-8

Check the following statements that apply to you:

O I know what I may not delegate to unlicensed assistive personnel according to my state's practice act.

O I know which parts of the nursing process I may safely delegate.

Although our diagram of the nursing process appears to be limiting, we want to make certain that you understand that parts of the processes of assessment, planning, and evaluation may also be delegated. When a new patient is admitted to any healthcare setting, it is common for the initial data assessment of vital signs, height, and weight, as well as chief complaint, be obtained by someone other than the RN. The LPN may perform additional interviewing and gathering of data for the RN to complete the assessment. The question of whether an LPN may perform a complete patient assessment remains an area of controversy. Arguments range from the opinion that the education of the LPN does not provide sufficient theoretical base for assessment to the opinion that an LPN can be taught basic assessment skills as long as the data are interpreted by an RN. Once again, the accountability of the assessment rests with the RN, and it is the RN who is best prepared through education and experience to assess the patient.

Planning is another area of the nursing process that may invite participation from the other members of the team. Nursing assistants

Thirty percent of the respondents in a nationwide survey of consumers were uncertain whether UAP were providing their care. Of those who correctly identified the caregiver, many admitted to guessing, based on assumptions of who should be doing the task. "I think nurses give the meds, but I don't really know," and "When they come quick, I believe they are aides," were some of the reasons offered (Lange & Polifroni, 2000).

The accountability of the assessment rests with the RN, and it is the RN who is best prepared through education and experience to assess the patient.

The RN's critical analysis will be necessary to determine if the nursing diagnosis is correct, if the outcomes targeted are reasonable, and if the patient is responding to the interventions that have been performed.

might have the opportunity to spend additional direct time with the patient and might learn information that would assist the RN in best planning the care for the patient during hospitalization or while under the care of the agency. A home health aide who visits the home frequently will certainly have valuable input for the RN who makes only a monthly visit.

Evaluation involves the interpretation of data to make judgments regarding the effectiveness of the interventions, and it rests primarily with the RN. Again, the other members of the team might have observations and other information that will assist the RN in the evaluation, but the responsibility for the judgment belongs to the RN. The RN's critical analysis will be necessary to determine if the nursing diagnosis is correct, if the outcomes targeted are reasonable, and if the patient responds to the interventions that have been performed. This systematic process involves the coordination of all members of the team and requires the organized skill of the RN.

The bar graph in **Figure 3–2** illustrates the overlap of the performance of the various components of the nursing process by the four levels of nursing personnel. This study involved a survey of over 15,000 providers, randomly selected from all states, by the Research Services Division of the NCSBN (NCSBN, 1994). The purpose of the study was to obtain data to delineate the roles of the four levels of personnel and to facilitate the delegation of nursing activities to unlicensed personnel. A complete report of this study was distributed at the Delegate Assembly in August 1994. The survey demonstrated a specific pattern regarding the performance of the activities of the nursing process. The frequency of each component is ranked as follows:

NAs and LPNs: implementation, assessment, analysis, planning, evaluation

RNs: assessment, implementation, analysis, evaluation, planning

Nurse Practitioners: assessment, implementation, analysis, planning, evaluation

From this study it is apparent that NAs and LPNs report spending more time implementing care, whereas RNs and nurse practitioners spend more time in assessing the need and type of care to be given. As of 2007, no additional study of this type has been conducted by the NCSBN. We

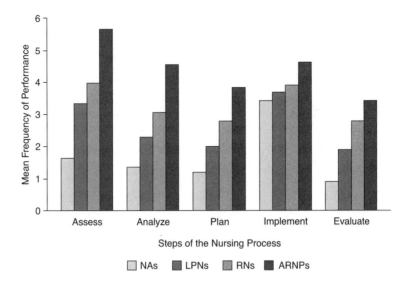

FIGURE 3-2 Average mean frequency of performance values for nursing process activity statements, by personnel category. *Source:* Reprinted with permission of the National Council of State Boards of Nursing, Chicago, Illinois.

continue to include it here as a seminal work that gives insight to the use of the nursing process and in hopes that further research will be done in the future as a comparison.

CONCLUSION

In this chapter we have discussed the fundamental knowledge of the nurse practice act that is necessary to determine if the delegation you are considering will truly "put your license on the line." Understanding the limitations of your practice act, as well as the purpose and the powers of the board of nursing, are key factors in dispelling the fear of responsibility for the actions of those with whom you work. No single individual can provide all things to all people, and the risks involved in relying on others can be minimized with the knowledge of legal definitions and expectations.

You are encouraged to seek the resources available to you: Obtain a copy of the nurse practice act in your state, request any advisory opinions that have been issued on the subject of delegation, and contact your board of nursing to learn more about the process of ensuring the safety of the public through the regulation of nursing practice. Better yet—get on the Internet and access the National Council Web site or any number of professional organizations that now have a Web page for your continued professional development. It's your license—protect it!

ANSWERS TO CHECKPOINTS

3–1.   c

3–2.   d

3–3.   d

3–5.   c

3–6.

1. initial direction/periodic inspection

2. unsupervised

3. continuous supervision

4. never delegated

3–7.

1. The LPN may or may not be allowed to delegate nursing tasks. Check your state's nurse practice act for the correct answer in your state.

2. There is a difference. (There should be!) This difference should be apparent in the job description, the system of care delivery, and the reporting and documentation expectations of the LPN.

3. I do know the limitations of the LPN in this state. (If you do not, do you feel safe in delegating to an LPN?)

REFERENCES

American Nurses Association & National Council of State Boards of Nursing. (2006). *Joint statement on delegation*. Retrieved April 14, 2008, from https://www.ncsbn.org/Joint_statement.pdf

Behrens, M. (2007, March–May). *Wyoming Nurse, 20*(1).

Donahue, M. P. (1985). *Nursing, the finest art*. St. Louis, MO: CV Mosby.

Hansten, R., & Washburn, M. (1990). *I light the lamp*. Vancouver, WA: Applied Therapeutics.

Hansten, R., & Washburn, M. (1995). *Land in sight*. Children's Hospital Workshop Syllabus. Seattle, WA, p. i.

Heschel, R., Crowley, A., & Cohen, S. (2005). State policies regarding nursing delegation and medication administration in child care settings: A case study. *Policy, Politics, and Nursing Practice, 6*(2), 86–98.

Lange, J. C. W., & Polifroni, E. C. (2000). Nurses and assistive personnel, do patients know the difference? *Journal of Nursing Administration, 30*(11), 512–513.

Murphree, J. (2007, March). *ASBN Update, 11*(2).

National Council of State Boards of Nursing. (1994). *Preliminary report: Role delineation study of nurse aides, licensed practical/vocational nurses, registered nurses and advanced registered nurse practitioners*. Chicago: Author.

National Council of State Boards of Nursing. (1995, December). Delegation: Concepts and decision-making process. *Issues*, 1–4.

National Council of State Boards of Nursing. (2005a). *Working with others: A position paper*. Chicago: Author.

National Council of State Boards of Nursing. (2005b). *Practical nurse scope of practice white paper*. Chicago: Author.

National Council of State Boards of Nursing. (2006). *Executive summary: Job analysis of medication assistants*. Chicago: Author.

National Council of State Boards of Nursing. (2007). *2006 LPN/VN practice analysis linking the NCLEX-PN exam to practice*. Chicago: Author.

Person, C. (1997). Delegation: Risk management implications for nurses. *Creative Nursing, 3*(1), 12.

Reinhard, S., Young, H., Kane, R., & Quinn, W. (2006). Nurse delegation of medication administration for older adults in assisted living. *Nursing Outlook, 54*(2), 74–80.

Smith, J. E., & Crawford, L. H. (2002). *Report of findings from the 2001 practice and professional issues survey, spring 2001* (NCSBN Research Brief, Vol. 2). Chicago: National Council of State Boards of Nursing.

Know Your Organization: What About Where I Work?

4

CHAPTER SKILLS

+ Identify 3 components of union representation in an organization.
+ Assess your organization to determine its support of the delegation process and professional practice.
+ Discuss positive and negative impacts of the use of assistive personnel.

RECOMMENDED RESOURCES

▶ Read the mission statement, vision, values, and nursing philosophy of your organization.

▶ Review the job descriptions/skills checklists of the members of your team.

▶ Check out the organizational policies regarding delegation at your facility.

▶ Interview your nursing leaders regarding their ideas for advancing and promoting nursing in the community.

"My manager is always talking about the mission and values of this organization. Big deal. All that seems to really mean is how much work can they get out of us without paying us any more. They keep changing things and talking about this wonderful quality program at the same time they're taking our jobs and giving them to assistive personnel."

Historical Development—Or, How Did We Get Here?
Ruth I. Hansten and Marilynn Jackson

In the previous chapters we have begun to create a foundation of knowledge regarding the legal support you have as a practicing professional. At the same time we have discussed some of the primary reasons for the constant state of change that many organizations are experiencing, with the intention of offering you some basis for understanding what you as an employee might be experiencing. We must now take our assessment one further step and take a clear look at the environment in which you work so that you might not feel the way the individual does in our example above.

Those of you who are groaning at the idea of a little history, please stay with us on this one as we explore a quick review of organizational development to better appreciate the framework of the healthcare system as it has evolved today. It is unusual for many of us to question why things are the way they are. For most, if the environment in which we are working is challenging, unfulfilling, or supportive, we don't question the rationale but seek instead to make changes or to be grateful for what we have in terms of a job and make the best of it. But why are you in a top-down, chain-of-command system? Or if you are in a more progressive style of participative management, complete with administrative support for multidisciplinary team building, why is your organization making this change? If you are a student thinking about future career options, what work setting would fit you best?

CHECKPOINT 4–1

Are the following statements true or false?

____ 1.   There is only one style of organization, and the administrator always controls the decisions.

____ 2.   There has been little change in the way healthcare professionals are treated as employees.

____ 3.   Most healthcare organizations have a mission statement and have always had one.

____ 4.   Unions are involved in all healthcare facilities and have been since hospitals first opened.

____ 5.   Employer policies are more important than the nurse practice act.

See the end of the chapter for the answers.

How did you do with the previous checkpoint? As we continue our discussion, keep these questions in mind. We will review the role of unions, mission statements, and policies in the evolution of the health-care system from its humble beginnings to the challenges of today. Most important of all will be the process of delegation as part of your changing work environment and the role the organization plays in the process.

IN THE BEGINNING

If we were to go back before Nightingale's day, we would discover that health care was not an organized system. There were few hospitals, and the general expectation was that the women of the family would provide most of the ministering to the sick. There were few effective medicinal resources, and society as a whole had not fully organized its system of work.

The industrial revolution, the progression of medicine, and the advancement of technology brought significant changes to the newly forming hospital system. Almshouses and military and public hospitals offered the only early options for health care outside of the home. With the advent of anesthetics and septic technique, the demand for hospitals increased. It was no longer desirable for physicians to perform surgery at home on the far from sterile kitchen table, where many had demanded surgery be done and where people had once felt safer than they would risking their lives to the high level of infection at the hospital.

The world continued to change rapidly as transportation made it easier for families to be mobile and industry became more organized in its structure. Salaried management emerged in all industries, and administrators and professors joined the ranks of universities. In hospitals, however, the decision-making power was shifting to the physicians, who were more and more in control of the admissions to a hospital. Boards of trustees were being replaced by medical boards, who held controlling authority over the administration of the hospital. It was not unusual for physicians to own small private hospitals and to employ a management team to enact their decisions. As the hospital setting grew and physicians were able to belong to several hospitals, their needs for administrative services increased as well. Administrators were empowered with increasing authority to oversee the employees, ensuring that the hospital ran smoothly internally so that the physicians could perform their services. Hospital management then followed the mainstream of scientific management principles, and a top-down, controlling approach was embraced.

Hospital management then followed the mainstream of scientific management principles, and a top-down, controlling approach was embraced. In the meantime, nursing was advancing quickly, organizing nursing schools, setting minimum standards for licensure, and responding to the needs of the people in the community in addition to the institution. Lillian Wald was an exemplary leader in the late 1800s, developing the Henry Street Settlement and advancing the system of public health. Under her direction, the first system for nurses in public schools was created, and nursing services for insurance policyholders were initiated (Christy, 1984). Nursing was defining its role in many arenas outside the hospital, but it was the hospital that remained the benchmark for the healthcare system.

Hospital development was rapid throughout the 20th century, responding to many diverse sociocultural events. World Wars I and II, the Great Depression, and the changing face of disease from polio epidemics to demands for organ transplants kept the hospital system in constant turmoil. The treatment of employees, including nurses, became more controlling as hospital management adopted policies and systems to strengthen their control over an internal environment in response to increasing public and federal involvement. Unions found their place in health care after World War II, representing nurses and other healthcare workers who fought for employee protection and the assurance of individual rights.

The Unionized Organization and Delegation
Karen A. McGrath

What could unions possibly have to do with clinical delegation? Whether you are considering or already working in a facility where nurses are represented by a union, it is important to understand the role of the union in ensuring a fair and reasonable work environment.

Since before the turn of the 20th century in this country, workers have struggled to assert some measure of control over working conditions. Leaders came from the ranks of employees in a number of trades or industries; they included miners, garment workers, auto workers, and longshoremen. They understood the workplace and what was needed to prevent abuse and exploitation of employees. They worked to educate and unite workers, to establish equitable wage standards, and to generally improve the quality of work life.

Healthcare employees are relative newcomers to the union movement. Federal laws—the Railway Labor Act of 1926 and the National

Labor Relations Act (or Wagner Act) of 1935—were enacted to protect workers' "right to self-organization, to form, join, or assist labor organizations, to bargain collectively through representatives of their own choosing, and to engage in concerted activities, for the purpose of collective bargaining or other mutual aid or protection" (National Labor Relations Act, Section 7). Until 1974, however, private, not-for-profit healthcare institutions were exempt from union coverage. Individual states passed laws governing collective bargaining rights for public sector employees.

> Unions found their place in health care after World War II, representing nurses and other healthcare workers who fought for employee protection and the insurance of individual rights.

Other laws that advanced unionization included the Taft-Hartley Act (or the Labor-Management Relations Act) of 1947, which further defined the rights and duties of both labor and management, and the Landrum-Griffin Act (or the Labor-Management Reporting and Disclosure Act) of 1959, which spelled out the rights of union members. These measures went a long way toward eliminating abuses and corruption that had come to light.

The American Nurses Association (ANA) and its constituent state nurses associations (SNAs) had, since their inception in 1896, been addressing employment standards for nurses, and until the mid-1940s they had achieved only limited success. The approach had focused on educating nurses and consumers about matters affecting the recruitment of qualified nurses. In 1946, the ANA House of Delegates took a bold step by approving a plan for a national economic and security program. A key piece of the program called upon the SNAs to act as collective bargaining representatives for nurses. Many of the SNAs began to build their own programs with trained staff to meet this challenge. Today, about half of the SNAs have full economic and general welfare (or labor relations) programs that are responsible for representing nurses in a variety of work settings.

In addition to the SNAs, many other unions represent healthcare employees, including nurses. During the 1970s and 1980s, the economy in the United States began to shift away from the manufacturing sector to a growing service sector. Health care, as a large part of the service industry, became fertile ground for organizing, and unions looked to bolster shrinking membership numbers by shifting their attention to this arena.

> In 1946, the ANA House of Delegates took a bold step by approving a plan for a national economic and security program. A key piece of the program called upon the state nurses associations to act as collective bargaining representatives for nurses.

No matter which union a group has selected as its representative, knowing some basic principles will maximize your own union experience (if you work in a facility where the employees are represented by a union) and make it work for you and your patients. Remember those key phrases from the Wagner Act: collective bargaining, mutual aid and protection, and concerted activity? They assume people are working together toward a common goal. It begins with a secret ballot election in which an identified employee group decides if and by which union it wants to be represented. The group becomes a bargaining unit and proceeds to elect local leaders from within its own membership. The new leaders' task is to seek out and represent the needs and desires of the membership. The union provides experts in labor relations and industry trends and standards to guide and advise the leaders as they negotiate a collective bargaining agreement (a contract) with the employer.

For all of this to be successful, the membership has certain rights and responsibilities as well. The union has the legal responsibility to represent all members fairly, and the members are expected to join and support the union they have selected. This is one of those instances where the old axiom about the house divided truly applies. The union is the membership and functions democratically. The members give direction to leaders by participating in meetings and voting on matters of concern. To be an effective member, you must be informed and involved. Your degree of involvement will depend on your own desires as well as other personal and professional demands on your time. Attending meetings, reading the literature, volunteering for committees, and becoming a unit representative are degrees of involvement that are open to you as a union member.

When dealing with management, the most successful bargaining units are able to demonstrate unity and credibility. An adversarial relationship is not necessary and is often counterproductive to reaching mutually acceptable solutions to problems. Management representatives who recognize and respect the collective bargaining relationship are also most often successful in maintaining a measure of what is known as labor peace.

> The union has the legal responsibility to represent all members fairly, and the members are expected to join and support the union they have selected.

The process lends itself to the popular thinking of participative management: total quality management (TQM) and continuous quality improvement (CQI). The difference in the unionized setting is the balance of power. The assistance of the union in dealing with the management structure is intended to level the playing field.

But what does all of this have to do with clinical delegation?

One of the committees that is very important for nurses is the nursing practice committee.

An employment contract typically covers such topics as wages, premium pay for unusual or extra shifts, holidays, vacations, insurance benefits, seniority, work schedules, and a grievance procedure for dispute resolution. In addition, contracts covering nurses very often speak to staffing and patient safety concerns and establish joint labor–management committees designed to open communications. One of the committees that is very important for nurses is the nursing practice committee.

This committee is composed of nurses elected by members of the bargaining unit who meet from time to time with representatives of nursing administration to discuss issues of concern with policies and procedures that affect patient care delivery. The issues can be raised by either the nurses or managers, are thoroughly researched, and require a written response from administration detailing what is to be done to resolve the issue. In most cases a joint solution can be found.

Now, let us see how the system works in three practice settings.

Setting 1: Sunshine Community Hospital

Sunshine Community Hospital has announced to the staff in its Friday newsletter that nursing will be changing in a very innovative way. It is the wave of the future and will free the nurses from such mundane tasks as bathing and feeding patients, walking patients, changing dressings, and administering medications. A two-week training program has been developed, and the first trainees will begin on Monday. For the past 15 years, nurses have functioned in a primary care delivery model, with a few LPNs on some of the units to help with the heavier patients.

Mary Ann has worked at the hospital for five years and never felt the need to join the union. She is not alone here; less than half of the nurses belong. Her nurse manager tells her not to worry: they have researched these new delivery models and know what they are doing. "Just trust us."

The local leaders contact the union office to find out what to do. The staff representative advises that they need to request a meeting with management to ask questions and gets a letter out immediately. Management reluctantly agrees to meet but firmly states that the plan is already in place and moving along. The Nursing Practice Committee has not met for some time because the leaders could not find nurses who were interested or willing to invest the time. The first meeting to discuss the change in staff mix is difficult because not everyone knows everyone else. The nurses are angry, and management is defensive of its plan. At the second meeting, the nurses are able to articulate their concerns about the new plan and begin to ask questions about such things as the new care partners, the training program, and the acuity of the patients in relation to the new staff model. The third meeting yields an agreement to conduct a study of the effect of the new plan on patient satisfaction.

This process has taken three months. In the meantime nurses have begun to work with the new care partners and have found it difficult to relinquish many of the bedside activities that have been so much a part of their daily routines. They complain to leaders that this new model has doubled their patient load while not giving them much more help, and they demand to know what the union is doing to stop this. Mary Ann is among several nurses who resign rather than practice this way.

Setting 2: Northern Visiting Nurse Service

Northern Visiting Nurse Service has been experiencing a growth spurt. Referrals are up as patients are discharged from hospitals sooner, often needing nursing follow-up. Maureen finds herself going home later and more tired, even though she loves home care and still feels professionally challenged. She has been an SNA member since graduation but has never really paid much attention to the contract. The raises have been nice, and she enjoys a fairly good relationship with Jean, her supervisor.

A memo from the director of patient care services warns staff that the current use of overtime is excessive and must be reduced. This results in increased grumbling in the office, and Maureen is worried. Jean's response is that the directive is from upstairs and there is nothing she can do. Posted on the bulletin board, next to the overtime memo, is the list of bargaining unit officers. The same day, she locates the chairperson, John, and asks if the union can do anything about the mounting pressure. She expresses her frustration with an administration that appears to have lost touch with the facts of direct care. John is very understanding and reports that nurses have been calling him all day.

As they talk, it becomes apparent that the problems are sicker patients who require more time, more paperwork, and orienting new nurses without an adjustment of workload. John invites Maureen to a meeting of the bargaining unit to discuss the issues. She is able to repeat her concerns, and John leads a discussion of possible solutions to be presented to administration. At the next labor–management meeting, John presents the issue along with a time study done by several of the nurses. Administration's initial response is that the nurses just have to dig in and bear with it until the new nurses are able to make visits independently. John continues to discuss the solutions developed by the group, concentrating on the enormous amount of paperwork required. As he describes the different forms and their purposes, it becomes clear that some contain redundant information and are simple enough that clerical employees could transcribe the information from reports that the nurses complete. The nurses have calculated that approximately one hour per day is spent by nurses on an activity that could be done by current clericals, saving the agency a significant amount in overtime costs or lost visits. The director is impressed and commits to examining the issue further, looking at the paperwork to determine if a report is really needed and, if so, who could fill it out. John reports that Maureen will head a bargaining unit task force to examine the agency's preceptor program with a goal of maximizing the orientation experience while being sensitive to the workload of the preceptors. The director states that she is eager to see the results.

Setting 3: Toowell Memorial

Across town, at Toowell Memorial, the Nursing Practice Committee is meeting at its usual time this month, and the nurses see a new item on the agenda. The director of nursing describes a new staff mix model they have been interested in trying. She shares material from professional journals on trends in nursing management that point to a delivery model incorporating nonlicensed nurse extenders to free nurses to be more involved in the care management of patients. Sharon is the local unit's chairperson. She is able to report on concerns expressed by staff nurses at a recent symposium sponsored by the union. It is agreed that supervisors and the union's leaders will conduct meetings with staff nurses in the next two weeks to detail the proposed plan and listen to the nurses' concerns and suggestions.

At the conclusion of these meetings, the committee reconvenes to try to work on the nurses' concerns, and several changes are made to the plan in response. At Sharon's suggestion, the committee agrees that the plan will be better received if it is examined again by the staff nurses. A pilot program is planned for a volunteer unit, with criteria established for measurement. The nurses will be provided training in delegation skills, an expert from the SNA is invited to discuss the practice act implications of the new care partners, and the training program for care partners is jointly developed. The experiment goes well, with only a few modifications to the plan needed. Regular progress reports are published in the union's newsletter to the nurses.

The presence of a union is not a guarantee that employment is secure and that no changes in your practice will ever be made. As with any process, you have to make it work.

Three months later, Sharon and her local unit colleagues on the Nurse Practice Committee assist staff nurses from the pilot unit to present the results to the local unit's members. Ninety percent of the hospital's staff nurses are members and attend the meetings to vote. The plan is overwhelmingly approved, and the nurses leave the meeting looking forward to having the new staff mix plan introduced on their unit.

As you can see, the presence of a union is not a guarantee that employment is secure and that no changes in your practice will ever be made. Selecting a union can be important, but it is not enough. As with any process, you have to make it work. It is a little like buying a car. Without one, you might take a bit longer to get around, but it does not do any good just left to sit in the garage. For managers, having a union is not a sign of failure. It can provide a vehicle for discussion and change. A contract provides structure that everyone can understand and work with to resolve problems.

CHECKPOINT 4-2

1. Union representation

    a) is available in all states

    b) is required in all hospitals

    c) has always been available for healthcare employees

    d) relies on membership participation to be effective

2. Being a member of a union

    a) means that I will always have a job

    b) is required by my licensure

    c) provides me with an additional opportunity to join with fellow employees in an organized fashion to discuss working conditions with management

    d) is prohibited by my nurse practice act

3. I can be involved in changes in care delivery that result in my need to delegate nursing care by

    a) being an active union member and attending nurse practice committee meetings

b) participating in the management of my (nonunion) work setting by attending staff meetings and serving on committees and task forces that plan changes in care delivery and staffing

c) keeping myself informed and updated on trends in nursing practice

d) all of the above

See the end of the chapter for the answers.

Assessing the Healthcare Organization
Ruth I. Hansten and Marilynn Jackson

THE NONUNION ENVIRONMENT

If you aren't in a union environment, never fear! In many states or locales, nurses are not represented by a union, nor do they feel a need for one. When management practices in a participative fashion, with true empowerment of all staff, such as in shared governance or self-directed work teams, staff nurses' concerns are equally important and valued. Wise administrators develop staff through education and encourage autonomy in decision making regarding patient care. Wise staff become involved in committees or task forces (whether union or not) that develop policies and procedures and plan for innovative practice that will ensure quality and cost-effective care. "If anything has emerged over the last 30 years of organizational research, it is the understanding that effective human relationships in the workplace are essential to sustaining the purposes and agenda of the organization" (Porter-O'Grady, 2002). It is your responsibility as a professional nurse to uphold those relationships by being involved in your employing organization.

Whether the facility you work for has union representation for its employees or not is only one part of the picture. Several factors must be assessed as we continue our knowledge of the organization.

THE MISSION STATEMENT

Today's contemporary healthcare facility carries with it the history of intensifying social demands and the increasing involvement of federal policy. The focus of any healthcare organization must shift from a

> ... effective human relationships in the workplace are essential to sustaining the purposes and agenda of the organization.

singular perspective to a systems approach or global perspective on patient and client needs. Traditional roles and traditional management techniques will no longer be effective in the reformed system. Organizational systems are emerging in which the employees are truly valued members of the team and in which it is believed that the employee is responsible to think and achieve. With this major shift in premise is the need to begin at the root of the organization—the mission statement.

Having received a wake-up call from a public that has loudly voiced its dissatisfaction with the healthcare system, organizations are reexamining their values and mission statements to make certain they are guiding the shift from a product emphasis to a service approach. Mission statements of the early hospitals in the mid-1800s focused on primarily religious and moralistic objectives. It was not unusual for a hospital to identify its mission as one of providing homes for the orphans or the poor and creating a Christian environment. The advent of surgery and the relief of acute illness caused many hospitals to redefine their mission in terms of medical objectives, and the emphasis shifted from a moral stance to an approach that clearly identified the purpose as the treatment of disease and injury (Starr, 1982, p. 158).

The healthcare organization of today has broadened its perspective, integrating the social, moral, and medical objectives in a more holistic expression of the mission of the institution. For example, the Web site for Florida Hospital Heartland Division (http://www.fhhd.org/AboutUs/Mission/tabid/2512/Default.aspx) describes their mission as:

> ... to serve our community by providing quality healthcare services and promoting wellness and healthful living.

- We seek to deliver our services with compassion and understanding.
- We strive to deliver our services efficiently, using the highest level of technology available to us and keeping in mind our customers' need for cost containment.
- To ensure the best possible outcomes, we will promote quality cost containment and service excellence among all who are involved in serving our customers.
- Our services will be provided to all in need of medical assistance without discrimination.

◆ We offer our services in an environment where physical, mental and spiritual healing are promoted and where everyone is treated with courtesy and respect.

We will fulfill this mission with a Christian spirit and to the best of our abilities.

The components of quality, cost-effectiveness, and accessibility are common to most mission statements today. Most will also include a component relating to the employee, and the statement might look something like this: "To promote the continuous professional growth of each employee within a supportive environment." Stephen Covey (1991) said it best years ago when he suggested a universal personal and professional mission statement: "To improve the economic well being and quality of life for all stakeholders."

In addition to a mission, the statement can include a "vision," a direction or focus for the organization. This can specifically outline an area of the community, an aspect of service to be provided, or a specific age group to be emphasized, as in this statement from an East Coast hospital: "As part of a regional health system, we specialize in quality, family-centered services, with emphasis on a continuum of care for those adults 50 years of age and older. We will be an active partner in improving the health of the communities we serve."

The mission statement can also be supported by a list of values, those fundamental beliefs that form the framework of the culture of the organization. There is a growing body of research regarding the connection of personal, professional, and organizational values It is apparent that when there is a disconnection between any of these, there is opportunity for dissatisfaction and stress. McNeese-Smith and Crook (2003) studied 412 RNs in three hospitals and determined that "supervisory relations" is the highest-rated value, underscoring the importance of a positive working relationship with a supervisor who is "fair and with whom one can get along." As we discuss delegation and its counterpart, supervision, it is a good idea to remember this value and understand that assistive personnel will appreciate the same value, looking for someone who is fair in delegation decisions and understanding.

Representing extensive and lengthy research, the list that follows describes the 15 values defined by D. Super (as cited in McNeese-Smith & Crook, 2003) and the contextual definition of each. Think about this list in terms of your own organization, your personal values, and those of the assistants you might supervise.

VALUE	DEFINITION: WORK THAT . . .
Achievement	Gives one a feeling of accomplishment
Aesthetics	Allows one to contribute to the beauty of the world
Altruism	Enables one to contribute to the welfare of others
Associates	Has connections with fellow workers one likes
Creativity	Permits one to develop new ideas
Economic returns	Pays well and enables one to have the things desired
Independence	Allows one to work at one's own pace, in own way
Intellectual stimulation	Provides opportunity for learning and independent thinking
Management	Allows one to plan and direct work for others
Prestige	Evokes respect from others
Security	Provides one with job certainty
Supervisory relations	Is done under the direction of someone who is fair and congenial
Surroundings	Is performed in pleasant conditions
Variety	Provides an opportunity to do different jobs
Way of life	Permits one to have the life one desires

Source: Adapted from McNeese-Smith & Crook, 2003.

Understanding the mission and values of the organization for which you work is essential in understanding and safely implementing the process of delegation. Another key ingredient of the organizational framework is the nursing philosophy, usually a statement or compilation of statements that represents the beliefs of the division of nursing within the organization. It is important that nursing leadership oversee this draft, but it is equally important for staff nurses to participate in its creation. Again, we emphasize, the relationship you are developing with your employer needs continual nurturing!

The following is an example of a nursing philosophy created by the staff nurses and their leadership:

WE BELIEVE . . .

- Nursing is the pivotal, fundamental component of the acute healthcare team, working collaboratively with all other disciplines.
- Nursing is a professional role that is driven from within, demonstrating evidence-based clinical excellence, action orientation, and accountability.
- Providing nursing care with excellence requires that we be cognizant of our own well-being and needs.
- Our patient focus is outcome based, considering the needs, rights, education and care of each individual/family according to the Patient Bill of Rights as established by the American Nurses Association.

Source: University of Texas Health Center at Tyler. Reprinted with permission.

CHECKPOINT 4–3

Knowledge of the mission and values of my employing facility is important in delegation because:

a) They are not important because no one follows them anyway.

b) I'm not sure because I have never seen the mission statement.

c) They clarify the basic premise of the agency and will enable me to assess what value the organization places on employee involvement, particularly in redesigning the care delivery system.

d) The mission will tell me if I'm in the right place or not and if I need to join a union to improve the working conditions.

See the end of the chapter for the answers.

Congratulations! You've made it this far, and we promise you that the following discussion will be firmly focused on contemporary issues (except for a brief reminder of history!).

By now you know that we are emphasizing the importance of the nursing process and continually applying it to our discussion of delegation. A clearer understanding of your organization, or the one in which you will work, requires the assessment of several factors that directly affect you in working with, delegating to, and supervising other healthcare workers.

Knowing the answers to the questions in the four major areas of assessment outlined in the assessment tool in **Exhibit 4–1** will help you to be able to practice professionally and safely, to the fullest potential of your license. A brief discussion of each area should be helpful in completing your knowledge base.

THE ORGANIZATIONAL STRUCTURE

Whether the setting in which you work is an acute care hospital or any one of a number of alternative healthcare facilities, there will typically be an organizational chart that describes the reporting relationships of personnel. Although traditional frameworks are continually changing, we have not yet found a substitute for the "snapshot" provided by a chart showing the titles of positions and/or departments/units and their relationship to everyone else in the agency. This chart serves only as a road map of the facility: it might identify landmarks but will not describe everything about each location. Unlike earlier organizational charts that demonstrated the traditional top-down hierarchy, today's chart might resemble the one in **Figure 4–1**.

Although the chart might provide the framework for the agency, it leaves several questions unanswered. You will need to further assess the degree of RN participation on committees, particularly collaborative practice and interdisciplinary committees, which might not be represented on any chart. These informal groups can be very instrumental and powerful in planning changes in personnel and care delivery.

As we discussed in Chapter 3 and will review in subsequent chapters, when an RN delegates, he or she is responsible for supervising the delegate and taking any corrective measures that might be necessary as a result of the delegate's performance. Clearly defined reporting mechanisms and systems that facilitate the fulfillment of this responsibility of the RN are necessary ingredients for the organization that expects the RN to delegate nursing tasks.

Congruency between personal and organizational values is essential for positive job satisfaction and performance.

THE IMPACT OF REDESIGN

Since as long ago as the 1980s, healthcare organizations have been creatively attempting to respond to the turbulent changes in our society. Increasing costs,

---

EXHIBIT 4-1   Assessment Tool: Organizational Support of the Delegation Process

Yes   No

Organizational Structure

____ ____   1. Is there an organizational chart?

____ ____   2. Are there clearly defined reporting systems for RNs who supervise delegates?

____ ____   3. Is there sufficient communication among the various units?

____ ____   4. Is the mission visible to everyone, and is it followed?

____ ____   5. Are there interdisciplinary committees in which RNs participate?

Quality

____ ____   1. Is a quality program currently in place?

____ ____   2. Does the model focus on outcomes?

____ ____   3. Is it supported by management and staff?

____ ____   4. Are nurses actively involved in the process?

____ ____   5. Do RNs participate in determining the criteria for measuring quality?

Safety in Practice

____ ____   1. Are there policies that address standards for appropriate staffing?

____ ____   2. Is there a nurse advisory committee involved in addressing problems related to staffing?

____ ____   3. Are the policies that directly affect nursing evaluated for their consistency with state regulations?

____ ____   4. Do RNs have responsibility and autonomy for continually appraising the care delivery system and implementing changes as needed?

____ ____   5. Are assistive personnel roles created or enlarged without the input and evaluation of nursing?

Educational Resources

____ ____   1. Are unlicensed assistive personnel adequately trained and oriented (using validated competencies and measurable outcomes)?

____ ____   2. Is there a system for providing additional skill development for assistive personnel when the need is identified by an RN who supervises an employee?

____ ____   3. Are RNs offered frequent educational opportunities to develop supervisory skills?

____ ____   4. Is there a documentation process for establishing competency in all skills required by the job description?

____ ____   5. Is there a mentorship or preceptorship program for all new licensed personnel?

____ ____   6. Is information regarding new changes in health care and healthcare regulations, including the nurse practice act, readily available?

OUR PATIENTS &

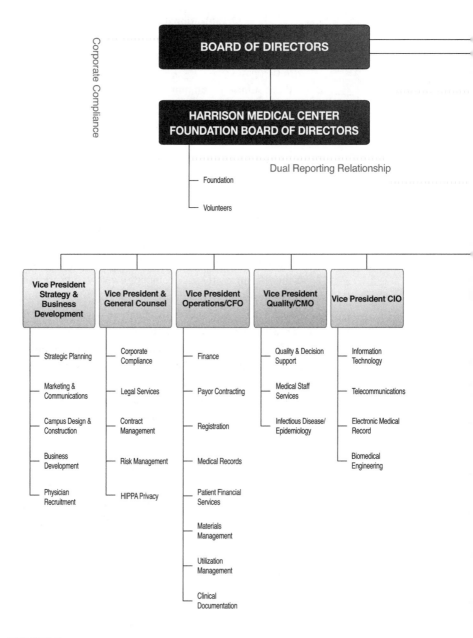

FIGURE 4–1 Harrison Medical Center Organizational Chart. *Source:* Harrison Medical Center Organizational Chart as of November 1, 2007, Bremerton, WA.

THEIR FAMILIES

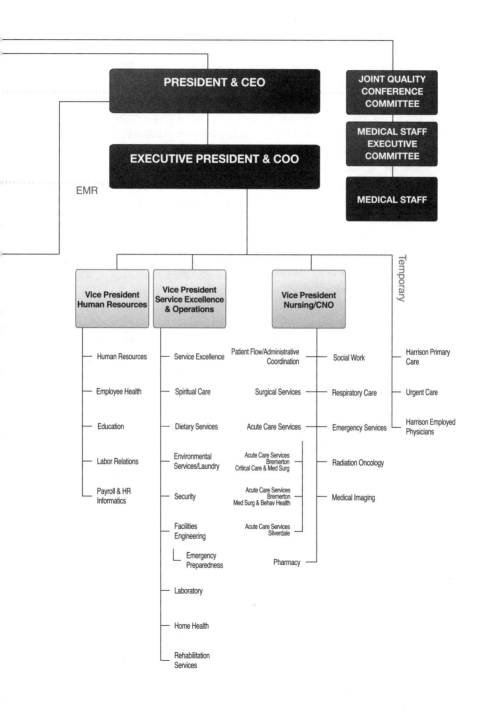

Clearly defined expectations and accountabilities, in addition to systems that facilitate the fulfillment of the responsibility of the RN, are necessary ingredients for the organization that expects the RN to delegate nursing tasks.

consumer demands, decreasing insurance coverage, an aging society, and so on are all contributing factors to the ongoing movement toward a more cost-effective delivery system. Because nurses make up over 60% of the care providers in this system, it is not surprising that we are seriously affected by any organization's efforts to modify the way care is delivered.

One of the most common forms of redesign has been the addition of unlicensed assistive personnel (UAP), more recently referred to as "nursing assistive personnel" (NAP), to the healthcare team. "Ninety-six percent of 1455 RN respondents to an *American Journal of Nursing* survey reported working with UAP, and two of every three RNs favored this practice" (Bernreuter, 1997, p. 49). In 1999, nurses in Hawaii reported an 11% increase in the use of UAP since 1995. In addition, 32% of the nurses were delegating work to UAP, up from 25% in 1995 (Kido, 2001). Because the licensed skill mix fell slightly during the last decade, licensed nurses reported doing more supervisory tasks in 2000 than in 1991 (Unruh, 2003).

In a landmark national study by *NurseWeek* and the American Organization of Nurse Executives (Domrose, 2002), approximately half of the respondents reported that so many nonnursing tasks dominate their time that they had little time for nursing work. Relating to the organization, only 40% said that opportunities to influence workplace decisions were good, very good, or excellent. Addressing the issue of operational failures, Tucker and Spear (2006) determined that nurses experience an average of 8.4 work system failures (those involving medications, orders, supplies, staffing, and equipment) per 8 hour shift and spend 42 minutes of each 8 hour shift resolving operational failures. Clearly there is work to be done!

With this steady increase in the use of UAP, are nurses satisfied? Are there any significant improvements in care? Seeking to add statistical significance to a dearth of studies in the area of UAP, the NCSBN completed a qualitative study to determine the effect of UAP delegation on patient clinical outcomes (Standing, Anthony, & Hertz, 2001). The narrative responses of 148 licensed nurses were analyzed for negative and positive outcomes. While this is a very limited sample set for a national survey, the results do conclude that positive outcomes result when there is clear communication with the UAP and follow-through to assure task completion. Positive outcomes included enhanced

Studies repeatedly support the necessity for the RN to provide clear communication to the UAP. If the organization expects and supports delegation of care, the RN must communicate and follow through to assure positive patient outcomes.

client well-being, prevention of poor outcomes, and enhanced unit functioning. Conversely, negative outcomes were often a result of poor communication between nurse and UAP and included skin injury, falls, family upsets, potential falls, worsening conditions, and other injury. Hospitals are actively seeking ways to measure satisfaction

"If the UAP did their job as stated in the job description, it would be very helpful; but you have to tell them everything to do, or do their job for them, and that's not helpful."

of both staff and patient and to relate to such variables as staffing and who delivers the care. The ANA has developed a core set of quality indicators to assist in this quest for standardized data collection and will continue to advocate for research on staffing and outcomes using these identified criteria. Among the indicators selected are nosocomial infection rate; patient injury rate; maintenance of skin integrity; patient satisfaction with pain management, nursing care, education, and care in general; nurse satisfaction and staffing mix; and total nursing care hours per patient day.

Narrative descriptions to most studies are very telling in terms of satisfaction. "If the UAP did their job as stated in the job description, it would be very helpful; but you have to tell them everything to do, or do their job for them, and that's not helpful." And, the RN must now "be responsible for everything and can not assume anything" (Barter, et al., 1997, p. 33).

The survey completed through the *American Journal of Nursing* in March 1996 involved over 7000 nurses who echoed these negative comments. The greater use of UAP is a cause for concern when coupled with decreasing lengths of stay, increasing acuities of patients, and changing technology. Declining morale and increasing readmissions, work-related injuries, and nosocomial infections add to the overall negative impact of a rapidly changing environment in which the use of assistive personnel is only a part of the total picture.

CHECKPOINT 4-4

Knowing the organizational chart of the employing agency can tell me

a) everything I need to know about the chain of command

b) nothing because my facility does not have a chart

c) the framework of the reporting relationships of units/departments/ or supervisors

d) the committee I should join to discuss delegation

See the end of the chapter for the answers.

Despite the negative reports, there are positive studies that have demonstrated increases· in staff and patient satisfaction and increased professional growth through thoughtful, judicious redesign. At Pennsylvania's Medical Center, RNs noted increased time spent in assessment and evaluation of care and the addition of patient education to the top 10 functions performed by the RN. Prior to redesign, charting took most of the RN's time, in addition to bathing, patient assessment, and medication assessment. After the change in skill mix, RNs spent more time on patient assessment, professional judgment, and medication assessment than they did on charting (Pedersen, 1997). When Community Hospitals of Central California added multiskilled workers in a partnership model of care, the time the RN spent in performing direct professional nursing activities increased from 43 percent to 60 percent (Davis, 1996, p. 1). Reporting on two med–surg units that have partnered an RN with a patient care technician (PCT), Barnes-Jewish Hospital in St. Louis found that "knowing your patients" scores improved for RNs by 12%–28% (Potter & Mueller, 2007). The addition of multiskilled workers to Griffin Hospital in Derby, Connecticut, had the following positive results:

+ Medication errors decreased 30%.
+ Eighty-nine percent of the nurses say they've seen a positive effect in their practice of nursing.
+ Eighty-six percent of the nurses report greater professional satisfaction.
+ Patient satisfaction is exceeding the 93% target and approaching 100%.
+ Ninety-six percent of the patients prefer current patient care design to the prior delivery system. (Hansten & Washburn, 1997)

The jury is no longer out as continued studies validate the positive impact of the presence of an RN to lead the care team (Domrose, 2002; Rosenfeld & Harrington, 2003). There is statistical validation for what we have known all along: An RN is essential for leading the healthcare team, planning and coordinating patient care, and delegating the work to those most appropriate to perform it.

> There is statistical validation that the RN is essential for planning and coordinating patient care and delegating the work to the most appropriate team member to get the job done.

THE QUALITY PROGRAM

When 56% of the hospitals surveyed in 1989 by The Joint Commission received contingencies for quality assurance activities, CQI and TQM programs were implemented with great zest (Curtin, 1992). Responding to market changes and increased competition for the patient, more healthcare agencies shifted their focus to emphasize a service approach. The race was on to improve systems and to streamline the delivery of care in any way possible.

> The key here is participation. If you want to question the data and the results of a TQM and/or CQI survey at your work site, get involved in the process.

Unfortunately, many nurses report that they have not been included in the loop when it comes to quality improvement programs. They remain ignorant in many cases, not fully understanding and certainly not participating in the new programs that have resulted in many of the changes that directly affect nurses.

Let's briefly review the change in quality focus and see where it has taken us so far. When The Joint Commission created its Agenda for Change in the late 1980s, one of the major guiding concepts served to foster the rapid growth in a new idea of quality. Driven by increasing consumer demands to demonstrate results and value for the dollar, The Joint Commission stated that "continual improvement in the quality of care should be a priority goal for a health care organization" (1990, p. 2). The opinion was expressed that the assurance of quality was an unrealistic expectation and that a continuing effort to improve quality was more achievable. Greater emphasis was and will continue to be placed on outcomes rather than on the structure or process for attaining those outcomes.

We can all remember the somewhat punitive flavor of the quality assurance program, which seemed to be little more than a search for who was doing something wrong. This search-and-punish approach made staff members unwilling to participate in quality programs because they felt they had more than ample opportunity to serve as targets for blame. The movement toward the creation of a "just culture environment" is rapidly replacing the adversarial approaches of past quality assurance efforts. Researcher and assistant professor at the University of Illinois Dr. Terry L. von Thaden explains, "A just culture organization takes a fair and balanced approach to event reporting, learns from mistakes, and holds individuals or the organization accountable where appropriate. While rules and processes are an important basis for organizational safety, the way an organization runs and the way its people interact truly define whether or not it's a safe and just working environment" (Pastorius, 2007). Replacing the traditional punitive approach with the more positive program of analysis of an entire event, and looking for ways in which to improve the outcome of that event rather than pointing the blame, invites the participation of nurses who are concerned for the improvement of patient care.

Although this rationale for the shift in emphasis to results, or outcomes, makes a lot of sense, the point must be made that success for any healthcare improvement plan will require the involvement and support of all employees, as well as commitment from management. Involvement is a major issue, and nurses will need to seek out that involvement if it is not readily offered. Decisions made that affect the delivery of patient care in an attempt to improve the quality of the outcome must include the nurse executive, stipulates The Joint Commission standard. Through this standard, nursing leaders have received the support for their integration into healthcare facilities' administrations and now have an opportunity to involve staff nurses in all clinical improvement efforts, including the creation and use of assistive personnel. Participation on your part is essential. We have spoken with numerous nurses who have not been involved in their quality program and then question the credibility of the data when the survey results are posted. "Yeah, but they don't post the real data," has been a comment heard too often. If you want to know the real truth and suspect there is not an accurate reporting, or that what's really important is not being measured, the message is clear: get involved.

CHECKPOINT 4–5

Are the following statements true or false?

1. The emphasis on quality is now on structure and process.

2. CQI stands for continuous quality improvement, a tool used to facilitate the monitoring of outcomes and look for ways to improve them.

3. The Joint Commission does not support the involvement of nursing in quality improvement efforts.

See the end of the chapter for the answers.

SAFETY IN PRACTICE MODELS

We now come to the very significant issue of staffing. In our collective years of nursing experience, we heard more times than we can remember that staffing was "unsafe" or "insufficient" and that the quality of care, not to mention the safety of the patients, was being seriously jeopardized. It is a problem that has plagued nursing since the beginning, when Florence Nightingale realized that one night nurse could take care of four times as many patients if they were all in one room. Nurses have studied, quantified, computerized, centralized, and decentralized the process of care delivery in an effort to ensure that the staffing levels in any healthcare setting are safe and adequate. Through both nursing shortages and abundance, always driven by the constraints of the budget, we have strived to create workable solutions to the ever-present dilemma.

Solutions to the issue of adequate and safe coverage by nursing personnel include the development of policies that describe the procedure and, in many instances, quantify different levels of care that depend on available staff. In acute care and extended care settings, we have noted policies in place that determine the actions to take for providing optimum care, good care, and essential care. This prioritization of levels of care is one method by which the nursing division plans for variances in staffing and clearly outlines the expectations of performance in a given situation.

Many nursing committees have developed tracking mechanisms, similar to the tools used in a continuous quality improvement (CQI) program, to monitor patient acuities and staffing levels and their relationship to the achievement of various desired outcomes. Nurses can complete "assignment despite objection" forms that record and alert management to staffing concerns when they feel that levels of personnel are not sufficient for the degree of care required.

Because of the high degree of variability of patient needs, minimum standards of staffing from a regulatory standpoint are often difficult to make. California was the first state to pass a law mandating staffing ratios, and as of 2004, med–surg units must have only six patients per nurse, further reducing that ratio to one nurse per five patients by 2005 (Clarke, 2003). In 2002, a total of 17 states introduced legislation regarding staffing plans and ratios, and Texas enacted that legislation (Runy, 2003). Such minimum standards take away the flexibility of both the employer and the nurse, argue many administrators, and the controversy continues. Currently 18 states have introduced staffing legislation, and the RN Safe Staffing Act was reviewed by both the 109th and 110th Congress (Keeler & Cramer, 2007). Clearly there is a growing national concern about nurse staffing and safety issues. For a detailed overview

The employer who would take the RN out of this loop of the decision process is not following regulations that provide the RN with the ultimate decision regarding the appropriateness of delegation.

of the proposed federal policy, which is beyond the scope of this text, we recommend reading Keeler and Cramer's policy analysis.

In addition to the fundamental issue of how many staff, there is the very real question of what kind of staff should be utilized to provide the best care. For many of the reasons we have discussed elsewhere, assistive personnel continue to be added to the patient care team. The list is extensive, including assistants that many of us have never heard of but might at some time be delegating care to in the future. Medical technicians, hospice aides, orthopedic physician assistants, psychiatric technicians, geriatric assistants, personal care aides, and many more have joined the ranks of assistive personnel. By the mid-1990s, the majority of hospitals reported using some kind of assistive personnel (Krapohl & Larson, 1996), and as the current nursing shortage worsens, creative approaches to care will expand.

The use of assistive personnel not only continues, but their roles have been expanded to include many additional tasks such as blood glucose monitoring, phlebotomy, catheter insertion, and in some settings, medication administration (Kido, 2001). As these new positions are created and utilized in the work setting, it is imperative that RNs be involved in determining how the assistants are trained and supervised. The employer who would take the RN out of this loop of the decision process is not following regulations that provide the RN with the ultimate decision regarding the appropriateness of delegation.

CHECKPOINT 4-6

1. Standards of staffing

   a) are difficult to establish due to the variability of patient needs

   b) might limit the flexibility of the employer and the healthcare provider

   c) have been set in California to address the critical care areas

   d) all of the above

2. New positions for healthcare assistants

   a) have increased significantly during recent years

   b) are decreasing as employers recognize that an all-RN staff is the best

c)   must be delegated to by the RN if the employer says so

d)   none of the above

See the end of the chapter for the answers.

EDUCATIONAL RESOURCES

We have repeatedly noted that the RN is accountable for ensuring the competency of the individual to whom he or she delegates any nursing task. To fulfill that responsibility, certain factors must be in place. Employers who do not provide for the adequate screening and orientation of employees are placing themselves and their patients at risk. RNs need to assess the facility for such tools as skills checklists, performance-based job descriptions, periodic update and renewal of specific skills, and provision of continuing education. Accrediting agencies (The Joint Commission, American Osteopathic Association, etc.) and regulatory bodies (the state department of health) have various requirements to ensure competency of employees.

After they are hired, personnel need to be oriented, with a plan for evaluating their performance and skill levels at periodic intervals. The RN must make certain this process is in place to be able to provide the supervision of the delegate that is required. What department is responsible for overseeing the orientation process? Are nurses involved in precepting or mentoring? This is a time-consuming responsibility, and not one that nurses have traditionally been trained in, so the availability of preceptorship training is valuable and demonstrates the importance the agency places on the program. New employees who are expected to perform on the day of hire and are not partnered with anyone place everyone at risk.

The majority of respondents to a survey conducted by *RN* magazine in 1996 noted that the UAP at their organization received fewer than three weeks of training.

> Quite to the contrary, UAPs are more a source of worry than support: 42% of readers believe that UAPs don't receive enough training. Another 21% went so far as to say that their training was woefully inadequate . . . even more—30%—take issue with the type of training they receive, indicating that it wasn't commensurate with the degree of responsibility that unlicensed personnel assume. (Ventura, 1996, p. 41)

Currently, training time often expands or contracts based on availability of staffing.

> You can't do what you don't know how to do.

The NCSBN continues to recognize this challenge, addressing it in their position paper "Working with Others" (2005):

> The variation in the preparation, regulation and use of nursing assistive personnel presents a challenge to nurses and assistants alike. Consistent education and training requirements that prepare nursing assistive personnel to perform a range of functions will allow delegating nurses to know the preparation and skill level of assistive personnel, and will prepare nursing assistants to do this work.

In addition to the focus on training of the UAP, there must be training for RNs who are experiencing changes in their roles. The NCSBN survey of nursing narratives concluded that "not all nurses had a clear conceptualization of delegation" (Standing, et al., 2001). A survey of 14 hospitals that had completed redesign revealed that "staff nurses often had to assume greater management responsibilities without additional training" (Walston, 1997). The very important issue, then, is education. Make sure you take steps to get the information you need to organize, plan, coordinate, and supervise the care of your patients.

Putting It All Together in the Professional Practice Environment

As a response to the nursing shortage of the 1970s, a study was completed to identify organizational characteristics that were favorable in recruiting and retaining nurses. The research completed in 1983 revealed 14 factors that were to become the "Forces of Magnetism" as part of the ANCC Magnet Recognition Program Since its inception, the program has become the standard of excellence in hospital environments, with the number of organizations who have achieved such an honorable stature now exceeding 230 and an additional 250 hospitals preparing for the journey (Triolo, Scherer, & Floyd, 2006). While all 14 forces contribute to a successful professional practice environment, eight have been singled out by RNs as "Essentials of Magnetism" for quality patient care and job satisfaction (Kramer & Schmalenberg in Ulrich et al., 2007). Among these eight are issues that we have discussed as indicative of an organization that supports successful clinical delegation: clinically competent coworkers, control over nursing practice, adequate staffing, support for education, autonomy, and a culture emphasizing the primary importance of concern for the patient.

Of the 14 forces, three address components that determine the establishment of a professional practice environment (PPE): force 2, organizational structure; force 5, professional models of care; and force 9, autonomy. The concept of a PPE is to define attributes that, when in place, allow the professional nurse to practice with accountability, making independent and interdependent care decisions that advocate for the patient (Arford & Zone-Smith, 2005). We agree that the presence of a supportive organization with an emphasis on professional development is essential for ensuring the success of the patient/client/resident in addition to allowing the nurse to achieve satisfaction in her or his practice.

We encourage you to further explore the organization in which you work and to hold its structure and culture as key elements in your success. It is important to know whether or not the organization you work for has achieved Magnet certification. If not, find out if its application is in process and if it identifies with and ascribes to the 14 forces that will enhance and support your practice. For more details on the certification process, visit ANCC's Web site at http://www.nursecredentialing.org/magnet/forces.html.

YOUR ROLE IN ORGANIZATIONAL SUCCESS

We have taken a detailed look at how to assess the organization in which you work in terms of its "delegation friendliness." Certain factors, such as the policies that define reporting relationships and staffing levels and the measures taken to validate the competency of employees, are critical to the success of the RN in practicing delegation. Also critical to the success of the delegator is his or her level of involvement in the organization. Participation on committees, task forces, and so forth, whether union or not, is an important component of professional control over changes in patient care.

Simply understanding why the organization is managed the way it is and why decisions are made is not enough. The RN has a real opportunity to shape practice in the working environment by being actively involved in assessing, planning, and evaluating the decisions that are made regarding the delivery of patient care. Support for this involvement comes from the regulating and accrediting bodies, as well as from the progressive movement of quality improvement programs. Missions and values are the driving forces of the assessment, and congruency with the professional values of the practicing RN will assist in the attainment of a satisfying partnership from which the patient benefits.

ANSWERS TO CHECKPOINTS

4–1.

1.   False. Organizational styles have changed over the years, from physician ownership, physician led, to large corporate structures with governing boards and administrative teams. There is a variety of organizational structure available, based on the size, mission, and intent of the organization.

2.   False. Some who have been in practice for over 20 years may argue that this is true, and if you have been with the same organization for more than a decade, it may be difficult to realize and appreciate any changes. However, managers and leaders have worked hard to support the employee and to make changes that create better working environments: better healthcare benefits, long-term disability programs, insurance for families, and changes in paid time off structures are just a few examples.

3.   True. Yes, do you know what the mission of your organization is?

4.   False. Union representation is only available in approximately 25% of healthcare organizations and did not start until the 1920s.

5.   False. As you learned in Chapter 3, the nurse practice act is the legal foundation for nursing practice and employer policies must be in agreement with the statutes.

4–2.

1.   d: Active membership is essential for the success of a union, but it is not available in all states, nor is it required by all hospitals, and has been available only since the 1920s.

2.   c: Union membership is another opportunity for collegial connection, but it does not guarantee employment, is not required by licensure, and is not prohibited by the state practice act.

3.   d: All of the actions listed are excellent ways to be involved.

4–3. c: Missions do clarify the purpose and intent of an organization; leadership, management, and employees do follow the mission
and values (although perhaps not everyone practices them!). If you have
not seen your mission statement, be sure to look it up on your organization's Web site or ask your manager. The mission does not really indicate
your need for union representation; the working conditions and satisfaction of your fellow employees would be better indicators.

4–4. c: The organizational chart will give you the framework from
which to find out more about the chain of command and who you
might ask about committee membership. If you do not think that your
organization has a chart, be sure to ask your manager or the human
resource department or look in your policy book.

4–5.

    1. False. While structure and process are very important
    contributors to quality, the outcome is the key indicator.

    2. True. CQI is one process for measuring quality.

    3. False. The Joint Commission has been an active supporter
    of nursing involvement, recognizing the important role that
    nurses play in contributing to the quality of patient care.

4–6.

    1. d: Staffing standards will continue to be challenging due
    to variability and flexibility and the need to serve two masters:
    the patient and the employee. More states will adopt staffing
    standards as an attempt to address this challenging issue.

    2. a: The demand for healthcare assistants continues to rise as
    we struggle with a continuing shortage of licensed healthcare
    professionals.

REFERENCES

Arford, P.H., & Zoe-Smith, L. (2005). Organizational commitment to professional practice models. *Journal of Nursing Administration*, 35(10), 467-472.

Barter, M., et al. (1997). Registered nurse role changes and satisfaction with unlicensed assistive personnel. *Journal of Nursing Administration*, 27(1), 29–38.

Bernreuter, M. (1997). Survey and critique of studies related to unlicensed assistant personnel from 1975–1997, Part 2. *Journal of Nursing Administration*, 27(718), 49–55.

Christy, T. (1984). Portrait of a leader: Lillian Wald. Pages from nursing history. *American Journal of Nursing*, 84–88.

Clarke, S. (2003). Balancing staffing and safety. *Nursing Management, 34*(6), 44–48.

Covey, S. (1991). *Principle centered leadership.* New York: Summit Books.

Curtin, L. (1992). Of commissions, omissions, and just plain missions. *Nursing Management, 23,* 7–8.

Davis, S. (1996). Adapting to the accelerated health care evolution. *Reengineering the Hospital, 3*(1), 1–4.

Domrose, C. (2002, August 5). Changing tides. *NurseWeek,* 17–19.

Hansten, R., & Washburn, M. (1997). Multiskilled technician's role: Making it work. *Successful Restructuring, 1*(3), 5.

Joint Commission on Accreditation of Healthcare Organizations. (1990). *The Joint Commission's agenda for change.* Oakbrook Terrace, IL: Author.

Keeler, H., & Cramer, M. (2007). A policy analysis of federal registered nurses safe staffing legislation. *Journal of Nursing Administration, 37*(7/8), 350–356.

Kido, V. (2001). The UAP dilemma. *Nursing Management, 32*(11), 27–29.

Krapohl, G., & Larson, E. (1996). The impact of unlicensed assistive personnel on nursing care delivery. *Nursing Economics 14*(2), 99–110.

McNeese-Smith, D., & Crook, M. (2003). Nursing values and a changing workforce: Values, age and job stages. *Journal of Nursing Administration, 33*(5), 260–270.

National Council of State Boards of Nursing. (2005). *Working with others: A position paper.* Chicago: Author.

Pastorius, D. (2007). Crime in the workplace, part 1. *Nursing Management, 38*(10), 18–27.

Pedersen, A. (1997). A data-driven approach to work redesign in nursing units. *Journal of Nursing Administration, 27*(4), 49–54.

Potter, P., & Mueller, J. (2007). How well do you know your patients? *Nursing Management, 38*(2), 40-48.

Porter-O'Grady, T. (2002). Guest editorial: Building trusting organizations. *Nursing Administration Quarterly, 26*(3), viii–ix.

Rosenfeld, P., and Harrington, C. 2003. Nursing counts. *AJN,* 103(5), p. 115.

Runy, L. (2003). The health care workforce. *Hospitals and Health Networks, 76*(8).

Standing, T., Anthony, M., & Hertz, J. (2001). Nurses narratives of outcomes after delegation to unlicensed assistive personnel. *Outcomes Management for Nursing Practice, 5*(1), 18–23.

Starr, P. (1982). *The social transformation of American medicine.* New York: Basic Books.

Triolo, P., Scherer, E.M., & Floyd, J.M. (2006). Evaluation of the Magnet Recognition program. *Journal of Nursing Administration, 36,* 42-48.

Tucker, A., & Spear, S. (2006). Operational failures and interruptions in hospital nursing. *Health Research and Education Trust,* 1–20.

Ulrich, B., et al. (2007). Magnet status and registered nurse views of the work environment and nursing as a career. *Journal of Nursing Administration, 37*(5), 212–220.

Unruh, L. (2003). The effect of LPN reductions on RN patient load. *Journal of Nursing Administration, 33*(4), 201–208.

Ventura, M. (1996, September). Workload, UAPs and you. *RN,* 41–45.

Walston, S. (1997, August 16). Reengineering hospitals: Evidence from the field. *Healthcare Leadership Review, 7,* 6.

Know Yourself

Ruth I. Hansten and Marilynn Jackson

5

CHAPTER SKILLS

- Determine your level of clinical development from novice to expert.
- Using the critical thinking skill of reflection, list your personal barriers to team leadership.
- Apply the grief process to changes you encounter in your daily work.
- Define the possible benefits to practicing with excellent team leadership skills.

RECOMMENDED RESOURCES

- Read a good resource on emotional intelligence: Merlevede, P., Bridoux, D., & Vandamme, R. (2003). *7 steps to emotional intelligence.* Williston VT: Crown House Publishing; or any book by Daniel Goleman such as *Primal Leadership* or *Social Intelligence.*
- Ask your coworkers, family, or friends for some feedback on your leadership style, with a question like, "What would you say are my strengths when I am functioning as a leader? What would you suggest I do differently?"
- Bridges, W. (1991). *Managing transitions: Making the most of change.* Reading, MA: Addison-Wesley.
- Patterson K., Grenny, J., McMillan R., & Switzler, A. (2002). *Crucial conversations: Tools for talking when stakes are high.* New York: McGraw-Hill.

"Do I dare ask June to take care of that complaining patient when she has so much seniority here? If she says no, and I press her further, will the manager back me up? Besides, if I don't do the care myself, I'm sure I'll forget how to be technically proficient! How can I remain a real nurse and still supervise some of the care? We are so short that I can't really spend the time learning to delegate and supervise!"

Delegation in a clinical setting is essentially a complex interaction of very personal relationships. Your personal relationships and communication with your supervisor, your coworkers, and those you supervise are absolutely fundamental to providing safe and effective care for those you serve. But your relationship with yourself is the cornerstone of the process. Your own thought processes and the words you say to yourself, your "self-talk," determine your ability to perform the delegation process and whether or not you take the risks to supervise effectively. Being able to reflect on the emotions that fuel our behavior offers an opportunity for mastering our practice as professionals. The Gallup organization measures employee engagement and has found that those employees who are connected and work with excitement are healthier than those who are actively working out their unhappiness by undermining others (Gallup, 2005). Actual clinical results that are correlated to the nurses' feelings about their jobs show that nosocomial infection rates were 18 times higher and patients were 54 times more likely to get surgical site infections on units in which nurses were not engaged or connected to their work (Gallup, 2004a, 2005). Hospitals with the least engaged nurses have paid more than $1.1 million annually in malpractice claims (Gallup, 2004b). Cardiac units where the nurses' general mood was "depressed" had a death rate among comparable patients 4 times higher than comparable units (Schneider & Bowen, 1995). There's plenty of research that encourages us to pay attention to ourselves, our internal environment, and how we frame our external environment to create our own best practice.

CHECKPOINT 5–1

Employee engagement has been found to affect clinical outcomes. What results have been noted in units with the least employee engagement or connection to their work?

CHECKPOINT 5-2

What condition in registered nurses increased the cardiac patient death rate fourfold?

Your progress along the journey from novice to expert clinical practitioner also affects your ability to work effectively with others in a team. The thoughts previously expressed show that this supervisor or charge nurse will certainly not feel confident to assign June part of the care of that patient or client.

Hundreds of nurses throughout the United States have expressed their concerns about the delegation process and their ability to supervise other personnel. Their anxieties are a product of several realities: the remarkable interpersonal nature of risks inherent in the delegation process, unique personal barriers known to each individual, lack of experience or education regarding delegation in the clinical arena, concerns about finding the time to delegate and supervise, and a climate of unrelenting change.

Often compounding the personal barriers surrounding the delegation process is the fact that many nurses first recognize the need to delegate in response to comprehensive changes in their organization. They might first discover that they need to learn to delegate when they are told that they will be working in new care delivery models, often with additional unlicensed assistive personnel (UAP) working in the team. Unit closures, mergers, or reconfigurations, leadership changes, or perpetual personnel shortages can impact best practices. New regulations, initiatives, and electronic records or other technology alter the workplace with little notice. The whole idea of delegation and improving professional practice then becomes tainted with the anger and fear surrounding other stresses that nurses are experiencing. However, sometimes the barriers are related less to changes in the organization than they are to the level of experience of the nurse. For those readers experienced and comfortable with delegation in their practice and those training as preceptors and mentors to others, we encourage you to read this chapter with consideration of your own professional development as well as where other team members might be arrested in their development.

CHECKPOINT 5-3

Why is reflection an important part of the delegation process?

LEVEL OF CLINICAL EXPERIENCE: FROM NOVICE TO EXPERT[1]

One model of the professional development continuum that is very familiar to the nursing world is Patricia Benner's model of From Novice to Expert (Benner & Benner, 1984). Her adaptation comes from the groundbreaking work done by Dreyfus and Dreyfus (Garland, 1996) in their studies of skill acquisition by chess players and Air Force pilots. As more experience and education are attained, an individual can progress through recognizable stages of development, with marked differences in approach to decision making, problem solving, organization, and work efficiency. However, as Benner reminds us, "Some persons will tend to settle in a competent or proficient level because of personal learning styles, personal concerns, or organizational constraints that cause them to plateau at a level of practice" (Benner & Benner, 1991). Individuals who have been locked into the same job for many years and are reacting negatively to changes in the workplace might not have been advancing to expert professional development. We will explore some of the organizational and personal barriers that might have impeded this development later in this chapter.

While Benner has adapted the Dreyfus model to nursing, we suggest that the general implications are applicable in all fields of care providers. Nurses who take the test in Appendix 5–A will begin to understand whether their lack of experience is getting in the way of delegating and working as a team. An understanding of this development will assist managers in planning what first steps might need to be taken to support staff nurses' progression along the scale and in determining if the available staff members are prepared to lead the way.

The journey from novice to expert can influence the ability of a nurse to see the patient as a whole. A novice or advanced beginner might find his or her level of experience to be a temporary barrier in identifying patient outcomes, deciding what task can be matched with what person, and communicating the overall plan when supervising others.

Stages of Development

Level I: Novice. Beginners, because they have no experience with the situations in which they are expected to perform, must depend on rules to guide their actions. Following rules, however, has limits. No rule can tell novices which tasks are most relevant in real situations or when to make exceptions. These individuals might profit the most from the decision-making tools we have included in this book.

---

[1]Adapted from Hansten and Washburn, *Toolbook for Health Care Redesign*, 1997, pp. 32–37.

Implications: Beginners organize work by task, become disorganized easily, and might not be able to identify patient outcomes and communicate these readily in collaboration with the patient or other team members. Managers can't expect that these individuals will be able to lead a team appropriately (Hansten, 2005). Consider this comparison to a person attempting to put together a jigsaw puzzle. A novice does not yet have access to the picture on the top of the jigsaw puzzle box but tries to put the puzzle together by fitting piece into piece, task by task.

Advice to Novice Nurses: The use of delegation aids or supports such as the delegation decision-making grid (see Chapter 6, Exhibit 6-3, NCSBN Delegation Decision-Making Process, and Figure 6-1, RN Delegation Decision Tree) will be helpful. Conceptual information (how the process of delegation works and what the state regulations consist of) will be essential for you.

Level II: Advanced Beginner. Advanced beginners have coped with enough real situations (or have had them pointed out by a mentor) to recognize some of the recurrent meaningful aspects. They need help setting priorities because they operate on general guidelines and are only beginning to perceive recurrent meaningful patterns. The advanced beginner cannot reliably sort out what is most important in complex situations. Again, a decision-making tool is helpful at this stage because nurses can use it to assist critical thinking by practicing scenarios in assignment making and discussing other clinical situations, such as errors or mistakes that have occurred in their department.

Implications: In stable situations, advanced beginners follow orders and procedures; they get disorganized in unstable situations and have a naive trust in standard protocols. The advanced beginner does not yet have the picture on the top of the jigsaw puzzle box, but they know whom to ask to determine which pieces to fit together first.

Advice to Advanced Beginner Nurses: Use the decision-making tools (Chapter 6), or ask a charge nurse or other more experienced nurse for help when you are in a complex delegation situation. Practice using scenarios for assignment making.

Level III: Competent. Typically, a nurse at the competent level has been in practice 2 to 3 years. This person can rely on long-range goals and plans to determine which aspects of a situation are important and which can be ignored. The competent individual lacks the speed and flexibility of the person who has reached the proficient level, but competence is characterized by a feeling of mastery and the ability to cope with and manage many contingencies of clinical care. These individuals find identification of patient goals to be easier, but they might still require some assistance in thinking through critical situations they have not yet experienced.

Implications: Competent nurses work with preset plans and goals that are personally identified, are less naive about protocols and coworkers, and develop their own way of doing some things. These nurses have seen an overview of the photo on the top of the jigsaw puzzle box.

Advice to Competent Nurses: (We assume all of you are competent, but we are referring to those who score at this level in terms of the novice–expert test!) Begin to focus on patient outcomes and what they mean to the assistive personnel you lead. Discuss these with the patients and team members. When faced with very complex situations, ask for help from supervisory personnel. You can still benefit by working through scenarios and might feel ready to mentor novice nurses in their delegation skills.

Level IV: Proficient. Proficient individuals perceive situations as wholes rather than in terms of aspects. With holistic understanding, decision making is less labored because the individual has a perspective on which of the many attributes and aspects present are the important ones. The proficient performer considers fewer options and homes in on an accurate region of the problem. These individuals find identification of patient outcomes to be second nature and might be able to plan care and organize a team to work with challenging patients without anxiety. A proficient nurse owns the jigsaw puzzle box, sees the top of the box clearly, and the pieces are put together so the picture makes sense.

Implications: Proficient nurses read situations better and set priorities according to the situation as it unfolds.

Advice to Proficient Nurses: Set the pace and mentor others who are having difficulty in delegating. Help others discuss patient outcomes in reports from shift to shift (acute and long-term care). Share any tools you have developed in terms of delegation and supervision, such as mental anchors, lists, or "brains" sheets.

If you are new at delegation but have been proficient in your nursing in a solo care situation, the process of delegation should come quite easily to you. When you understand the concepts, some practice will be required to feel comfortable, but your understanding of organizing a group of patients and focusing on patient goals will serve you well!

If you are new at delegation but have been proficient in your nursing in a solo care situation, the process of delegation should come quite easily to you. When you understand the concepts, some practice will be required to feel comfortable, but your understanding of organizing a group of patients and focusing on patient goals will serve you well!

Level V: Expert. The expert no longer relies on an analytical principle (rule, guideline, maxim) to connect understanding of a given situation to an appropriate action. The expert individual with an enormous background of experience has an intuitive grasp of the situation and zeroes in on the accurate region of the problem without wasteful consideration of a large range of unfruitful possibilities. These jewels are able to lead a team effectively and efficiently and will be able to organize their work and the work of others while supervising them effectively. An expert nurse does not need to visualize the top of the jigsaw puzzle box to get her/his tasks done. Practice is innate, and the jigsaw puzzle pieces that don't fit are easily discarded.

Implications: Experts are fluid and skillful in managing and attend to both the most salient aspects as well as those that go unnoticed by less experienced staff. Experts sometimes find it difficult to break down their intuitive, rapid thinking processes into steps so that they can clearly describe them to teach others.

Advice to Expert Nurses: We wish that we could clone you! However, if you are new to the idea of delegating, refer to the comments in the proficient level section and follow them. Expert nurses will soon be able to discern what tasks can be delegated to others when they understand the roles of coworkers. Your gut-level understanding of what needs to be done (intuition) will help you work effectively in a team configuration, but it might be necessary to reflect on what thinking processes you use to be able to explain your methods to others.

Nursing Expertise Self-Report Scale

Gayle Garland, a nurse educator in England, has developed a survey tool for the beginning assessment of professional development (Appendix 5–A). It makes an effective first step in analysis of clinical performance. We are delighted to have the opportunity to include this tool and encourage your connection with Gayle as you gather data. Gayle Garland requests that those who use the Nursing Expertise Self-Report Scale forward a copy of their findings and any comments to the address given. She also can be contacted for assistance.

EXPLORING BARRIERS

It's not uncommon for us to teach delegation skills to nurses throughout the country and find at the end of the workshop that several people have not absorbed a word of what was said. We've discovered that these folks are so caught up in their negative feelings about staffing shortages or other stresses occurring in their organizations that they've been unable to listen. Some do not feel that nurses should be leaders at all. Some are perfectly comfortable with the idea of delegation and are expert at skills, but they discover that their care delivery models do not support best practices or that too scarce assistive personnel do not comply with their requests when they do delegate. To readers who are feeling negative about the whole issue or are being required against their will to read this book, we recommend that they spend some time considering their personal barriers to delegation in some detail.

When you think of delegating to other healthcare workers, what feelings/thoughts enter your mind? Write them down now as you reflect.

_____

_____

_____

_____

Here are a few that have been shared with us:

+ fear
+ anger
+ loss of trust in management
+ loss of control
+ loss of achievement
+ concern about quality
+ burnout
+ stress
+ feeling overwhelmed
+ lack of enjoyment in work
+ decreased job satisfaction
+ confusion
+ feeling betrayed
+ feeling abandoned
+ excitement
+ ambivalence
+ apathy
+ loss of security

CHECKPOINT 5-4

We've now established that knowing oneself more intimately, understanding and acknowledging one's barriers and strengths in the delegation process, will help each nurse work more effectively with assistive personnel. The bonus for each nurse? A better work life! Safe care for patients! Feeling more "in control."

What's in it for me? Why do I care about how I feel about the delegation process?

a) I need to understand myself to be able to interact appropriately with those I supervise.

b) Dwelling on my negative emotions and feelings is a great way to avoid learning about this topic altogether.

c) If I can work more effectively with others, I'll feel better about work and about myself, and care for my clients will be improved.

d) I don't care. All this assistive personnel junk is a plot to get rid of nurses and give terrible care.

See the end of the chapter for the answers.

If you have been delegating to unlicensed healthcare workers for some time and this is not a new experience for you, recall your first emotions and concerns when you first began to try to tell others what to do and actually supervised their work. Do any of the feelings described in the previous list apply to you at that stage? Expert delegators will likely be asked to teach or precept novice staff and will find this exercise to be helpful.

We hear the same emotions repeated throughout the United States and internationally as we travel and discuss delegation, care delivery models, and critical thinking with nurses. We've determined that many of these feelings are related to a nurse's individual responses to the changes in his or her work life and the method by which the change took place.

In organizations in which economics demanded immediate action and changes in staffing configurations, the culture did not support a measured and educational approach, and/or staff participation in developing the roles of assistive personnel was discouraged, and anger, fear, and distrust were expressed vehemently. In multiple organizations in the past, the addition of unlicensed workers to a skill mix was accompanied by redeployment of nursing personnel. When this occurred, the rage and pain were often nearly debilitating. Most nurses who are experiencing the 21st century's nursing shortages are relieved and happy that assistive personnel are present, but their systems for utilizing team members effectively are often described as less than optimal. Whether you are furious, confused, frustrated, or merely uncomfortable, the fact remains that each of us must find a method of dealing with negative emotions to be able to provide effective patient care. (For anyone who is contemplating a change in care delivery models, please see the discussion of the process in *Toolbook for Health Care Redesign*, Hansten and Washburn, 1997, and www.HanstenRROHC. com.) Whether you have experienced a change in your work life or system of care delivery or believe you need to improve your current system, or whether

> In organizations where changes in care delivery systems and use of assistive personnel were implemented with a larger degree of employee involvement and participation and in which staff were educated and understood the rationale for the change, the intensity of negative emotions was apparent to a lesser degree.

you've always delegated effectively to other healthcare workers but discovered noncompliance or resistance from the delegates, negative emotions can be a huge stumbling block to effective supervision. Whether anger or apathy, these emotions can override your best intentions to communicate clearly when assigning tasks to the patient care associate who was quickly hired and oriented because of a worker shortage.

Nurses often discuss the grief process in their daily work. In home health, acute care hospitals, or long-term care, the stages of the grief process that are experienced by clients or their families provide a model to use in our interventions. Just as we might recognize Mr. Brown's anger as a part of the grief process as he watches his wife die, rather than personalizing the anger that was directed at the nursing staff, we must step back and superimpose the grief process model on our personal or unit care plan for knowing ourselves and our emotional barriers.

Our first step to overcoming our emotional barriers is complete: that of naming our emotions. Identifying our emotions allows us to use a replenishable resource, our brains, to harness our emotional energy. Emotional intelligence is considered to be a hallmark of success in life. It is subdivided into Intrapersonal Intelligence and Interpersonal Intelligence (Merlevede, Bridoux, & Vandamme, 2003). In this chapter we are asking the readers to stop and reflect on how their moods or emotions affect them and to consider their ability to manage the resulting behaviors. In later chapters we will spend more time on interpersonal or social intelligence and how we manage interpersonal relationships through identifying emotions in others, empathizing, and communicating with them. Let's go through the steps of the grief process and determine how we can use our energy in a productive manner for our own self-care.

CHECKPOINT 5-5

Emotional intelligence is often subdivided into two competencies: Name them and explain what those competencies would have to do with delegation and supervision.

Denial

The first step of the grief process itself is denial. At this stage, we haven't fully realized the impact yet, but soon we'll be ready. The negative, destructive side of denial is acted out by people who refuse to pull their heads

> Denial is a great emotion. It allows us some time to garner our internal fortitude and get ready to deal with the onslaught that's just around the corner.

out of the sand. Having one's vision blinded will not allow one to react appropriately, learn the necessary skills, and adapt to changes.

This stage of the grief process is often exemplified by seminar participants who write on their evaluations, "I refuse to delegate. I don't have time to delegate. I'm finding a job where I don't have to delegate because we never have enough staff." Amusingly enough, it seems that these nurses have been unable to hear that they were already presumably delegating to someone in their present roles. As professional nurses, they were supervising a secretary, new personnel, perhaps students. The only place we could determine would be an appropriate setting for someone who refuses to delegate would be private nursing practice in a sand dune in the Sahara desert—a perfect place for placing one's head in the sand, so this would be a fitting alternative work assignment!

For those who remain in the denial stage, it might be helpful for coworkers to point out the studies that show positive outcomes for nurses who delegate some of the care, and in many areas of the country, personnel shortages preclude an all RN staff. It might also be appropriate to note that the nurse practice acts, the National Council of State Boards of Nursing, and even the Code for Nurses discuss delegation as a part of nursing practice. For example, the American Nurses Association (ANA) Code for Nurses states:

> The nurse exercises informed judgment and uses individual competence and qualifications as criteria in seeking consultation, accepting responsibilities, and delegating nursing activities to others. . . . The nurse must assess individual competency in assigning selected components of nursing care to other nursing service personnel. The nurse should not delegate to any member of the nursing team a function for which that person is not prepared or qualified. (American Nurses Association, 1976, 1985, p. 1)

The updated ANA Code for Nurses similarly asserts that "The nurse is responsible and accountable for individual nursing practice and determines the appropriate delegation of tasks consistent with the nurse's obligation to provide optimum patient care" (American Nurses Association, 2001). Since this code was established in 1976, reaffirmed in 1985, and updated in 2001, apparently a few nurses have been using this code to guide them in delegating for the last several decades!

Nurse practice statutes and rules, as noted in Chapter 3, often specify that delegation is a part of nursing practice. The Massachusetts Board of Registration in Nursing states that the functions of a registered nurse (RN) include delegating:

A registered nurse, within the parameters of her/his generic and continuing education and experience, may delegate nursing activities to other registered nurses and/or healthcare personnel, provided that the delegating registered nurse shall bear full and ultimate responsibility for: 1) making an appropriate assignment 2) properly and adequately teaching, directing and supervising the delegate and 3) the outcomes of that delegation (244CMR: 3.02, effective March 11, 1994).

It's hard for even the most recalcitrant person in denial to avoid the fact that delegation is a part of nursing practice by law! Even if the past practice on your nursing unit has meant "the assistants do their jobs and we do ours" with little ongoing contact, you now know better: RNs must supervise other workers. Even if your care delivery model has not supported that process, it's now clear to any reader that practice must change.

As we further explore the stages of the grief process, we can also consider the individual's usual response to change. In the Pacific Northwest, the coming of winter is often heralded by the first storm from the Pacific Ocean. Some people enjoy the hallmark event by visiting rocky beaches when the storm is far off. One nurse might see the storm clouds approaching and leave. Others might decide to stay on the beach, but no matter how hard the winds and waves roar and crash, they are determined to dig in their heels and stay in their accustomed spots. When the first waves pound the shore, these nurses are flung onto the barnacle-encrusted boulders and emerge between waves, bruised and bleeding. Others, seeing the storm clouds and waves on the horizon, outfit themselves with a wetsuit, gauge the waves' rhythm and the wind's velocity, and dive right in! These nurses body surf to the shore, gently gliding to the ground at the ebb of the wave. While we are not recommending body surfing in a Pacific Northwest storm, the image recommends observing the climate of health care and responding proactively to emerging realities.

Consider yourself: Are you the nurse in denial who is continually bruised and broken by changes, the nurse who tries to dig in and keep your heels in one place while sands shift around you? Or are you one of the nurses who sees the turbulence coming, judges the best method of adjusting, and survives the storm? You might never be able to love or to welcome change, but do realize that it is a fact of life. Change can't be controlled, but your response to it can be.

Anger

Anger is a formidable emotion. It is a very powerful, normal part of the grief process. It is not wrong to be angry, but it is maladaptive and downright destructive for us to use our anger against each other or ourselves.

Some of us move into anger early on in our career and remain in this stage for lengthy periods of time. Nurses aren't used to dealing with their anger effectively. Instead we often try to deny it because we don't believe it's nice to be angry. We say instead that we are "upset" or "burned out" or "worried about patient care."

One of the operational definitions of anger is "unmet expectations." If you or someone you know is angry, which expectation has been left unmet? Were you told that the only way to be a "real nurse" was to do all the care yourself? Was it your school of nursing's expectation that graduates would always be nurses who do "total patient care"? Those expectations caused a fair amount of frustration and job dissatisfaction with new graduates who worked in long-term care, rural hospitals, and home health, where supervising others has always been a standard piece of the job description. Was your vision of practice based on working with one or two patients as a student nurse?

Were you expecting that your preferred type of practice or routine wouldn't be altered? Although you've known healthcare reform has been needed for years, did you hope you wouldn't be affected? We often meet nurses who have avoided (denial again?) any current literature or healthcare news as they focused only on their clinical area and improving their expertise. We do recommend staying abreast of research in your clinical area, but venturing to a broader current events focus will help prepare for changes in work and life. Were you hoping that your administrative people or your unit shared governance council would have asked for more input before implementing a new care delivery model? Would you like to have been involved? These are valid expectations, certainly, but often the people in administrative posts are reacting to rapid change while trying to preserve their own jobs. Perhaps they didn't have time based on emerging finances, or they didn't know how to effectively engage your input, or they didn't think staff wanted to be involved.

Did you think there wouldn't be a nurse shortage when you went to school, and did you hope to remain unaffected? Unmet expectations, whether based on fact or fantasy, are another valid reason to be angry. Depending on the vagaries of the marketplace and what happens with healthcare reimbursement, in a few short years of your career, we can expect myriad changes to occur. Whether in the midst of "the perfect storm" of a

Anger = unmet expectations

nurse shortage or during periods of unemployment, one begins to think more about how to continue to be marketable in one's skill, maintaining flexibility.

If you have been angry, or even depressed, which expectations seem to be the foundation of your anger? Determine the expectations and write them down now.

_____

_____

_____

_____

_____

_____

_____

Think about it: Are your expectations still reasonable? Where did these expectations come from?

_____

_____

_____

All of the previous unmet expectations are commonly expressed. Remember, anger is normal. All of that great energy must not be wasted, though. Be angry, express it, and then use it to make things work out better for yourself and your patients.

Be aware of where your anger is percolating! Is the energy going home with you and being discharged at your family? Are you finding yourself on a short fuse with your coworkers? (Be particularly aware of negative emotions toward those who are new to the workplace, such as new graduates and assistive personnel. They came looking for a job to support themselves, not to upset you or your habitual way of work.) Or have you noticed that you find less joy in the things you used to like about your job? This might be the burnout that occurs when people turn their anger inward. Serious depression might ensue. Remember, express the anger and then get on with it! How can you best adjust, learn, cope? How can you make certain the care that is given works the best for the patients and other consumers? Use your energy to be involved in creating the best methods of supervising the added personnel.

> The energy from anger is often misplaced and ends up in depression, burnout, and poor team relationships.

Bargaining

"Today I don't have time to teach Helen to chart the intakes and outputs. I'll do it myself. But tomorrow, I'm sure I can find the time to assign it properly."

Bargaining, like denial, buys some time for the individual to adjust. We might bargain with ourselves, with other staff, with management. However, after the first few bargains, nurses can find themselves back in maladaptive denial and anger. Usually, our bargains don't work so well for our own adjustment. We often hear of nurses who stay at work overtime repeatedly because they are in the bargaining stage of the grief process. They don't ever find the time to do the supervision part of their jobs properly.

Another common bargaining statement goes something like this: "Well, I'll see how this delegation and care partners idea works out in the next month. And if I don't see major improvements in quality of patient care, I'll find another place to work." This nurse is slipping into the denial stage once again.

Bargaining, like all other stages, is normal. It allows for adjustment and adaptation as nurses begin to try out their new skills. But if it continues, it will strangle the bargainer's ability to delegate safely and effectively.

As we return to our first example, the bargainer avoids teaching the assistive person, Helen, how to do a routine task because it will take too much time, yet she might be on overtime doing the intakes and outputs herself. She might have the added satisfaction of seeing every drop of urine herself, thus meeting her own (and perhaps her nursing instructor's) expectations; however, the delegate (Helen) does not fulfill her own expectations of her role. There will be anger from Helen at some point, as well as anger from the exhausted RN. The maxim that "if you give a person a fish, you feed him for a day, but if you teach a person to fish, you feed him for a lifetime" applies here. Encouraging personal growth is one of the foundations for personal empowerment.

So bargain if you must, but force yourself to continue to expand into your role as a supervisor. Both you and your delegates have the opportunity to be empowered.

Depression

Here's where anger rears its flaming head again. That anger that wasn't expressed, that energy that wasn't channeled to help you and those you serve, is revisiting itself on your life. Depression is anger turned inward. When you are depressed, all problems that would normally be a part of your day now seem to be insurmountable mountains. You don't even go to the beach to see the waves; you are at home trying to get yourself out of bed and off to work.

Depression is anger turned inward.

We are convinced, as we work with nurses everywhere, that burnout as experienced within our profession is a by-product of the difficulty we have experienced collectively in dealing with anger. It's okay to be angry. It's normal. But determine which expectation you had that wasn't met. Decide whether that expectation is still operational and realistic. If you decide that it is not, your anger won't be as acute. If it is, then use the energy to quit whining and be involved in sculpting what you want out of the future.

We aren't psychologists. If you find yourself to be clinically depressed and unable to function normally, or if you know someone who is, urge him or her to contact a mental health professional for help. Many organizations offer Employee Assistance Programs (ask at your Human Resources office). But if you have mild depression related to work issues, we are certain you'll feel better if you take just one step to do something to adjust to the changes. We think reading this book and working out the exercises might be one of those action items that will help. Follow up with unit governance committee work or a discussion with your boss or your coworkers about what things are bugging you and what you think can be done about them. But whatever you do, GET INVOLVED! It's a sure cure and far less expensive than antidepressant medication.

Acceptance

The last stage of the grief process is acceptance. This term needs to be clarified a bit because people often believe that accepting the whole idea of never-ending change within their organizations or accepting the role of supervisor within their jobs means a real leap of faith. Some readers are already excellent delegators and perceive they have no issue with delegation and supervision; they are already comfortable with supervising teams. If so, please read our recommendations for future reference in mentoring others in developing their leadership skills.

Some may shout, "Yes, yes, hallelujah, I have seen the light! Let me work alone with a hospital full of patients and be the only licensed person on duty! Let me be the only public health RN in our town! Let me be the only RN in our long-term care facility!"

This idea of "life-altering" acceptance is not realistic for many nurses. However, it is possible for nurses to overcome their barriers to delegation and to actually enjoy working with a group of people to achieve their goals. Many tell us they find more job satisfaction and many other benefits, but for now, recognize that acceptance is a gradual process. Some nurses might first accept that, yes, change is needed. Some nurses go back and forth through the stages of the grief process as is normal in other grief situations. They might offer initial direction and feedback to an assistant one day and receive a negative response and not try again until a manager reviews her practice and offers to role-play giving feedback. Another nurse might then accept that it probably is necessary to deliver care with assistive personnel because without them there would be fewer people to help the patients. Still others might first accept that they might be able to master the process and later feel safer and more in control. All of these incremental steps in acceptance will lead the nurse to effective delegation. We treasure the stories nurses tell us about a "problem" nursing assistant with a "bad attitude" who now works effectively as a team member. These are success stories for nurses, assistants, leaders, and patients and families.

For those readers who are still having difficulty with the idea of this process and who are still in an earlier stage of the grief process, the most basic acceptance is this: It is possible to learn to delegate effectively and deliver safe, effective nursing care. We've considered the emotions that are often present when nurses first begin to delegate. Although some of these emotions depend on the manner in which care delivery system changes are introduced, there is a great similarity of emotions expressed across the country, ranging from excitement to anger to apathy. Some hospitals are using more assistive personnel due to the nurse shortage and have not supervised care closely in the past. Using the best team practices in professional nursing is a new concept to staff as well as managers. Using the grief process and the concept of change as a model, we have asked you to identify your own emotions and the stage of the grief process. We have explored the positive and negative sequelae of the stages and the emotions and encouraged you to consider your own set of circumstances and feelings about working closely with team members.

1. Use your brain power to harness and identify your own emotions.
2. Determine the stage you or your coworkers are experiencing.
3. If you feel angry, decide which expectation you've had that hasn't been met.
4. Consider whether your expectation is still realistic.
5. Use your emotional energy for action: by reading this book, by using skills, by being a part of task forces or discussion groups.

Occasionally a new set of administrators will herald more leadership job vacancies as a new executive team is formed, and staff confusion about rules or expectations creates a sense of mistrust in an organization. Staffing shortages can create frustration, disappointment, anger, and stress. When employees begin orientation believing that they could retire happily without ever leaving this organization, trusting that their financial future is secure, organizational redesign, unit mergers, or job changes come as a very rude awakening. Once again we are faced with the unmet expectations that cause anger and loss of trust. Feelings, however negative, cannot be erased or ignored. We have often visited organizations as "damage control" experts and have winced at the staff's hopelessness and hurt that is immediately evident in their interactions with one another and their patients. These feelings are a by-product of the situation and an individual's personality, past experiences, and current concepts and perceptions, and they must be dealt with so that the negative effects of these behaviors don't destroy what we have set out to do for our patients.

CHECKPOINT 5–6

Which stage of the grief process is being experienced by the following nurses?

1. Nurse Powell sits reading the paper with her back turned to the manager as the manager tries to discuss the rationale for the changes in the care delivery model and additional assistive personnel.

2. John, the charge nurse, decides to take on a larger patient assignment today because he doesn't think the other nurses have the time to supervise the nursing assistants.

3. Pat has agreed to be on the task force that is clarifying the expectations of each of the new roles. Pat has seen other roles being used in various ways in other health departments in other cities where she's been employed.

4. Sharon, a new graduate, has been calling in ill frequently the last two months. She says she's having trouble getting out of bed at 10 p.m. and feels overwhelmed by the supervisory role she must play with the assistive personnel at the rehab center.

5. Tom turned in his resignation today. He said he wanted to find a job where nurses were allowed to practice "professional nursing."

See the end of the chapter for the answers.

First, we recommend that organizational changes be done with sensitivity and with staff participation in the planning, if possible. Then the organization must provide for grieving and facilitation of emotional release, including such group processes as a "wake" for the department or people lost (Noer, 1993, p. 128) or facilitated venting sessions (Noer, 1997, p. 34). Changes build upon additional rapid changes, and change weariness occurs. Dealing with the feelings will certainly help them come out in full force; don't be afraid of those emotions that are "out there." Be fearful of what will happen with the strength of those emotions if they are not expressed openly but instead run underground, squelching creativity and producing depression.

The organization can also assist staff in learning about what might be an unhealthy or codependent attachment to their job roles, more often noted in the senior generations of workers. As much as we all seek fulfillment in our work and find satisfaction in why we are doing our jobs (our purpose), the job itself and that particular organization are not the only ways we can express our talents. Leaving behind a belief that our employer has replaced our loving parents and has become our family is a necessary component of life in this millennium. Entitlement beliefs (e.g., you'll keep your job and collect regular paychecks no matter how much you add value to your organization or no matter what happens in healthcare reimbursement) only serve to make us dependent, resentful, and vulnerable (Bardwick, 1995, p. 22).

> Don't be afraid of those emotions that are expressed, but be wary of those that are not.

Recognizing the new realities of the workplace can vary from feeling that "no one values what I do anymore personally because of needing any warm body to fill staffing needs" to the proactive attitude of "I realize the rationale for changes here and have a clear internal understanding of my value as a professional and the impact I make with patients and families, whether employed by this organization or any other."

Your organization can help empower and use your talents fully by:

+ recognizing the new employment contract
+ being clear on accountabilities and the rules of the road
+ sticking to its word
+ keeping information flowing
+ helping all staff to be involved in the organizational growth

Your part is to be there to participate fully.

Dealing with Resistance to Change and Grief

For nurses to be able to thrive in the midst of ongoing recurrent changes in their work lives, each individual must be able to work effectively with those negative emotions that might stifle abilities to work most effectively with patients. Why should an individual give up the possibility of exciting, fulfilling work and become a nurse (in name only) who drags herself to work hating every moment of what she does, often creating a negative work environment for all who relate to her during her shift? We sometimes call these people "RIP" or "retired in place."

Based on our work with numerous nurses and other healthcare professionals who have been slogging in the muck of these negative feelings, we have been able to develop some practical strategies to deal effectively with negative emotions. Incorporating some of William Bridges' work with transition and change in helping with this process (for more information and tools, see Hansten & Washburn, 1997, p. 24), staff members can describe their feelings in metaphors, or word pictures, and identify what has changed, what they feel they have been forced to alter, and what each person needs to do to make the changes successful for him or her. The real crux of this matter is what people need to let go of, to get through this difficult time.

Sometimes the personal barriers are in the form of resentment toward others, the concept

Individuals who have moved to professional independence see themselves as performing part of their personal mission and growth plan (which they have fully developed) within the organization right now; they network with their professional organizations, and they have many support systems outside the workplace.

that time would never alter their team or department, their fear of the future. Being certain never to let go of personal purposes such as "making a difference in patients' and families' lives," each professional can begin to build again from the bedrock of their choice of profession. Further work includes developing clear role accountabilities and assisting managers and staff in realizing the true benefits of an empowered, engaged workforce.

For you, personally, here is a plan for dealing with constant workplace change.

PLAN FOR DEALING WITH CONSTANT CHANGE

1. Develop a personal mission statement. Why do you do what you do?
2. Develop a plan for your career. Does it include working at the same job in the same organization for the next 30 years? If so, reevaluate reality.
3. Identify the feelings that might be stalling you. Relate:
   - a metaphor, or word picture, that describes your feelings
   - what's been lost
   - what you feel you've been forced to give up or do (the real issues that are problematic for you)
   - what you want to hang on to no matter what (the bedrock of your personal beliefs about your profession)
   - what you feel that you need to let go of to make this job successful— then let go of it!
4. Determine what you have expected your organization to provide for you in the past. Are these requests reasonable at this time?
5. Make a list of connections and supports you can access, both professionally and personally.
6. Be involved in making things better. This might be in the form of task forces, leading or participating in staff meetings, or communicating concerns to those who have the organizational authority to make a difference. Feel the power that is there for you if you choose to use it! If you find that anger or other emotions are still a barrier, review the steps for dealing with emotions and the grief process and read on about other barriers you might be experiencing that are related to working as a team.

OTHER BARRIERS

Personal feelings about implementing a new system of care or about the constant changes in health care themselves are often barriers to effective clinical delegation, but many other personal barriers might be present within each nurse. Some of these can be related to past experiences, whether from undergraduate education, life experiences, training, or clinical realities that nurses have faced during their careers. Let's examine these and determine which might be operational in your own life.

Take the self-assessment quiz in **Exhibit 5–1** to determine how much these barriers challenge you in implementing the clinical delegation process.

EXHIBIT 5–1   Delegation Self-Assessment

Answer the following with Strongly Agree (SA), Agree (A), Unsure (U), Disagree (D), or Strongly Disagree (SD).

___1. I hate risk: I don't think risk of any kind should be present in health-care delivery.

___2. It's very difficult for me to trust the people I work with. How can I be sure they'll do what I want them to?

___3. Letting go of the tasks I like to do is impossible for me. I get all my positive feedback from doing my clinical tasks exceptionally well.

___4. There's so little I can control about my daily work that I find it very difficult to lose the control I gain by doing it all myself. How can I control others enough to be certain everything is done my way?

___5. I'm finding that overcoming my old habits of doing it all myself is more difficult than giving up (choose one) cigarettes, or chocolate, or fine wine. Giving up things that are comfortable for me and are a part of my daily life is not my cup of tea.

___6. I feel very little achievement when someone else does the nuts and bolts of the care. I want to do that myself so I can feel the satisfaction of crossing tasks off my list.

___7. If everyone else does the tasks on the care plan, I'm confused about what's left for me to do.

___8. When people tell me they have time to help me, it's difficult for me to tell them what they can do to help. I could use some help with organizing my work.

___9. I do all the work in my area better than most people. I am an expert clinician, and I would hate for the clients to receive an "inferior" product if I am not the person actually performing that care.

____10. I really hate to make people mad when I assign them work. I'd rather do it myself than give out a bad assignment.

____11. There are a few people that work as hard as I do. I often find myself with the most challenging assignments. I rarely ask for help. Often, I'm behind doing my charting after the shift is over while the "slackers" go out for pizza.

____12. I am uncertain about what can be delegated to the personnel in our department. The roles are unclear, and I'm not comfortable with the state regulations and rules.

____13. I hate to even think about delegating care to anyone else!

____14. If I don't do the tasks I'm used to doing, I wonder if I will still be a real nurse? I've worked too hard to become a clinical "has-been."

____15. I've never seen or worked with anyone who is a good delegator. I wouldn't know what it's like.

Look at the items for which you agreed or strongly agreed. These will most likely be your highest barriers. Those that are marked "unsure" might also crop up as problems for you in learning and implementing clinical delegation skills. Let's dissect each of these in more detail.

Barrier 1: Risk Aversion

We certainly aren't advocating that you take risks with your patients' lives! However, when we delegate to others, there is always some risk.

> You cannot absolutely guarantee that the delegate will not err (just as you might err yourself) or that all will be completed exactly the same way you'd prefer. Following the delegation process correctly will minimize the negative aspects of the inherent risk.

Think about the risk involved in not having assistive personnel available to help you do the work. There's some risk there as well.

Barrier 2: Being Able to Trust Others

We aren't encouraging you in any way to trust implicitly all the people with whom you work or even those within your personal life. It doesn't make sense, and this kind of blind, trusting approach is the same that allows charlatans and con artists to take advantage of the elderly.

> In delegating aspects of care to others, some degree of trust must develop. Delegates must trust that you'll be there to help with problems. You must be able to trust delegates to do what they say they will do and to communicate changes in the patient's condition.

How does trust develop? In all relationships, trust develops from risking enough to establish the relationship and then by experiencing the objective results of that relationship. If your expectations are fulfilled, you begin to develop an image of that person as one who can be trusted. When one problem occurs in which that trust is violated, it's difficult to regain the same ease of communication and positive relationship. For example, Pat, a licensed practical/vocational nurse (LPN/LVN) had been working with Jo, an RN, for several weeks, and during that time Jo had always telephoned physicians promptly for changes in orders. This time Pat thought that Mrs. Smith's condition was worsening quickly and told Jo. Jo, however, did not come to check on the patient promptly and did not call the physician promptly to discuss the changes in condition. Even though Jo might not have considered the changes to be important enough, the message she gave to Pat was loud and clear: She didn't think that Pat's input was important. It will take a long time for Jo to regain Pat's trust.

When we talk to assistive personnel (and we do this nearly every week), we hear that they would truly appreciate some respect for what they do and some discussion about what you expect of them. As a nursing assistant wrote in a letter to the editor of *American Journal of Nursing*, "Just because the 'numbers' and 'mix' are correct doesn't mean the patients are getting good care. Some RNs are very defensive when an unlicensed person dares to tell them something should be done about one of their patients; others are too busy discussing their social life to be bothered about the patients. Some lack experience, some are burned out, some just shouldn't be RNs" (Robbins, 1997, p. 17). It sounds like there's room to develop trust on both sides!

Barrier 3: Letting Go

Letting go of those tasks that have been important to you in the past is difficult but necessary for growth to occur.

> Is it reasonable to expect that our nation is willing to pay, for example, $45 per hour for you as an RN to empty retention catheters and trash cans when someone else can be paid $18 per hour to do the same work?

In an era of limited resources, yours must be used to the fullest extent. If you aren't doing the professional role of the RN, who is? When we lead a seminar, a nurse occasionally will remark, "But I like to do the baths and bed changes! That's why I went into nursing!" If that is true for you, it's time to think about why you are in this profession and what else you are doing, or could be doing, during that task. Is there anything within the professional role of the RN that would also give you some satisfaction? For example, if you became an RN because you wanted to help people or to make a difference in people's lives, then you can certainly do a better job using all your skills, going beyond the merely technical to the intellectual. (For more information, see Chapter 6 regarding the PTA model.)

Barrier 4: Fear of Loss of Control

Nurses would like to be able to control a lot more about their work. We can't control what kind and acuity of patients are admitted through our emergency departments. We can't control our caseload in home health or the number of Alzheimer's patients that become residents at our long-term care facility. At the beginning of our shift, it's difficult to know how our best-laid plans might be upset by the inevitable human factors we might encounter, so we try to control everything we can.

> We can only control ourselves and our own behavior, including the decisions we make when delegating.

When we delegate care to others, we can't control their every move. No one expects that we will be able to control our coworkers like robots.

However, as we now understand the process of delegation more fully, we know that we can control how we delegate: how we assess ourselves and our barriers; how we appraise the strengths, weaknesses, motivation, and preferences of our delegates; how we match the task to the delegate; how we communicate; and how we evaluate and give feedback to those we supervise. There is more control than we expected!

Barrier 5: Overcoming Old Habits

As we've already discussed, the rate of change is increasing at a dizzying speed. It's probably more difficult to change the way we work than to change some of our personal habits. We often spend more time at work than with our families!

> "Doing it all myself" sometimes seems like the best way to make certain it is done correctly. But when there isn't enough of you to go around, when it's impossible for you to do it all, give yourself a break. Try to use the delegation process.

Just as some nurses find it is easier to give up that piece of cheesecake after lunch little by little, some nurses find that overcoming the old habits engendered by earlier care delivery systems can be done in stages. If you decide to go "cold turkey," remember to be kind and supportive to yourself and those with whom you work.

Barrier 6: Needing to Cross Tasks Off a List

Some nurses are so task oriented that they rush through their "morning work" and get all their "work" done by noon. Their work, they announce, is the bed/bath/assessment ritual on their unit. Changing your to-do list to include such things as discharge planning and coordinating care for each patient is less concrete and, to some, less satisfying. If you see this as one of your barriers, begin new lists that focus on processes or patient and family centered outcomes rather than tasks. Include such items as "getting report" and "giving feedback to each delegate." Nurses have stated that this strategy has helped them overcome the nebulous feeling of having achieved very little each shift. We recommend it as long as nurses remember first and foremost that the patient's short-term and long-term outcomes must be in mind before they make out the process (rather than task) list. When clients or patients achieve a goal with your help, celebrate it! The outcome for the patient or family is the most important achievement of the entire team!

Barrier 7: What's Left for Me to Do?

This barrier is closely related to barriers 3, 5, and 6. If you've delegated tasks and can't see the implications of your professional role, we recommend that you read the discussion of the PTA model in Chapter 6. The healthcare system needs you as an RN to do your professional job well so that clinical outcomes can be realized. Also, think about those things that you've wanted to complete but have been unable to because you've had to deal with so many details of care before (patient education, emotional support, coordination of all healthcare disciplines, family conferences, discharge planning, communication with other professionals).

Begin to think about how you add value in your organization. Why are you needed? Why does the chief financial officer think that the correct complement of nurses must be present to ensure that patients receive optimal care? (Or does he or she think unlicensed personnel, LPNs, and RNs are interchangeable?) Why does a physician sigh with relief and state, "Thank goodness I put my patients in this extended care facility instead of any other! The nurses here really make the difference!" (What difference do you make?) We are convinced that the most important jobs you do, those that make a difference to the patients' end results and the care they receive along the way have to do with those things only an RN can do.

Barrier 8: Needing Help with Organization of Work

We know you recognize the phenomenon: a nurse who is excellent at performing discrete tasks or processes but has difficulty seeing the forest for the trees. He or she might be unable to break down the overall work to be done into manageable pieces. Learning to be more organized is difficult; however, we've seen some successes. If this is a barrier for you, talk to the nurses you find to be the most organized. Ask them to show you how they divide up their work. Sometimes one work sheet or method of organizing will work better for one nurse than another. Keep asking until you find one that makes sense to you. Often a visit with your manager or clinical instructor will be useful. He or she might even authorize some time for you to shadow or work with someone who is efficient in delivering care. You might want to review your scores on the Nursing Expertise Self-Report Scale found in Appendix 5–A. Perhaps you just need some more time to develop that "big picture."

Barrier 9: The Supernurse Syndrome

It's great to know you are out there caring for us and our families! Being an expert in your area and being extremely conscientious about your work are certainly positive qualities. However, it is tough for a supernurse to let others grow in their skills. After all, those served might not receive the highest quality of care while these others (UAP) are developing their skills.

> Unfortunately, supernurses cannot be everywhere at all times, particularly in this environment of cost containment. Supernurses who find themselves unable to delegate will also become overwhelmed and burned out as they try to do it all.

If you are a supernurse, find some examples of care given by others that is satisfactory, maybe even good. Keep looking for those examples so that you will feel less guilty about the care you weren't able to deliver alone.

Barrier 10: Wanting to Be Liked

Who will be happy to take the assignment of the abusive patient who is throwing stool and is having diarrhea and needs constant perineal care? Which nurse wants to manage the case of the patient with multiple personalities who likes to talk about child abuse exploits? If you are the person in charge of making those types of assignments, you wonder what will happen if you assign your best friend to care for these challenging patients. What will he or she slip into your coffee at the next coffee break? Will anyone ever ask you to go out for social time after work?

> One of the most difficult aspects of being in a supervisory position is the struggle over the question: Is it more important to be liked or to be respected?

You, through your nurse practice act and by virtue of your job description, must take a leadership role. Would you rather like your supervisors and leaders or respect their decisions and leadership abilities? Think about how others earn your respect. Respect is generally earned through performing supervisory duties faithfully. You have been entrusted to ensure that patient/client/resident care is the highest quality possible. Making the best assignment for the difficult patient should not be based on who will be the most angry and vengeful. It should be based on the best match of assignment and delegate.

Barrier 11: The Supermartyr Syndrome

We've started a new group, Supermartyr Nurses Anonymous. It's a 12-step program, and the first step is to announce, "Hi, my name is Mary, and I'm a supermartyr nurse!"

Identifying the problem yourself is the first step. However, ask any of your coworkers: They already know who the supermartyrs are. (Some of them might have used your need to be needed and indispensable by giving you some extra work!) Ask your coworkers to help you limit yourself to doing what is reasonable and what is performed by others with your job description. You must take care of yourself so that you can take care of others. (For additional information, see *The Nurse Manager's Answer Book*, Hansten and Washburn, 1993, Chapter 16, on codependency.)

Barrier 12: Uncertain About Rules, Regulations

Nurses who don't want to delegate might be those who are still unsure about what is included in their roles and job descriptions. They might also worry about "putting my license on the line" when working with unlicensed caregivers. There are two main strategies for dealing with this barrier.

First, get some education. After you've read the information in this book, call your state board and get a copy of your nurse practice act or go online and download a copy. Ask questions of the board staff. Ask your facility to have a speaker from the state come and discuss your concerns.

Second, clarify roles within your organization. Ask to have a staff meeting to clarify who is supposed to be doing what. Find out what the assistive personnel can expect of you as well. What do they think their roles are? Where are you all in agreement? Where is there confusion? This is one of the most essential points for overcoming barriers to delegation. Clarify expectations. This discussion often goes beyond who should do what task and ends up discussing such things as being called by name, being asked with a please and a thank you, and who really should answer the phone or call lights or talk with physicians or other professionals.

As you clarify roles, you might also find you need to develop a skills or evaluation checklist for each role. We've seen many of these used to assist in overcoming the barrier of confusion about roles.

Barrier 13: Denial

Some of you might not even want to think about delegation! If this is the case for you or for some of your coworkers, it will be pretty difficult for you to learn how to supervise effectively. We suggest that you are remaining in the denial stage of the grief process. Review the information earlier in this chapter and continue to read on as we evaluate the potential benefits you can reap as you learn how to delegate effectively.

Barrier 14: Am I Still a Real Nurse When I Delegate?

Many nurses continue to harbor this fear even as they continue to do an expert job of delegation and supervising others. Because we have experienced this fear ourselves as we entered supervisory, management, and executive roles, we have struggled with the uncertainty and concerns about remaining "clinically expert."

The first step in overcoming this barrier is to consider why you went into nursing at all. When we ask this question, we get a wide range of answers. Think now about why you decided to be a nurse.

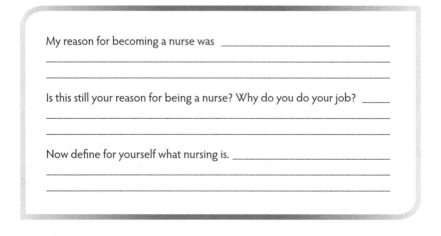

My reason for becoming a nurse was _____

_____

_____

Is this still your reason for being a nurse? Why do you do your job? _____

_____

_____

Now define for yourself what nursing is. _____

_____

_____

Can you still fulfill your definition of nursing and the reason you went into nursing if you ask someone else to do some of the tasks?

For example, if you went into nursing to make a difference in other people's lives, and to you nursing is a profession that uses the nursing process (assessment, nursing diagnosis, planning, intervening, and evaluating) in a holistic manner with patients, families, and social systems to aid the individual and his or her significant others to move toward their own definitions of health or wellness, then certainly you can use the help of others in performing your duties. We as nurses have done this since the days of Florence Nightingale.

If you still think nursing is only doing the tasks, it's time to think about what else might satisfy you within your new or emerging role. If you must still perform all the care to feel fulfilled, consider why you are doing your job. You won't feel fulfilled from the tasks that you do but from why you perform your professional role.

Barrier 15: No Role Models

We have asked groups of nurses how many of them have had excellent role models in the delegation or supervisory process, and very few have acknowledged delegation mentors. Perhaps this is because nurses weren't looking for this skill in others when it seemed less important. Perhaps it is because nurses determined that other nurses were highly organized, or efficient and effective, or just that things always went well, but they didn't connect clinical delegation skills with the end product: better patient care. Or perhaps there are expert nurses out there who can't find the time to mentor others.

If you don't have a role model, never fear! You will have all the information you'll need to be successful.

DETERMINING THE POTENTIAL BENEFITS

Each nurse might have a barrier or two to conquer, and all have multiple strengths they can use to overcome those barriers. Think about how we evaluate the problems or needs of our clients and families. We identify their strengths for coping and use them in our plan of care. Often the plan of care includes education and practicing new skills. That's our plan for you as you learn (or refresh your memory) about the process of clinical delegation.

To mobilize the energy to leap over these barriers, nurses need to visualize what's waiting on the other side of the wall. What outcomes can be expected?

If you are able to overcome your barriers, or at least prevent them from being a stumbling block on a daily basis, and if you become an expert at delegating and supervising others, what will the potential benefits be?

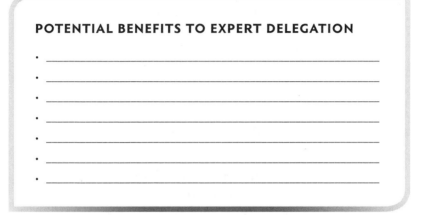

POTENTIAL BENEFITS TO EXPERT DELEGATION

- _____
- _____
- _____
- _____
- _____
- _____
- _____

When we began to educate nurses about delegation, we completed informal qualitative research with nurses from all areas of care delivery who had been delegating to assistive personnel for some time. We asked them what benefits had been realized from learning to delegate well. They told us the following had occurred:

- more time for myself (breaks, lunches)
- personal growth
- empowerment and growth of the assistive personnel
- making better use of my brain power and assessment skills
- more time for professional nursing (educating patients, emotional support, coordination of care, planning, communication with other professionals and family, discharge planning)
- less stressed out with "doing it all"
- more sense of team and support of each other
- collegiality
- someone to help gather data, answer lights
- less overtime
- job satisfaction
- better outcomes for patients (including nurse sensitive indicators such as fewer falls, fewer decubitus ulcers, shortened length of stay)
- improved job satisfaction for both assistive personnel and registered nurses

CHECKPOINT 5-7

There has been change in the care delivery model, and I feel pretty awful about it. All of us feel overworked and overwhelmed. All these new assistive personnel! I do get a bit resentful of those who left, though, because I note some of them are off this summer and one person even got a job with better pay. It's hard for me to get up and go in for my shift! The best plan for me is to:

a) Just put in the hours required. No one here is going to give me a gold watch for my years of service!

b) Focus on why I am a nurse and think about what I want from my career in the future, with the knowledge that my future might look very different.

c) Get involved in the redesign task force that is planning how to improve those systems that have never worked well at this hospital. I figure that now is our chance!

d) Go to the employee assistance counselor to discuss what I can do to feel better about my job. Maybe I need to see a mental health professional.

See the end of the chapter for the answers.

Nurse researchers have increased their emphasis on emerging care delivery systems and the impact of registered nurse hours on outcomes. For example, Blegen et al. (1992) at the University of Iowa began a study through the *American Journal of Nursing* in April 1991, asking nurses, "Who helps you with your work?" The study indicated that "nurses who reported delegating the routine aspects of patient care and those who planned by delegating most of the care were more satisfied with their jobs . . . than those who did all the care themselves" (Blegen, et al., 1992, p. 28).

Another study published in the *Journal of Nursing Administration* in March 1993 showed an improvement in patient satisfaction after assistive personnel were introduced (Neidlinger, et al., 1993). In the same journal, Lengacher and Mabe (1993) reviewed several models of nurse extender use and found differences in each. In a model in which RNs supervised nursing assistants, the following outcomes were discovered: "increased staff satisfaction, patient satisfaction, and unit pride, a visible improvement in the work environment, increased nurse–patient contact, reduced waste of supplies, and increased documentation in the patient record.

Staff members believed that they were more efficient and worked less overtime, and patients and physicians were more satisfied" (Lengacher & Mabe, 1993, p. 17). Aiken et al.'s work to correlate nurse staffing and patient mortality showed that patient care is positively affected by higher patient care ratios and that "patient mortality increased 7% for every additional patient in the average nurse's workload" (Kleinman & Saccomano, 2006, p. 163). In a study by Huston, increased registered nurse staffing as a percentage of staffing mix correlated to better pain relief in patients with nurse administered analgesia, and increased numbers of assistive personnel in relationship to RN ratios were correlated to increased pain in the patients (Huston, 2001). One wonders whether or not the nurses in this study were delegating and supervising appropriately! Better team relationships in a staff-developed patient care delivery model improved nurse and assistive personnel job satisfaction by 14% (Allen & Vitale-Nolen, 2005).

CHECKPOINT 5-8

We've discussed most of the potential obstructions to delegation and have focused on personal barriers. Look at **Exhibit 5-2** and determine your most sterling qualities. These strengths will give you the needed boost for expanding your delegation skills and bridging your barriers.

EXHIBIT 5-2 Assessing Strengths

_____ I understand my job description as well as the roles of those who assist me.

_____ I have studied the state nurse practice act and feel certain about its regulations.

_____ I am highly organized in doing my work.

_____ I am ready to overcome some old habits and learn some new ways of working.

_____ I look at nursing with a broader perspective than "tasks."

_____ I am willing to take some careful, calculated risks and slowly gain trust by supervising the assistive personnel.

_____ I am cognizant of my own strengths and weaknesses, and I am asking for feedback from my coworkers about my "supernurse" or "super-martyr" tendencies.

_____ I have delegated before, and it has been a great learning experience for me.

_____ I am focusing more on being worthy of my coworkers' respect than on being liked by everyone.

_____ I have learned from some excellent role models, or I can be a role model myself because I am already expert at this skill.

_____ I am willing to learn!

From our vast experience in working with different care delivery systems across the country for nearly 2 decades, it is evident to us that the manner in which care is assigned, whether or not clear lines of accountability exist, and the manner in which the RN leads the team, giving initial direction, calling periodic checkpoints and team meetings, and facilitating ongoing and reciprocal feedback, make all the difference in the success of any team system.

For more information about positive or negative effects regarding care delivery redesign in hospitals, refer to the hallmark commentary by Krapohl and Larson (1996) that evaluates 24 different studies of models of care delivery and to the Web site www.HanstenRROHC.com. We have personally worked with organizations that have implemented new care delivery systems or have merely improved the delegation skills of their RNs, and they have found the following benefits:

+ Patients are happier when they don't have to "bother" the RN for minor requests and when they know that someone is available to answer their call lights (acute and long-term care), resulting in improved patient satisfaction surveys.
+ Families are beginning to recognize the impact of professional nursing practice on their family member who is a resident in long-term care (or any area).
+ Organizations remain solvent financially from fiscally responsible staffing.
+ Physician and staff satisfaction improves as nurses are able to multiply their effectiveness and improve their communications

with one another and are helped with tasks, as evidenced by positive responses on nurse and physician satisfaction surveys.

+ Nurses with physical disabilities are able to continue to be clinically involved in a supervisory capacity.

+ Nurses are beginning to understand the full scope of their professional responsibilities and implementing their roles, resulting in more frequent, in-depth planning of care, evaluation of interventions, and practical, appropriate care pathways/plans (all areas).

+ Better discharge planning (acute, long-term, and community health care) occurs, resulting in decreased lengths of stay, fewer readmissions, and more effective and efficient use of resources.

+ There is better communication among healthcare disciplines (because RNs have time to coordinate care), and care planning is individualized and meaningful because all members of the team gather and share data, resulting in appropriate use of other disciplines' talents, streamlined institutionalized and home care, and fewer errors.

+ Charting reflects the patient status at more frequent intervals because more people are involved.

+ Better patient outcomes are accomplished: achievement of the individualized outcomes the patient and team have agreed upon as goals at the beginning of their relationship.

Whether or not the potential bonuses materialize in your work area will be determined, in large degree, by the energy you put into delegating effectively and making the system work the best for you and your patients.

CHECKPOINT 5-9

What positive results have been noted in research related to care delivery models using assistive personnel?

CONCLUSION

Delegation is a complex process that includes the scientific nursing process, critical thinking, and excellent communication skills. As the initiator of this process, your abilities are fundamental to the success of working in a team. As uncomfortable as it might be (for all of us!)

to objectively contemplate yourself, your ability to act effectively as an RN is enhanced by self-analysis and self-understanding. Recognition of personal emotions or beliefs that inhibit leadership will allow you to be clear about what's in the way and will free you to focus on the benefits of overcoming those barriers. What's in it for all of us? Improved morale, better teamwork, and better patient outcomes. It's worth it!

CHECKPOINT 5–10

This section has allowed nurses to evaluate themselves as an integral part of the delegation process. You have determined:

1. emotional barriers related to a change in care delivery system

2. other barriers to delegation

3. your strengths related to your ability to delegate effectively

4. potential benefits to overcoming the barriers

Have you determined how to deal with your emotional barriers and those of your coworkers? Have you chosen strategies to overcome your barriers to delegation, using your strengths to overcome obstacles? Keep visualizing the potential benefits for you and for your patients. After all, the real bottom line is delivering quality care for those we serve, achieving the outcomes we've planned together.

ANSWERS TO CHECKPOINTS

5–1.   Nosocomial infection rates were 18 times higher, patients were 54 times more likely to get surgical site infections, and hospitals with the least engaged nurses have paid more than $1.1 million annually in malpractice claims (Gallup, 2004a, 2004b, 2005).

5–2.   Depression (Schneider & Bowen, 1995). This evidence links the emotional state of the caregivers with clinical outcomes for the patient.

5–3.   Reflection is a key skill marking excellent critical thinking and clinical judgment and is necessary for personal development. In the delegation and supervision process, the registered nurse becomes the leader of the team, engaged in the crucial work of saving lives and making an impact on the health of our communities. Whatever we can do personally to review our thoughts, feelings, and behavior and make improvements in our ability to heal based on renewed self-understanding is worth the time, effort, and discomfort!

5–4.   a and c

5–5.   a) intrapersonal and b) interpersonal (social) intelligence. As we reflect on ourselves and our own skill level and gain intrapersonal knowledge, we are better able to manage ourselves internally and work more effectively with others.

5–6.

1.   anger, depression, or denial

2.   bargaining

3.   acceptance

4.   depression, anger

5.   denial, bargaining, or anger

5–7.   b, c, and d. Some individuals might need to seek professional help if they try all the steps but can't seem to shake the depression. Some might need to move on to another job if the negative feelings don't subside and they are unable to recapture the joy they once felt in their profession.

5–8.   Answer???

5–9.

• Better job satisfaction for nurses (Blegen, et al., 1992)

• Patient satisfaction (Neidlinger, et al., 1993)

• Improved job satisfaction by 14% for both nurses and assistive personnel in a staff-developed patient care delivery model (Allen & Vitale-Nolen, 2005)

• "Improved unit pride, visible improvement in the work environment, increased nurse-patient contact, reduced waste of supplies, and increased documentation in the patient record, more efficient, worked less over time, patients and physicians were more satisfied" (Lengacher & Mabe, 1993)

- Negative results have been shown based on RN and assistive personnel ratios (fewer RNs), in terms of poorer pain relief and patient mortality (Aiken et al., 2005; Huston, 2001; Kleinman & Saccomano, 2006)

Appendix 5–A

NURSING EXPERTISE SELF-REPORT SCALE

(Instructions for completion follow the scale.)
Please circle the answer that best describes you.

1. I am an:
   RN   Other
2. My job is:
   Staff nurse   Assistant Nurse Manager   Other
3. Length of time since graduating as an RN:
   Under 6 months   6 months to 3 years   More than 3 years
4. Length of time working on your unit:
   Under 6 months   6 months to 3 year   More than 3 years
5. Previous experience in nursing prior to graduating as an RN:
   Under 6 months   6 months to 3 years   More than 3 years

The following is a list of statements about nursing care. Please circle the number that best represents your agreement with the statement.

	Strongly Agree	Agree	Unsure	Disagree	Strongly Disagree
1. I often know ahead of time that my patient will take a turn for the worse.	1	2	3	4	5
2. I frequently draw on past experiences when making patient care decisions.	1	2	3	4	5
3. Quality nursing care results from strictly adhering to policy and procedure.	1	2	3	4	5
4. When I do patient care, only a few pieces of information stand out as critically important.	1	2	3	4	5
5. I am consciously aware of the process of decision making in patient care.	1	2	3	4	5
6. Emotional attachments get in the way of good nursing care.	1	2	3	4	5

Source: Reprinted with permission from G. Garland, Self-Report of Competence, *Journal of Nursing Staff Development*, Vol. 12, No. 4, p. 197, 1996, Lippincott-Raven.

	Strongly Agree	Agree	Unsure	Disagree	Strongly Disagree
7. When something goes wrong with my patient, I seem to know automatically what to do.	1	2	3	4	5
8. Sometimes I find it difficult to identify objective reasons for certain patient care decisions.	1	2	3	4	5
9. The best way to give good nursing care is to get close to the patient.	1	2	3	4	5
10. I find it time consuming to set priorities in patient care.	1	2	3	4	5
11. I make my best decisions about patient care when I remain objective.	1	2	3	4	5
12. In an emergency, things happen so quickly that I don't know what to do.	1	2	3	4	5
13. I base my patient care decisions more often on the rules that I learned in nursing school than on my experience in patient care.	1	2	3	4	5
14. It seems obvious to me what things need to be done first for my patients.	1	2	3	4	5
15. I use facts such as lab values and vital signs as my main source of information for making patient care decisions.	1	2	3	4	5
16. I usually require a lot of information about a patient care situation before I am comfortable with making a decision.	1	2	3	4	5
17. I do my best nursing care when I become truly involved with the patient.	1	2	3	4	5
18. I am comfortable with altering standard patient care procedures when I see the need.	1	2	3	4	5
19. Sudden patient care emergencies usually come as a complete surprise to me.	1	2	3	4	5
20. Most often I find myself relying on gut feelings when it comes to patient care.	1	2	3	4	5

INSTRUCTIONS FOR COMPLETING THE NURSING SELF-REPORT SCALE

Overview

The Nursing Expertise Self-Report Scale was developed from Patricia Benner's model of clinical competence described in Benner and Benner (1984). Benner described three changes in performance as the nurse progresses from novice to expert practice. One change is from the reliance on rules and principles to the reliance on past experience to guide performance. The second change is a transition from viewing the clinical situation as a collection of equally important features to viewing the clinical situation as a whole, in which only a few features are important. The third change is the passage from detached observer to involved performer. Unique to the expert level of performance is the element of intuition. This scale is designed to measure self-perception of these three transitions and intuitive decision making.

Self-report methodology is widely used in psychological and human subject research. Self-report methodology has the advantage of being versatile and direct in measuring feelings, values, opinions, and perceptions. However, the most limiting disadvantage is the concern for validity and accuracy of self-report. Therefore, the self-reported level of competence derived from the use of this scale may not correspond to the observed level of practice for an individual nurse. This scale is not intended as a substitute for observation and testing of competence in the clinical setting.

Potential uses for this scale include:

Designing educational offerings,

Discussion and planning for transitions in care assignments, and

Individual professional development planning.

Validity and Reliability

Reliability testing was done using a test–retest method. Content validity was reviewed by nurses in the practice of nursing staff development.

Scale Scoring and Interpretation

The Nursing Expertise Self-Report may be used with or without the demographic tool. Benner's model discusses a potential relationship between experience and expertise, therefore the design of the demographic tool.

Scoring—The Nursing Expertise Self-Report Scale has 20 items scored using a Likert scale from Strongly Agree to Strongly Disagree. For items 3, 5, 6, 10, 11, 12, 13, 15, 16, and 19, the Strongly Disagree response is identified as the Expert response. For the remaining items, the Strongly Agree response represents the Expert response. A value of 1 is given to the response that reflects novice practice. The expert response receives a score of 5. The potential minimum score, assuming a response on each item, is 20. The potential maximum score, assuming a response on each item, is 100.

There are no identified point values that demark any specific level of competence. Lower aggregate totals show self-perception reflective of novice practice. Higher overall scores show self-perception reflective of expert practice.

Copies of the original study may be obtained by contacting the author.

Gayle A. Garland
University of Leeds
School of Healthcare Rm 4.12
Baines Wing
LEEDS, UK LS29UT
Telephone: 0113 343 1300

Please e-mail your findings and how you apply them to Gayle at g.a.garland@leeds.ac.uk

Source: Copyright 1993, Gayle A. Garland

REFERENCES

Aiken, L.H., Halm, M., Peterson, M., Kandels, M., Sabo, J., Blalock, M., et al. (2005) Hospital nurse staffing and patient mortality, emotional exhaustion, and job dissatisfaction. *Clinical Nurse Specialist,* 19(5):241-51.

Allen, D., & Vitale-Nolen, R. (2005). Patient care delivery model improves nurse job satisfaction. *The Journal of Continuing Education in Nursing,* 36, 277–282.

American Nurses Association. (1976, 1985). *Code for nurses with interpretive statements.* Kansas City, MO.

American Nurses Association. (2001). *Code for nurses with interpretive statements.* Kansas City, MO.

Bardwick, J.M. (1995). *Danger in the comfort zone.* New York: AMACOM (American Management Association).

Benner, P., & Benner, R. (1984). *From novice to expert: Excellence and power in clinical nursing practice.* Menlo Park, CA: Addison-Wesley.

Benner, P., & Benner, R. (1991, July–August). Stories from the front lines. *Healthcare Forum Journal*, 69–74.

Blegen, M.A., et al. (1992). Who helps you with your work? *American Journal of Nursing, 921*, 28.

Gallup. (2004a). Paller, D. *RX for the nursing shortage.* Retrieved May 12, 2008, from http://gmj.gallup.com/content/13603/Nursing-Shortage.aspx

Gallup. (2004b). Paller, D., & Perkins, E. *What's the key to providing quality healthcare?* Retrieved May 12, 2008, from http://www.worldcongress.com/pdf/Whats_the_Key_to_Providing_Quality_Healthcare.pdf

Gallup. (2005). *Gallup study: Unhappy workers are unhealthy too.* Retrieved July 17, 2007, from http://gmj.gallup.com/content/14545/Gallup-Study-Unhappy-Workers-Unhealthy-Too.aspx

Garland, G. (1996). Self-report of competence. *Journal of Nursing Staff Development, 12*(4), 197.

Goleman, D. Boyatzis, R., & McKee, A. (2002). *Primal leadership.* Boston: Harvard Business School Press.

Hansten, R. (2005). Relationship and results oriented healthcare: Evaluate the basics. *JONA, 35*(12), 522–525.

Hansten, R., & Washburn, M. (1993). *The nurse manager's answer book.* Gaithersburg, MD: Aspen.

Hansten, R., & Washburn, M. (1997). *Toolbook for health care redesign.* Gaithersburg, MD: Aspen.

Huston, C. (2001). Contemporary staffing-mix changes: The impact on post operative pain management. *Payment Management Nursing, 2*(2), 65–72.

Kleinman, C., & Saccomano, S. (2006). Registered nurses and unlicensed assistive personnel: An uneasy alliance. *The Journal of Continuing Education in Nursing, 37*(4), 162–170.

Krapohl, G., & Larson, E. (1996). The impact of unlicensed assistive personnel on nursing care delivery. *Nursing Economic$, 14*(2), 99–122.

Lengacher, C., & Mabe, P. (1993). Nurse extenders. *Journal of Nursing Administration, 23*, 17.

Merlevede, P., Bridoux, D., & Vandamme, R. (2003). *7 steps to emotional intelligence.* Williston VT: Crown House Publishing

Neidlinger, S., et al. (1993). Incorporating nursing assistive personnel into a nursing professional practice model. *Journal of Nursing Administration, 23*, 33–34.

Noer, D. (1993). *Healing the wounds.* San Francisco: Jossey-Bass.

Noer, D. (1997). *Breaking free.* San Francisco: Jossey-Bass.

Robbins, A. 1997. Letter to the editor. *American Journal of Nursing.* 97, no. 7: 17.

Schneider, B., & Bowen, D. (1995). *Mood affects the cardiac care unit. Winning the service game.* Boston: Harvard Business School Press.

Know What Needs to Be Done

Ruth I. Hansten and Marilynn Jackson

CHAPTER SKILLS

+ Describe the role of the registered professional nurse in terms of what is visible, what is necessary, and what are the cornerstones of professional nursing practice.
+ List two measurable resources for nursing care delivery.
+ Make a decision on what to delegate based on job analysis, prioritization, and identified outcomes.

RECOMMENDED RESOURCES

▶ A listing of the 514 research-based nursing interventions can be downloaded from http://www.nursing.uiowa.edu/excellence/ nursing_knowledge/clinical_effectiveness/labeldefinitions.pdf.

▶ Obtain a delegation decision-making model from your state nursing regulations, your employer policies, or the ANA/ NCSBN Joint Statement on Delegation, which can be downloaded from https://www.ncsbn.org/Joint_statement.pdf.

▶ From *Silence to Voice: What Nurses Know and Must Communicate to the Public* (2nd ed.) by Bernice Buresh and Suzanne Gordon, published by Canadian Nurses Association (www.silencetovoice. com), has book excerpts, exercises, and speaker availability for workshops.

"Hi! I'm your supervisor for this evening's shift, and I'm making rounds to see how everyone is doing. Do you need anything, or is everything going okay?"

"I don't know—things are a little crazy. We've got admissions coming, a transfer from the unit, and two late discharges. Mary's upset because Dr. Jones just yelled at her in front of a patient, and we haven't

seen Steve for quite awhile. I wish he'd show up so we could get some work done. It looks like everyone will be working overtime just to get their charting done. I don't know how you could help."

The process of working with other people successfully requires a knowledge of the total picture, knowing what needs to be done in terms that are clearly defined. In the example at the opening of this chapter, the nurse responding to the supervisor has a general idea of the work waiting to be done but has not done an organized assessment or prioritized what's really happening on the unit. Without a plan, she can only react to the issues that are happening at the moment, and she is unable to accept or direct help when it is offered from the supervisor. The result can be a feeling of chaos and frustration for everyone involved that can be sensed by anyone walking into that kind of environment. The patients will certainly sense this as well, seeing the frenzied staff running in and out of the room and apologizing for not having enough time to spend with them right now.

Not everyone is organized by nature, and certainly we are not all equally endowed with the ability to see the whole picture. Fortunately, there are steps to take that will assist us in developing these skills so that situations like the one presented can be avoided. In this chapter we are going to discuss those steps by first exploring a model that delineates three major aspects of the nursing role. We will then discuss planning objectives for optimal conditions and the process of prioritizing those objectives when conditions and resources are limited in some way.

Despite all of our attempts and the multitude of systems created to date, nursing has not been carefully contained within a list of items that are to be done. In fact, as Marie Manthey (1991, p. 27) challenged us years ago, "Good nursing care. It's so simple, we all know it. The picture is brilliantly clear. But what are its boundaries? When can any nurse say, 'This patient has had enough nursing care.' The question seems almost sacrilegious. The answer seems to be, 'Never!' There is always one more thing a good nurse can think of for someone who is ill." Yet, resources are often limited, and boundaries must be set. Not having the ability to be all things to all people all the time, we must begin to define what needs to be done by first defining the role of professional nursing.

> "When can any nurse say, 'This patient has had enough nursing care'?"

DEFINING THE ROLE

Looking at the brief 100-year history of our profession, we can cite countless examples of nursing's amoeba-like progression. Many of us have heard the comment, "Get a nurse to do it if no one else will!" Throughout the course of history, nursing has willingly taken on work that no one else was willing to do. From mopping floors to sterilizing instruments, from cleaning contaminated wounds to caring for the highly infectious, nursing has been there to meet the need. As a result, we lack clear definition of what we do. Further, we are now training others and delegating to them tasks that have been a part of our scope of practice. Without a finite definition of our role, the idea of delegating any part of it invokes fear in many as they ask the question, "If I delegate all of these interventions, what's left for me to do?"

> If I delegate all of these interventions, what's left for me to do?

CHECKPOINT 6–1

As we've discussed so far, working successfully with others involves an understanding of what needs to be done in terms of the total picture and planning how that can be accomplished by delegating to the members on the healthcare team.

I can begin to do this by:

a) defining and clarifying my role as a professional nurse

b) relying on the supervisor to assist when things get tough

c) doing all things myself, meeting all of the patients' needs as they occur

d) letting members on the team do all of the work so that they can advance

See the end of the chapter for the answers.

Studies have been done that assist us in finding a clearer delineation of our role as nurses. Work sampling studies have validated the wide variety of our tasks, while one such study (Urden & Roode, 1997) has created a categorical description of our time. Various work sampling studies indicate that registered nurses (RNs) spend time as follows: 27.5% to 32.8% on direct patient care, 41.8% to 45% on indirect care activities, 15% in unit-related activities, and 13% to 20% in personal time. For purposes of these studies, the following category descriptors were used:

+ Direct care—All nursing care activities performed in the presence of the patient and/or family, such as assessment, medications, treatments, and procedures. Included was time spent communicating the plan of care, teaching patients/families, intervening, and evaluating.

+ Indirect care—All activities done away from the patient but on a specific patient's behalf, including communicating to others on the team, giving reports, gathering supplies, and preparing equipment and medications.

+ Unit-related activities—Activities for general maintenance of the nursing unit such as clerical work, ordering supplies, attending meetings, and running errands.

+ Personal activities—Activities not related to patient care, including meals, breaks, adjusting schedules, personal phone calls, and socializing with coworkers.

+ Documentation—All activities associated with documenting, reviewing, or evaluating patient condition and care, including the review of all patient data, correlation of interdisciplinary data and nursing judgment, and the action of documenting (Urden & Roode, 1997).

The ongoing work of Bulechek and McCloskey (2003), described in a three-volume set encapsulating years of research and development of the Nursing Interventions Classification (NIC) and the Nursing Outcomes Classification (NOC), moves us closer to that common language that clearly communicates what it is we do. Currently describing 514 research-based interventions and 260 outcomes, it is evident that the work of nursing is a complex role with multiple integrations from diagnosis to outcome. The latest edition of their work includes time estimates and educational levels necessary for performing the categorized interventions (Bulechek, Butcher, & Dochterman, 2007).

Professional organizations have also risen to the challenge of clarifying the practice of nursing and responding to the changing needs of the population through the creation of new roles and the qualifying of various scopes of practice. The Nursing Practice and Education Consortium (N-PEC) met in December of 2000 and proposed a new categorization of nursing, including four "scopes" (a–d) to respond to various populations of need (Floyd, 2001). The American Association of Colleges of

Nursing (AACN) has been busy as well, proposing a new role to "address the ardent call for change being heard in today's health care system." The clinical nurse leader (CNL) "designs, implements, and evaluates client care by coordinating, delegating and supervising the care provided by the health care team..." (AACN, 2007).

THE PTA MODEL

Consider looking at the nursing role as made up of three areas of practice in what we will call the "PTA model." In this model, nursing provides Professional, Technical, and Amenity care to a given group of patients or clients. Whether the setting is acute, long-term, or community care, the nurse can be described as functioning in one of these three areas. Let's look at this more closely to see what is meant.

Amenity

During the past 2 decades, this area of our role has received heightened attention as health care as a business became the issue and executives sought an element that would give them a leading edge over the health-care facility down the street. The "service mentality" was developed and promoted, and we educated our "consumers" to expect hotel-style treatment. Those who could afford to redesigned their interiors, making them more homelike and friendly, and hired marketing personnel to assist them in going the extra mile. Patient questionnaires were designed to help us to measure performance in terms of how hot and fast the meal was delivered, how friendly the nursing staff was, and how clean the rooms were.

Massages, wine with dinner, guest trays, and a vase for the flowers became important factors in "quality nursing care." The quality of our amenity service is highly visible to management and marketing, in terms of patient surveys, letters to the administrator expressing thanks or dismay, and the gifts of boxes of chocolates for the nurses. These were signs we had done our job well. The subtle education of the patient and family to expect the "amenities" of care was complete. This expectation extends to all areas of health care, from the homey, friendly labor/delivery rooms with the champagne dinners to the extended care center with the ice cream shop in the courtyard. (We think these amenities are nice touches and very important when you are ill, or aging, or experiencing a significant event in your life—but a note of caution should be made that this is not the primary function of the RN.)

Patient surveys often reflect a measurement of hospitality, not hospital care. What questions does your facility survey ask?

In this new century the trend toward more friendly and homelike environments has evolved into the creation of surroundings that support the spirit and foster a setting that promotes healing on all levels: body, mind, and spirit. We applaud this direction and appreciate the enhanced awareness that this development has brought to the forefront: the insight that nurses have understood since Florence's time, that surroundings have a compelling affect on our ability to heal. More than amenities, the newly designed environments of care provide spaces for all caregivers to meet the patients' needs in a more nurturing, caring, and supportive manner.

Technical

This is an obvious area of the nursing role and one we take pride in and fight to maintain. Examples of our technical expertise include cannulating a vein, catheterizing a child, irrigating the Blakemore tube, balancing the hemodynamic monitor, and giving a painless injection. These technical tasks are highly visible, and their outcomes are easily measured, making their performance obviously important. Quality improvement monitors, incident reports, medication error analyses, and patient complaints tell us how well we are performing in this area of our role. Physicians see the outcomes of these technical interventions and measure our effectiveness by the number of incidents they must deal with and the number of complaints from family members when physician orders to change their loved one's dressing three times daily have not been carried out.

Identifying the critical role that organizations play in creating systems and processes that support or impede technical performance, the American Academy of Nursing recently completed a study identifying more than 800 processes and over 1200 potential solutions to issues that currently interfere with the provision of efficient patient care. Areas studied for improvement include medication administration, communication and documentation, supplies and equipment, and care delivery and coordination. Inefficient work processes and environments are blamed for reducing the amount of time nurses spend at the bedside, which is currently estimated at only 30% (American Academy of Nursing, 2007).

The two areas of "amenity" and "technical" care contain many tasks that are readily delegated to other personnel. It does not take an RN to pass meal trays, deliver flowers, walk the dog in a long-term care center, or clean the room, and the increasing numbers of healthcare technicians offer many hands that are willing to be trained to perform the majority of our tech-

> These technical tasks are highly visible and their outcomes easily measured, making their performance obviously important.

nical duties. Licensed practical nurses (LPNs/LVNs) pass meds, change dressings, and start IVs in some states, and patient care assistants are also passing some medications, completing glucose tests, drawing blood samples, and providing all of the required hygienic care. With so much of our role clearly being done by others, what is left for the RN?

Professional

This part of our model presents the greatest degree of difficulty for many nurses. Answers to the question "if I delegate all of these interventions, what is left for me to do?" range from comments regarding attitude, image, and the number of years of education the nurse has completed. Yet we are not seeking to describe how we attain or present this part of our role, but rather what comprises the very heart of RN practice. What can you do, and do well, that cannot be delegated?

What ensures a high-value experience for the patient that is both efficient and effective? We hope you are saying to yourself that it is the implementation of the nursing process! For it is through your educational foundation, your ability to make assessments and plan the care, that you can effectively coordinate the efforts of the healthcare team and evaluate their effect. This collaborative coordination is essential to the successful functioning of any healthcare delivery system and cannot be eliminated or replaced. Tasks can be performed by anyone trained to do them; it is your ability to critically identify the need and evaluate the outcome that remains when all else is delegated. According to the National Council of State Boards of Nursing (NCSBN), delegation means "transferring to a competent individual the authority to perform a selected nursing task in a selected situation. The nurse retains the accountability for the delegation" (NCSBN, 1995, p. 2). Retaining that accountability through the implementation of the nursing process as we coordinate the entire picture of our patients' needs is the very core of our professional role.

Why do we find it difficult to articulate the professional component of our role? Realize that we tend to measure what we value. The inverse is also true in that we value what we measure. Notice that in the previous description of the professional area of practice we have not described any tools of measurement or discussed the visibility of performing the nursing process. As nurses, this is an area where we need to place more emphasis and not continue to allow others to dictate our practice in terms of measurement and value. Clinical errors and patient surveys have been our standard measurement tools in the past, keeping

What can you do as a licensed RN, and do well, that cannot be delegated?

> As nurses, we need to place more emphasis on making the nursing process more visible and not continue to allow others to dictate our practice in terms of measurement and value of tasks alone.

us at a task-oriented technical and amenity level of practice. However, beginning efforts are being noted as more nurses are tracking the impact of their case management and translating outcomes into terms that are highly visible to physicians, patients, the general public, and administrators alike. We must continue to shift our focus from those easily identified and measured parts of our role. Completing groundbreaking research at the Center for Health Outcomes and Policy Research at the University of Pennsylvania, Linda Aiken chairs a team that is clearly quantifying the impact of the professional component of nursing practice. Researching the concept of "failure to rescue" for the first time as a nursing outcome measure, their studies demonstrate the importance of 24-hour nursing surveillance in an acute care environment (Clark & Aiken, 2003). Further discussion and clarification of the term "failure to rescue" establishes the concept as a measurable indicator of nursing-sensitive measures (Needleman & Buerhaus, 2007).

Implementing the nursing process is relatively easy to describe on paper and to other nursing personnel. However, it is not visible in the same manner as giving a bath, changing a dressing, or starting an IV. It is visible only when connected to outcomes, when the whole picture of the patient's care is evaluated in terms of whether the plan of care was achieved in a timely fashion and no untoward results occurred. It is visible only when we make the connection, when we call attention to the fact that the length of stay for a specific critical pathway has decreased by one day due to consistent nursing planning and coordination of the care. It is visible only when we note that inappropriate readmissions to an acute care facility (less than 24 hours postdischarge for the same diagnosis) have been eliminated due to the discharge instructions, education, and follow-up provided by the nursing staff. It is visible only when we research the connection between our continuous teaching of diabetic foot care and the decrease of lower limb amputations among diabetics. Our professional visibility does not come from checking a task off a to-do list but from our continuous education of our publics regarding the outcomes of our interventions. Carol Lindeman, former dean of Oregon Health Sciences, reminds us,

> "Healthcare systems don't need a nurse who knows how to do those old routines. And more than that, they don't care how the person does something, as long as it produces the outcome."

"Healthcare systems don't need a nurse who knows how to do those old routines. And more than that, they don't care how the person does something, as long as it produces the outcome" (Lindeman, 1996, p. 8).

Yes, there is much to be done after you have delegated tasks to the other members of the team. What remains clearly defines you as an RN and is the "heartland" of our profession. As Adelaide Nutting challenged us so many years ago, "Perhaps, too, we need to remember that growth in our work must be preceded by ideas, and that any conditions which suppress thought, must retard growth. Surely we will not be satisfied in perpetuating methods and traditions. Surely we will wish to be more and more occupied with creating them" (Donahue, 1985, p. 366).

"Perhaps, too, we need to remember that growth in our work must be preceded by ideas, and that any conditions which suppress thought, must retard growth. Surely we will not be satisfied in perpetuating methods and traditions. Surely we will wish to be more and more occupied with creating them."

In looking forward to a blueprint of a model of nursing that will meet the needs of our future patients, Gail Wolf (2007) suggests that there are only four major roles that patients will be seeking: provider, partner, protector, and integrator.

- Provider—someone to meet the physical, emotional, and spiritual needs of the patient if he/she is not able to do so
- Partner—someone to assist the patient and family in sorting through the maze of healthcare information to make the best informed decisions about plan of care
- Protector—one who will advocate for the patient and assure safe passage through the often confusing and chaotic system
- Integrator—to be that conduit between all of the other members on the multidisciplinary team who will be needed to round out the picture of care

Beyond the Nursing Process

In addition to the overall coordination of patient care, which comes through the comprehensive nursing process of assessing, planning, intervening, and evaluating, there are other aspects to what RNs do that are worth mentioning. Consider this scenario.

The patient is in a clean bed, has a clean body, is relatively comfortable, has the right IV infusing at the right rate, has eaten the appropriate diet, has ambulated down the hall, and has had his dressing changed. What is there left to do? Some nurses will jokingly respond, "Take a break!" And deservedly so, for it is the coordinated efforts of the RN that have created such a complete and happy patient. However, a few aspects of care are not yet part of this picture. Discharge planning and patient/family

Discharge planning and patient/family teaching are essential functions of the role of the RN. Remember the list of functions that cannot be delegated? (See Chapter 3 for a review.) As Massachusetts Nursing Regulations remind us:

> It is the responsibility of the qualified licensed nurse to promote patient/client education and to involve the patient/client and when appropriate, significant others in the establishment and implementation of health goals. While unlicensed personnel may provide information to the patient/client, the ultimate responsibility for health teaching and health counseling must reside with the qualified licensed nurse as it relates to nursing and nursing services. (MNR, 1994)

Intentional Caring

When we ask nurses to describe what it is they do as RNs to provide value to the organization, they invariably respond, "I care for the patient." When you think back on a lot of marketing hype and those cute little items sold exclusively for nurses, you will remember that nurses give "TLC." (Remember the little red heart, or the bear with the banner declaring "Nurses give TLC"?) This "tender loving care" has been an essential aspect of who we are as nurses, just as much as the cure imperative has been for physicians. If we are to make visible this essence of nursing, we must have some definitive form of measurement. Nurse researchers have begun to build a database using measurable and identifiable actions to define caring. The Denver Nursing Project, funded by both state and national sources, is an example of measuring the impact of caring on patients with human immunodeficiency virus. In her discussion of this research and other actions related to caring, Karen Miller, RN, PhD (1995, p. 29), offers this definition: "Caring, then, may be defined as intentional action that conveys physical and emotional security and genuine connectedness with another person or group of people. Caring validates the humanness of both the care giver and the cared for." This deliberate and planned intervention is the cornerstone of what RNs do; without physical and emotional security a patient will not progress, cannot learn, and cannot move on successfully to the next level of independence within the healthcare continuum.

CHECKPOINT 6–2

Complete examples 2 through 4 of Exhibit 6–1, providing your own examples of professional, technical, and amenity care, noting who it is visible to and how it is measured.

See the end of the chapter for the answers.

EXHIBIT 6–1   Examples of Professional, Technical, and Amenity Care

The PTA Model	Professional "The Whole Picture"	Technical "Expert Skill Level"	Amenity "The Extra Touch"
Example 1	discharge planning	passing medications	changing linen
Visible to	colleagues	physicians/patient	patient/family
How measured	length of stay	medication errors	patient surveys/ letters
Example 2	diabetic teaching in the home setting	giving insulin injections	fixing a snack for the patient's family
Visible to			
How measured			
Example 3	medication instructions	changing a dressing	changing ice water
Visible to			
How Measured			
Example 4			
Visible to			
How Measured			

GETTING THE JOB DONE

Whether we are providing professional, technical, or amenity care, we must first establish what needs to be done. In our example at the beginning of this chapter, the head nurse of an acute care unit noted several issues that needed attention but was not certain how or by whom these issues would be resolved. What needs to be done in this example, and in every situation you face, is no different than the nursing process. (There seems to be no substitute for the nursing process—what a wonderful tool!) Let's take a look at how it applies here.

I. Assess

In any situation, whether in an outpatient clinic, a dialysis center, a home health agency, or wherever you practice, the first step in getting the job done is to assess the situation. You need as much data as possible to effectively plan what goals you can achieve, both for this shift and for the long term. Take a look at the information available. You might not be the one getting the information, but you must be the one to interpret what it means. Recall that in Chapter 3 we defined assessment from the RN perspective as "the initial phase of the nursing process, which involves the interpretation of the significance of the available subjective and objective data." From a critical thinking standpoint, you must be able to integrate your personal experience and assumptions with the facts presented to you to begin to determine potential and realistic outcomes.

Consider the following example of what can (and does!) happen when staff members focus not on outcomes but solely on tasks. This story is told by Dianna Mason in *Political Action Handbook for Nurses* (Mason and Talbott, 1985). While this story is over 2 decades old, we believe it is, unfortunately, a classic example of what can still happen in today's world. As you read, ask yourself what assumptions are being made and what data have been overlooked in the ongoing assessment of this patient.

> From a critical thinking standpoint, you must be able to integrate your personal experience and assumptions with the facts presented to you to begin to determine potential and realistic outcomes.

Mrs. Smith was a 90-year-old woman who had been admitted to the hospital from a nursing home for treatment of congestive heart failure. Her medical condition and the change in the environment exacerbated a problem with confusion accompanied by a loss of interest in eating. She was on a 40-bed medical unit that had a nurse–patient ratio of 1:8 to 1:12. The nurses were "too busy" to spend much time trying to feed her, particularly because she ate only small, frequent meals. They had sicker patients who demanded their time and attention, including a comatose patient on a respirator. As Mrs. Smith continued to lose weight, she became obviously malnourished and more confused. The physicians ordered that she be fed by nasogastric tube. When she tried to pull out the tube, hand mitts were ordered. The bolus tube feedings, for which the nurses now made time, gave the patient diarrhea, which quickly led to decubiti because the restraints prevented her from turning her buttocks away from the incontinent stool. As the diarrhea continued, she became more malnourished and finally died after suffering great humiliation and classic iatrogenic "unhealth" care.

Although many factors affect the nurse's decision as to how time is spent, none of these factors is as significant as the primary need to make all decisions based on clearly defined outcomes. What does Mrs. Smith want? What does her family want? Is this the kind of outcome they had in mind? If the staff had taken the time to determine the outcome for Mrs. Smith by more completely assessing her wishes, would there have been more emphasis placed on feeding her? Can this task be delegated if the nurses are "too busy"? Keep this example in mind as we continue our discussion of the process of what needs to be done.

II. Plan

Often we are so anxious to begin the shift that we do not recognize the value of planning. Remember that old adage Mom taught you (or was it an old nursing professor?): "Fail to plan, plan to fail." When you are tempted to skip this step and just jump right into the tasks at hand, be aware of the price you will pay in terms of feeling disorganized, moving from one job to another, and reaching the end of the shift with no clear sense of achievement. Your team members will no doubt share a sense of mounting frustration because they are not certain what to do next and will spend considerable time waiting for you to delegate or being overwhelmed at the confusion. As little as 15 minutes at the beginning of any shift reviewing the outcomes and determining what can be reasonably done and by whom will be much more effective than getting a quick report and going for it! (Further discussion of the communication process in delegation will be covered in Chapter 8.)

Fail to plan, plan to fail.

CHECKPOINT 6–3

Identify three optimal outcomes you might focus on at the beginning of your shift.

This planning step applies to all settings where you might be employed, from extended care centers where the emphasis is on long-term planning, to the ambulatory surgery center where you must consider the list of scheduled cases for the day and plan for who will be assigned to the patient, to the home health setting where there is much planning to be done to maximize the amount of time spent on each visit. Once again, focus on outcomes, on the results of your actions, not the actions themselves. Set your optimal goals by looking at what your ideal outcomes would be if you had no limitations: all patients/clients receive safe care, all medications and treatments are given on time and discussed with all patients to increase their knowledge and understanding of their care, all documentation is completed accurately, everyone is off duty on time (no overtime), and so on. These are very general outcomes; you should have specific outcomes related to the patient population and setting in which you are working.

When you have agreed to set aside the time to plan, a word or two must be said about the process. (Are you surprised? You didn't think we would just leave you to plan on your own, did you?) Planning requires not only determining outcomes but realizing that some prioritization must occur if resources are not unlimited. We propose the following steps.

1. Get the global picture. Don't limit yourself to just your assignment, but have an understanding of what fellow team members are also expecting to accomplish during this shift. For example, if you are working in ambulatory surgery, be aware of all the scheduled surgeries for the day, not just the ones assigned to your area. If you are in a home health agency, do you know what cases the other nurses on your team are carrying? On a skilled care unit in a long-term care facility, be aware of the assignments of the other team members on the floor, not just your assigned rooms. Expanding your awareness of the expectations of the other workers in your area will help you to offer assistance when you have time, or to know who might be called upon to help you, and to foster a sense of teamwork instead of isolation. The worst words we can ever hear (or speak!) are "It's not my patient." Establishing a global picture implies that we have an awareness of what's happening around us, not just with the patients immediately assigned to us.

   Often the perception or the mood of the unit or work setting is colored by the events of the previous shift or day. If the night shift in a corrective facility had a difficult time with an inmate who had to be "taken down," an under-tone of anxiety might be communicated and carried over to the next shift. An awareness of the events of the previous 24 hours will lend a better under-standing to what the "whole picture" of the time ahead will be. Perhaps things are not really as difficult as reported,

Beware self-fulfilling prophecies—get the whole picture and make your own assessment so that you can effectively plan your care and avoid reacting to one aspect of the situation.

and the team can move ahead, planning for outcomes with the understanding that the events of the previous shift have ended and that feelings carried over are now affecting the information shared. The weekend call coverage for a visiting nurse might leave a very lengthy message regarding the noncompliant attitude of the patient and his refusal to complete the medication regimen, but your phone call on Monday morning reveals a much calmer patient who is willing to talk about his IV therapy and consider completing the treatment plan. Beware self-fulfilling prophe-cies—get the whole picture and make your own assessment so that you can effectively plan your care.

2. Set optimal goals. Decide what you really want to achieve during this time in your work setting, given the best possible conditions. (No one is late to work, staffing is adequate, everyone is ready to work together, and so on.) As in our previous discussion, focus on outcomes, not on creating a laundry list of tasks to be done. What do you want the results of your professional efforts to be today? Remember, every action you take is a subtle form of education to your public (whether it is the physicians you work with, your fellow team members, the patients, or patients' families and visi-tors). What is the best impression you can make and the clearest message you can send regarding your professional ability?

3. Decide what is reasonable to expect. Part of planning involves being able to anticipate events and determine potential responses. What happens if a patient "crashes," one of the team members becomes ill, or you receive three unexpected transfers? Given limited and changing resources, what is reasonable to expect will be accomplished today? How do we let go of the ideal and optimal outcomes and be satisfied with less than the best? Can we give ourselves permission to do less than the optimum, and under what conditions is this acceptable? (See Chapter 4 for a discus-sion on policies and procedures in working with limited staff.)

4. Set priorities. Given limits to the resources we work with in terms of supplies, staff, and time, we must be able to determine those outcomes that are essential to achieve and prioritize our work. We can do this effectively by evaluating each desired outcome according to the following criteria:

- Life-threatening or potentially—Has the patient proven to be a risk to him- or herself and others, therefore requiring continual restraint and supervision? Has the patient demonstrated a labile response to medication, thereby requiring constant monitoring?

- Essential to safety—Was the code cart checked and restocked after the last code? Have you received the latest training regarding universal precautions, and do you take the time to practice them to protect your safety as well as that of your patient? Does the patient weigh 200 pounds and require two people to assist in moving? Does the resident require 24-hour observation because of a recent fall while unattended?

- Essential to the medical/nursing plan—Do the vital signs need to be monitored every 2 hours when there has been no significant change for the past 24? Is the monitoring of intake and output essential to the outcomes we have established for this patient? Does the lab work that has been ordered on a daily basis reflect the best therapeutic evaluation for this client? Does the 10-year-old really need to be awakened for a neuro check every hour when he's been stable for the last 24?

Often by asking these types of questions we can further assess the work to be done and prioritize according to the reasonable goals we have set. Failing to take the time to ask these questions continually keeps us in the task-oriented technical- and amenity-based roles of our position and does not allow us (or the patient!) to benefit from what we do best. We can continue to keep ourselves very busy, getting tasks done, not delegating appropriately, and therefore depriving the patient and our employer of the skills we are most needed to provide. It might seem far easier to cross "beds and baths" off a list, pass all of the medications, and complete the treatments than to assess the need for these interventions, plan who will do them, supervise the interventions, and evaluate their effect. However, because we are the professional nurses accountable for the total patient care for a given group of individuals, the implementation of the nursing process while delegating tasks to others is our primary responsibility.

III. Intervene

For many years, our focus has been on systems and processes, supported by criteria of The Joint Commission and state regulations. Beginning in the late 1980s, The Joint Commission developed its Agenda for Change, noting that there would be a shift in emphasis from systems and processes (tasks and how they are completed) to an emphasis on the outcomes of the service provided. Further support came from quality management programs: total quality management (TQM) and continuous quality improvement (CQI) replaced the traditional quality assurance (QA) monitoring departments found in most organizations. This change has intensified our need to be continuously aware of the cause-and-effect relationship our interventions have on the patients for whom we provide care. Successful practice requires that we as nurses change our focus too, always looking at the process outlined above: setting goals, realizing limits, prioritizing, and then implementing the plan, always with the patient's desired outcomes as our guide.

> Successful practice requires that we as nurses change our focus too, constantly looking at the process of setting goals, realizing limits, prioritizing, and then implementing the plan, always with the patient's desired outcomes as our guide.

CHECKPOINT 6-4

Prioritize the following tasks based on the desired outcome of providing safe and effective care for Mr. Bailey, a 68-year-old patient with a total hip replacement who is 2 days post op, alert and oriented, stable, and planning on being discharged in 2 days. Use the criteria (L) life threatening, (S) safety, (E) essential to medical/nursing plan, and (N) nice to do, but not a priority.

___ 1. administer medications as ordered for arrhythmia

___ 2. instruct patient regarding postdischarge care

___ 3. monitor vital signs every 4 hours

___ 4. order meal for patient's wife

___ 5. assist patient with ambulation after discussion with physical therapist

___ 6. place side rails up when patient has been medicated for pain

See the end of the chapter for the answers.

Job Analysis

With outcomes at the top of our list, having completed the previous steps to the process, we are ready to put the plan into action. Armed with priorities, we must determine who can best carry out the interventions necessary. This can be done by completing a quick "job analysis." (A note of caution here, so that we don't lose you entirely in a wave of disbelief— we know how busy you are on the job and realize that you will not have the luxury of spending precious time completing a job analysis when there is work to be done now. However, as you are reading this book, there is time to learn and understand the technique so that you can quickly apply the principles in your work setting, making the most out of the resources you have by delegating appropriately.) Supervisors often tell us that this is one of the most difficult skills to master and that if there were some way to help nurses organize their work and base the completion of that work on the resources available by getting the right person to do the job, they would be amazed. Although a job analysis sounds like something out of a personnel manual, we encourage you to read on to learn perhaps a new method for mastering that skill.

Giving a bath is only a task and can be done by anyone if the focus is only on the task. What is the outcome desired by giving the bath? Is it to make the patient feel more comfortable? Is it to assess the condition of the skin and to provide an opportunity to more completely assess the patient? Is it an opportunity to teach a family member how to complete range of motion exercises while also giving a bath? Knowing the desired outcome of the job to be done will have a significant effect on the selection of who should perform the task.

Current analysis of the work done by an RN has revealed that significant time is spent performing tasks that could be performed by someone else who does not have the knowledge and skill of the RN. Redesigns in care delivery are therefore focusing on isolating those functions that only an RN can perform and grouping the remaining tasks to be done by assistive personnel with minimal training. In many instances, the assistive person is then given a task assignment and not a patient assignment. This is a major difference from the team process of previous years.

A job analysis involves the following basic steps:

1. Break the job or jobs into parts. For example, if the job to be done is to start an IV, are there any parts to the process? Assembling the supplies, obtaining the proper IV solution, starting the IV, monitoring the administration, and documenting the procedure are all parts of the job.

2. Evaluate the job in the following terms:

    (a) Knowledge—What kind of knowledge is necessary to do this job? In the example of starting the IV, one needs to know the type of equipment required, how to use it, basic anatomy and physiology to select a site, the policy of the facility regarding the procedure, the potential effects of the fluid to be administered, and the physician's orders regarding rate and method of administration.

    (b) Skills—What skills are required to perform this task? Starting an IV requires the ability to be organized (having all supplies on hand before starting the insertion makes the process smoother!) and psychomotor ability to insert the cannula into the vein and attach the tubing.

    (c) Personal traits—What personal traits (personality characteristics) would be helpful? The ability to remain calm, appear confident, explain the procedure to the patient, and be reassuring is certainly helpful in starting an IV on anyone.

3. Match the job and the delegate. Given the analysis of the required knowledge, skills, and personal traits, who is the best person on the team to perform this job? In the case of starting an IV, the RN would be best qualified. However, the answer might change if the setting changes—consider a renal dialysis center where technicians have been trained to access a dialysis cannula or a radiology department where the radiology technician starts an IV for the administration of contrast media. In these instances, the technicians are performing a task with a specific, predetermined outcome and have been taught the skill of IV insertion and the potential complications of their specific application. The RN, however, will be more knowledgeable regarding the continual administration and monitoring of IV medications and fluids for therapeutic interventions. Once again, consideration of the outcome desired is essential in making the decision of who performs the task.

Let's see how the whole process of job analysis can be applied to the example given in **Exhibit 6–2.**

CHECKPOINT 6–5

Perform a job analysis of the following:

1. Assessment of a.m. vital signs of 12 patients on a med-surg unit in a local hospital:

    a) knowledge?

    b) skills?

    c) traits?

    d) who would do this job?

2. Teaching insulin administration to an insulin-dependent 60-year-old diabetic who lives alone:

    e) knowledge?

    f) skills?

    g) traits?

    h) who would do this job?

See the end of the chapter for the answers.

EXHIBIT 6–2 The Adult Day Care Center

You are the only RN working in an adult day care center. A rehab aide from a local staffing agency will be working with you today, and 17 clients are scheduled to visit, arriving at various times and staying until 4 p.m., when the center closes.

I. Assess What Needs to Be Done

This means supervising and providing for the physical needs of the clients while maintaining a safe and recreational environment. Diets will need to be monitored, medications given, and follow-up done with two of the families regarding their concerns.

II. Plan

a) The global picture—Seventeen clients will be visiting, spending various lengths of time. All 17 have been here before, and the report from yesterday's nurse states there have been no problems for the past three days. Mr. Darcy's family tends to want to stay and talk about how hard it is to care for Mr. Darcy at home. Perhaps he needs to be placed in a long-term care facility. Mrs. Morris complains about the food, saying it's not hot enough and there's not enough of it to make sure her bowels move. Her family is worried about her taking so many laxatives.

b) Optimal goals—To provide safe care in a fun environment, setting aside time to talk with Mr. Darcy and Mrs. Morris about their concerns, and to spend at least 10–15 minutes with every client to do a quick assessment.

c) Reasonable to expect—There might be at least one "walk-in," and there might be numerous phone calls about the program. One of the clients might be difficult (it seems like someone always has an "off" day!). The rehab aide has never been here before and will need some time for orientation.

d) Set priorities—Orient the rehab aide, pass medications, provide physical assistance to all clients, meet with clients as time allows (first with Mr. Darcy and Mrs. Morris).

III. Intervene

a) Break the job into parts—(1) physical care for the clients: assist to the bathroom, personal hygiene as needed, helping with snacks and meal setup at lunch, assisting with ambulation for exercise in the afternoon; (2) assess patients' current physical status, take blood pressures, weight, skin condition; (3) pass medications, review orders and supply of medications, assess clients throughout visit for any prn needs.

b) Consider knowledge, skills, and personal traits of available staff (a job analysis)—Interview the rehab aide, determining his background and experience in assisting with ambulation, hygienic care, blood pressures, and weights, and assess his personal traits for consideration in leading exercise group, card games, or other entertainment. (He says he has passed the medication administration course for nursing assistants and is allowed to do this at group homes—will you let him?)

c) Match the job to the delegate—RN will orient aide, pass meds, interview and assess each client, take phone calls to market the facility, follow up with Mr. Darcy and Mrs. Morris (could the aide follow up with Mrs. Morris at lunch, making certain her meal was sufficient and hot?). Rehab aide will assist with physical needs, ambulation, feeding, taking blood pressures, and talking to the clients, sharing information with the RN to complete the assessment of each client.

IV. Evaluate

Throughout the day, check with the aide as well as the clients to make certain all needs are being met, that the aide does not feel overwhelmed or bored (is there more that he could be doing as he gets more comfortable with the setting, or is he confused if he has never worked with geriatric clients before?), and that you are satisfied with your abilities to achieve the goals outlined for the day. If three new clients came in unannounced and Mrs. Morris had a reaction to the stool softener she was taking, were you able to reprioritize and let go of some of your expectations (perhaps rescheduling some of the assessments for later in the week)?

Decision-Making Models

Matching the right provider to the need, whether or not it is part of healthcare reform, is an essential component for safe delegation. Numerous tools have been developed to assist the RN in deciding who does what. Similar to the job analysis described previously, these models provide a road map for thinking and offer a guide to making the appropriate legal and safe decision of what to delegate.

The National Council Delegation Decision-Making Process. In their 1995 newsletter, the NCSBN suggested a framework for decision making to ensure patient safety in receiving delegated care. Their seven-step process is covered in **Exhibit 6–3** and offers a basic yet comprehensive pathway for evaluating the steps taken in delegation.

EXHIBIT 6–3 NCSBN Delegation Decision-Making Process

I. Delegation Criteria:
   A. Nursing Practice Act
      1. permits delegation
      2. authorizes task to be delegated or authorizes nurse to decide delegation
   B. Delegator qualifications
      1. within scope of authority to delegate
      2. appropriate education, skills, and experience
      3. documented/demonstrated evidence of current competency
   C. Delegatee qualifications
      1. appropriate education, skills, and experience
      2. documented/demonstrated evidence of current competency

Provided that this foundation is in place, the licensed nurse can enter the continuous process of delegation decision making.

II. Assess the Situation:
   A. Identify the needs of the patient, consulting the plan of care.
   B. Consider the circumstance/setting.
   C. Ensure the availability of adequate resources, including supervision.

If patient needs, circumstances, and available resources (including supervisor and delegatee) indicate patient safety will be maintained with delegated care, proceed to III.

III. Plan for the Specific Task To Be Delegated:
   A. Specify the nature of each task and the knowledge and skills required to perform it.
   B. Require documentation or demonstration of current competence by the delagatee for each task.
   C. Determine the implications for the patient, other patients, and significant others.

If the nature of the task, competence of the delegatee, and patient implications indicate patient safety will be maintained with delegated care, proceed to IV.

IV. Ensure Appropriate Accountability:
   A. As delegator, accept accountability for performance of the task.
   B. Verify that delegatee accepts the delegation and the accountability for carrying out the task correctly.

If delegator and delegatee accept the accountability for their respective roles in the delegated patient care, proceed to V.

V. Supervise Performance of the Task:
   A. Provide directions and clear expectations of how the task is to be performed.
   B. Monitor performance of the task to ensure compliance to established standards of practice, policies, and procedures.
   C. Intervene if necessary.
   D. Ensure appropriate documentation of the task.
VI. Evaluate the Entire Delegation Process:
   A. Evaluate the patient.
   B. Evaluate the performance of the task.
   C. Obtain and provide feedback.
VII. Reassess and Adjust the Overall Plan of Care as Needed.

Source: Used with permission of NCSBN. For a pictorial and detailed discussion of this process the reader is referred to the Joint Statement on Delegation, ANA and NCSBN, 2006, https://www.ncsbn.org/Joint_statement.pdf.

Many organizations have also created tools to support the RN in making decisions regarding who can do what. Swedish Medical Center in Denver, Colorado, created the pathway in **Figure 6–1** to assist in decision making.

The American Association of Critical-Care Nurses supported the decision making process with their framework of factors to consider, first created in 1990 (Evans, 1991, p. 17a) and updated this approach in their Delegation Handbook (2004). We offer it here as a good review of the more important questions to consider before delegating a task to anyone. Refer to **Exhibit 6–4.**

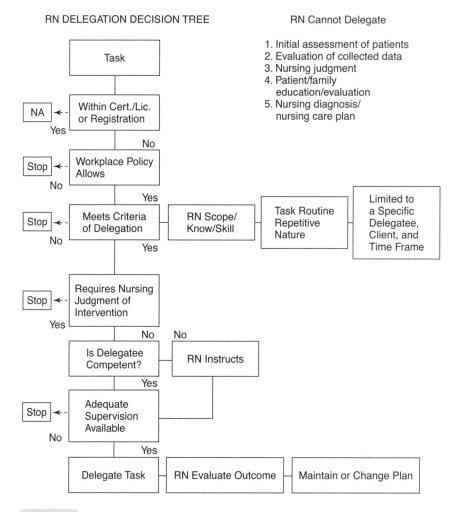

FIGURE 6–1 **RN Delegation Decision Tree.** *Source:* Used with permission of Columbia Swedish Medical Center, Professional Nursing Practice.

EXHIBIT 6–4   Factors on Which to Base a Decision to Delegate: The American Association of Critical-Care Nurses

- Potential for harm: What is the particular nursing activity's potential for harm?
- Complexity of the nursing activity: What psychomotor and cognitive skills are required to perform a particular nursing activity?
- Required problem solving and innovation: If a problem is suspected, does it require individualized problem solving to achieve a successful outcome?
- Predictability of outcome: How predictable are the outcomes of a nursing activity?
- Extent of patient interaction: Will delegating a nursing activity increase or decrease the amount of time a critical care nurse can spend with a patient and the patient's family?

Source: Data from *Heart & Lung*, (January 1991), Vol. 20., no. 1, p. 19A, © American Association of Critical-Care Nurses. Revisited in the AACN Delegation Handbook, 2nd ed., 2004. Retrieved November 19, 2007, from http://www.aacn.org/aacn/practice.nsf/Files/DBEd2/$file/1editedrevisedAACNDelegationHandbook%207-1-2004.pdf.

The Four Rights as a Model of Decision Making. Last, but not least, we present a rather simplistic but very effective approach for deciding what tasks you are prepared to hand off to another member of the team. For years, since 1990 in fact, we have borrowed from the mnemonic of the five rights of medication administration (do you remember the right med, right time, right route, right patient, right dose?). The four rights of effective delegation (Washburn, 1991) include consideration and determination of four major areas as described in **Figure 6–2**.

Using these four criteria as a guide, decision making can become a little easier and clearer. It is also important to note that the NCSBN (1995) used this approach as well, adding a fifth right, that of the right circumstances. (Refer to Chapter 3 for further discussion.) Their recommended list looks like this:

- Right task—one that is delegatable for a specific patient
- Right circumstances—appropriate patient setting, available resources, and other relevant factors considered
- Right person—right person delegating the right task to the right person to be performed on the right person
- Right direction/communication—clear, concise description of the task, including its objective, limits, and expectations
- Right supervision—appropriate monitoring, evaluation, intervention as needed, and feedback

The Four Rights of Delegation

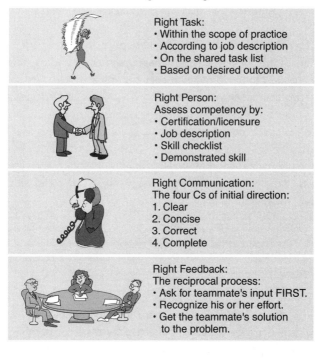

Right Task:
· Within the scope of practice
· According to job description
· On the shared task list
· Based on desired outcome

Right Person:
Assess competency by:
· Certification/licensure
· Job description
· Skill checklist
· Demonstrated skill

Right Communication:
The four Cs of initial direction:
1. Clear
2. Concise
3. Correct
4. Complete

Right Feedback:
The reciprocal process:
· Ask for teammate's input FIRST.
· Recognize his or her effort.
· Get the teammate's solution
  to the problem.

FIGURE 6-2 The Four Rights of Delegation. *Source:* Copyright © 1991, Marilynn J. Washburn.

CHECKPOINT 6-6

Would you delegate these tasks to an unlicensed caregiver?

1. Helping a stable patient walk

2. Evaluating patient response to pain medication (in an acute care setting)

3. Collecting intake and output data on 10 patients

4. Making rounds with physician

5. Assisting in activities of daily living (ADLs) with a homebound 70-year-old

6. Feeding a 2-year-old recovering from a spica cast application

See the end of the chapter for the answers.

Making Assignments

Another important part of implementing your plan involves making assignments to the members on your team. If your work setting is a facility that provides care for patients on a continuous basis, whether it is a psychiatric treatment center, a long-term care or extended care facility, an ambulatory care unit, or an acute care facility, you face the task of dividing up the workload and maximizing the resources available. In plain terms, this means making assignments, a skill that generally is not taught, but rather is learned "on the job." (Your charge nurse calls in sick, and you are asked to take her place, never having done so before. The supervisor says, "It's not so hard—all you have to do is make the assignments." Sound familiar?)

Institutional policies and The Joint Commission criteria provide the starting place for making assignments. Each work environment will vary, depending on the uniqueness of the patient population, but certain standards will apply in all settings. As of 1997, The Joint Commission no longer specifies detailed criteria to consider when making assignment decisions. In keeping with its approach toward flexibility and organizational choices, The Joint Commission now allows hospitals to define criteria of their own that support appropriate decision making in terms of assigning care providers to patients. However, we find the original criteria to be an excellent guide for consideration and include them here for your reference. Note: These criteria speak only to acute care settings; The Joint Commission does not make specific reference to the process in other settings such as home care or long-term care. However, we feel that these basic guidelines are important to keep in mind when making assignments in any setting.

NC.2.1.2 Assigning responsibility to nursing staff members for providing nursing care to patients is based on consideration of the following seven elements:

1. Complexity of the patient's care—How involved is the care that is required? Is this a multisystem failure or a primipara post delivery?
2. Dynamics of the patient's status—How often is the patient's condition changing? Is this a brittle diabetic with blood sugars all over the map or a stable post appendectomy waiting for discharge instructions?
3. Complexity of assessment—What is required to completely assess the patient's condition? Can the assessment be

performed quickly, involving a stable patient, or is this an emergency admission involving a motor vehicle accident that resulted in numerous injuries?

4. Technology involved—Is this patient being monitored for cardiac dysrhythmias, on a PCA pump, with two infusion pumps, and renal dialysis daily? Or is the patient on a psych unit, stable physically but severely depressed, not requiring any technological intervention?

5. Degree of supervision—What level of supervision is required by the nursing personnel based on their skill and competence? Are the members of the staff experienced and able to work together without difficulty, or is there a new team member who has never provided care for this type of patient before?

6. Availability of supervision—Is the appropriate nursing supervision available to provide the degree of supervision determined in number 5? Is there someone on the unit who is responsible for overseeing the actions of the team and assisting and evaluating when necessary, or is this the night shift in a long-term care facility and the director of nursing is available by phone?

7. Infection control and safety precautions—To what degree are universal precautions enforced? Are all staff members trained in safety issues, CPR, etc., or is someone being assigned to provide care who has not yet received this type of instruction? (The Joint Commission, 1994, pp. 12–13)

Hopefully, you included some of the following factors in your list:

+ Location—No one likes to run from one end of the hall to the other if it can be avoided. This has traditionally been one of the major criteria for making assignments, and it is still used today because some units have wings, pods, or blocks of rooms that make up their assigned area. Likewise, in a community setting, no one wants to drive from one end of town to the other, so most nurses are assigned to specific regions or districts.

+ Continuity of care—As rapidly as patients are moved through any system, it is essential that some degree of sameness be provided. If you had the patient yesterday, it would be nice to care for him or her again today. This is more than a nicety; familiarity with the patient assists in planning and evaluating his or her progress. Continuity of staff in terms of team composition is important for the same reasons; developing working relationships with a consistent team member makes it easier to plan and delegate work. Too often, the person making assignments is concerned only with the numbers of patients or clients assigned and not with protecting the integrity of the team. The

> Too often, the person making assignments is concerned only with the numbers of patients or clients assigned and not with protecting the integrity of the team.

assistant you worked with yesterday might be assigned to another RN today to "make the assignments even," and you will spend part of your shift bringing your new assistant up to speed.

+ Personal preference—It is nice if we can all have the opportunity to do what we prefer, and hopefully you have matched your preference with your job setting. If surgery is your thing, you probably are more skilled in this area and would be best on a surgical unit or in an OR suite. Beyond this, we all have certain types of patients we prefer (see Chapter 7, "Know Your Delegate"), and considering this when making an assignment is beneficial to the patient and the employee.

+ Acuity system—Many facilities employ a system for determining the acuity levels of all patients so that the work can be distributed more equably among the team. Past systems have ranged in sophistication from the most detailed computer process to the basic 1 through 4 categorizing of needs. We have yet to find a perfect system, and we continually emphasize that this is a dynamic, not a static, environment, with continual changes in patient needs that must be consistently met. Be wary of the importance that is placed on this system; it can be a very divisive tool as members of the team argue about how many "acuity points" they were assigned. It can also be a very useful tool for monitoring staffing needs and the changing demands of the patient population.

+ Care delivery system—Whether your work setting uses a case management system, primary care, team nursing, or any one of a number of new systems being currently created, this will influence how assignments are made. As with continuity of care, this is a criterion that might be quickly forgotten as we struggle to make certain everyone has an equal load. We have observed "team nursing" (acute care) in which the nursing assistant (NA) will report to four or five different RNs as the patients are divided up among the staff. This is not a team model and will serve only to ensure that chaos and frustration are the rule of the day, as the assistant struggles to meet the demands of numerous bosses.

Keeping all of these factors in mind, refer to the assignment exercise in **Exhibit 6–5** and see what you can do.

EXHIBIT 6–5 The Assignment

The following patients are on the unit during the day shift:

101: 65 yo total hip, day 2, has hyperal, is confused, family problem, very unhappy with care.

102: 35 yo bowel resection, day 3, very happy that cancerous bowel was removed, ready to begin to learn home care.

103: 82 yo cholecystitis, day 1, patient admitted by daughter because she wanted to go on vacation. Physician furious that ED physician admitted him. Patient is very stable and fun to take care of. Requires little care, will probably be sent home, or to another place if tests okay. Doubt pain is cardiac.

104: 35 yo total hysterectomy, day 2, very stable, requires little care, ready to go home in a.m.

105: 29 yo motor vehicle accident, day 3, multiple lacerations, bruises, dressings and wound care with saline/peroxide flush, takes about one hour to do wound care.

106: 19 yo motor vehicle accident, day 3, girlfriend of patient in 105. R/O fx pelvis, R/O possible pregnancy. Family upset, patient screams with pain, pain meds being held due to ? pregnancy, some arguments with physician and family. R/O drug dependence.

107: 81 yo TURP, day 2, patient from group home for disabled, ready to return tomorrow. Alert, friendly, understands instructions.

108: 74 yo TIA, day 1, CVA now evident, extending, family discussing code decision with physician, very unstable vital signs, on q 15" neuro checks.

109: 71 yo with abd pain, new admit, probable diverticulosis, has had hx in the past, stable. Language problem, speaks only Vietnamese.

110: 42 yo pneumonia, day 4, on 2 IV antibiotics q 4–6 hours.

Plan your assignment with the following staff:
Yourself (RN Charge Nurse):
LPN (LVN):
Nursing Assistant:

Source: Reprinted with permission from Ruth I. Hansten, Marilynn J. Washburn, Loretta O'Neill, and Washington Organization of Nurse Executives, © 1990.

We hope that you took the time to try your hand at making this assignment. Even if you do not currently work in an acute care setting and never have the opportunity to make assignments, it is a good method for getting the global picture and understanding what your fellow colleagues experience. It is also an excellent tool for prioritizing and performing a job analysis so that you become more skilled at matching the job to the delegate.

Often, when we use this exercise in our workshops, many individuals will look at us expectantly, waiting for the "right" answer. There isn't one. Those of you who are responsible for making assignments know this to be true. If you were to use this exercise in a small group of your coworkers or at a staff meeting, you would quickly find that everyone has a slightly different idea regarding how the work should be assigned. What is important here is the ability to define outcomes, organize the work flow, and justify the choices you have made.

CHECKPOINT 6-7

What other factors do you consider when making assignments?

Let's discuss some of the more typical responses to this exercise because we have noted that although individual approaches vary, there is a pattern of assignments based on the criteria we discussed earlier in the chapter. The primary factor for consideration seems to be the type of care delivery system the charge nurse is most experienced with and is therefore likely to implement in this exercise. Other factors of room location, personal preference, continuity of care, and the acuity system are not fully applied because that information is not provided in the information given in the exercise. However, the criteria of The Joint Commission, particularly the complexity of the patient and the availability of supervision, should be considered.

Keeping these criteria in mind, we often see an assignment that gives the charge nurse the most "difficult" patients, while the LPN is asked to do the treatments and medications on all patients and the NA is expected to do the typical "beds, baths, and answer the call lights." That assignment would look like this:

RN: 101, 106, 108, 109, all IVs, discharge planning for 103, 104, and 107
LPN: all treatments, all meds except IVs, 102, 103, 104, 105, 107, 110
NA: beds, baths, vital signs on all patients, answer call lights, assist where needed

This pattern reflects the idea of "equity," where the charge nurse feels she must carry at least as many patients as the LPN, and often more, to justify her position and to make certain everyone knows she is not just "working the desk." Does this reflect the best utilization of resources to meet the desired outcomes? Have we even thought about outcomes, or are we merely performing a task-oriented function? What outcomes would you determine are reasonable before you make the assignment? (Remember our process as described earlier in the chapter, and refer to **Exhibit 6–6** for a list of potential outcomes.)

EXHIBIT 6–6   Potential Outcomes for Patients 101–110

101:   Short-term outcome: to determine the source of the confusion and take steps to correct the underlying problem; by the end of the 24 hours, a reoriented patient who is ready to undertake the long-term outcome of going home and has the ability to ambulate with a one-person standby assist.

102:   Short-term outcome: patient will learn first steps of procedures for home care, with discharge planned for next day.

103:   Short-term outcome: review of lab tests will rule out pain from other sources. Dietary/medication home regimen will be completed. Patient's disposition will be to home with home health assistance or respite care.

104:   Outcome for today: patient will have bowel movement, ambulate, and verbalize home care of incision and bowels, medications such as hormonal replacement. Will probably go home today with family to assist since no one is allowed to wait for the a.m. for discharge unless fever or other variances occur.

105:   Outcome for today: plan for home care will be discussed, wound will show evidence of beginning granulation. Home assistant will begin to learn wound care procedure. Referral to VNS completed.

106:   Outcome for today: determine pregnancy status with blood test, family/MD/patient/hospital care team will set up conference for devising longer term plan, discuss question of drug dependence and rehabilitation. Patient will be pain free.

107:   RN or assistant from group home will receive instructions for discharge care, patient will verbalize home care plan.

108:   Code status will be discussed and a decision made as quickly as possible. Depending on the decision, the most likely outcome is that patient will receive terminal care, family will receive grief counseling.

109: Patient's history and assessment will be completed through use of interpreter. Origin of pain will be determined and treated so that patient will be pain free. Discharge plan will be initiated depending on information obtained about normal health and ADL support if needed.

110: Origin of pneumonia will be discovered and treated. (Is patient getting better on current regimen? Have cultures and sensitivities been done if he is not? If treatment is working, how long will it be necessary?) Discharge plan will begin based on prognosis and current respiratory status. (Is this patient a candidate for home IV antibiotic therapy?)

What is different about what the RN might do with the patients she has assigned to herself as compared to those who are not directly assigned to her? If the RN is assigned "patients," how many is she really responsible for? Can the LPN be solely responsible for a patient assignment? What plans, if any, are made for an emergency—are there any other tasks that can be delegated?

Another assignment we often see reflects the practice of "care partners," where the care delivery system involves the pairing of a licensed and unlicensed caregiver to provide for the needs of a given group of patients. This assignment would look something like this:

RN: 108 (to discuss transfer to another unit), 109 (to obtain translator from family member or staff roster), all IV medications
LPN: 101, 102, 103, 104, 105, 106, 107, 110
NA: 101, 102, 103, 104, 105, 106, 107, 110 (working with LPN)

This same rationale can be used to make the following assignment, pairing the NA with the RN and leaving the LPN to function as a provider of total patient care. In this case, the RN must assess the patients assigned to the LPN:

RN: 101, 105, 106, 108, 110
NA: 101, 105, 106, 108, 110 (NA can be trained in doing clean wound care for room 105, can assist with frequent monitoring of 108)
LPN: 102, 103, 104, 107, 109

A functional care delivery system would result in the following assignment and might provide the best opportunity for each individual to do what he or she knows best:

RN: all initial assessments, all IVs, discharge planning on 102 (with teaching of home care) and 104, rounds with physicians, family and physician conference regarding code status of 108, resolution of complaints of 101, placement of 103, and discussion with family and physician of 106; would also plan for all transfers and admits.

LPN: all medications (except IVs), all treatments, postop teaching of 104

NA: hygienic care on all patients; vital sign monitoring; assist with transfers, admits, and discharges; provide total care for 103 and 104

All staff share the answering of call lights.

As in any personal relationship, it is often the little things that make the difference, affecting whether the relationship will be successful and positive or doomed to difficulty because of assumptions regarding who is or is not doing his or her share of the work.

A word about call lights: in many instances we have seen this to be a major stumbling block to the work flow on any unit. As in any personal relationship, it is often the little things that make the difference, affecting whether the relationship will be successful and positive or doomed to difficulty because of assumptions regarding who is or is not doing his or her share of the work. If this sounds familiar to you, a frank discussion at a staff meeting or with the members on your shift will be necessary to clear the air. Is it reasonable to expect the NAs to answer all of the call lights? (We are making no judgments here; the answer will depend on your particular environment.) What is the perception of everyone on the team regarding this expectation? Do the NAs see the nurses sitting at the desk or having friendly conversations with visitors and physicians while call lights are ringing off the wall? If you are transitioning from an all-RN staff and adding unlicensed personnel, make certain that these seemingly benign issues are discussed at the beginning of your working relationships (see Chapter 7 for a complete discussion of role clarification). Taking time for this kind of discussion will make the task of making assignments easier and result in a smoother working relationship for everyone.

IV. Evaluate

Okay, so you've taken the time to assess the needs, plan and prioritize the outcomes, and implement your plan through careful job analysis, matching of the job to the delegate, and making the assignment based on specific criteria. Wow! What's next? The final step of the nursing process as we know it involves the evaluation of what we've done. Considerable discussion will be provided on this topic (see Chapter 11) as it relates to the process of delegation. What needs to be covered here relates specifically to the evaluation of whether we did the right things (effectiveness) and did them correctly (efficiency).

Once again, the true measure of our success goes back to the outcomes we determined to be our goals in the first step of our assessment. Did we achieve what we set out to do? (You would be amazed at how many nurses do not ever ask the question!) We wonder: If you never stop to evaluate your outcomes, how do you ever know if you have achieved them? How do you measure success? Or, to put it one more way, we took the time to determine where we were going; shouldn't we take the time to determine if we got there?

The use of two criteria, effectiveness and efficiency, makes our evaluation process simple. Let's look at efficiency first (because we know this to be one of those terms met with disdain by many nurses). Every nurse realizes the importance of doing things correctly. Few professions carry consequences as serious as those resulting from an incorrect healthcare procedure or intervention. Unlike manufacturing or the provision of retail goods and services, health care deals directly with people's lives, and mistakes carry a high price. Doing things right is tantamount to every nurse's professional standard and receives the appropriate emphasis in all of our training. Beyond the correct performance of a procedure, however, is another question regarding efficiency: Did the right person do the job? We have repeatedly stated that "things ain't the way they used to be," and this certainly applies to the resources available to us as healthcare providers. It is imperative, then, that we make every effort to determine that the individual who best meets the requirements of the job to be done is the one assigned to do the job. As nurses, it is our responsibility to the patients we care for to ensure that they receive the best that we can offer by delegating wisely.

Effectiveness, or doing the right things, will be apparent when outcomes are what we desired them to be. Reducing length of stays, eliminating readmissions 24 hours postdischarge, reducing the need for amputations due to poorly managed foot care of diabetics, and restoring autonomy to patients who have been dependent on others to meet their basic needs are all outcomes we can plan for and achieve.

If periodic evaluation (we recommend daily) does not reveal the desired results, review each of the steps of the process that you used to determine what needed to be done and by whom. In your analysis, be sure to consider input from other members of the team, as well as the patients.

ADDITIONAL SAMPLES FOR PLANNING CARE

Often it is necessary to take the time to review and practice the process of making assignments and planning care. As noted previously, this is not usually a skill that is taught, other than through the sharing of some time-honored principles regarding equality ("give everybody the same number of patients" and "be sure to assign breaks"). Yet this initial act of planning will have a significant impact on work flow and patient and employee satisfaction.

CHECKPOINT 6–8

Review how you currently start your shift on the job. Do you set aside time for planning? Who do you include in this time? Are there ways that this could be improved, or do you feel satisfied with the information received, and are you able to plan effectively and be organized regarding what needs to be done?

We have included here a number of sample patient populations (see "Shift Your Focus" box) and a tool for determining who does what based on outcomes planning (**Exhibit 6–7**). This is a significant cultural and procedural change for most RNs practicing today and will require continued support if we are to move from being slaves to a task list toward full realization of the role of the professional RN. Note: If the sample patient lists are not similar enough to yours, try taking a sample from your own population and using the outcomes-based planning tool to plan work for the members of your team. This makes a good exercise for a charge nurse (resource nurse, team leader, care coordinator, etc.) meeting or a staff meeting. It is amazing how everyone feels capable of commenting on assignments made, but most are unwilling to take over the job! And more amazing is our need to cling to a to-do list and overlook the real work of coordinating the care of the patient based on the results desired by the patient, the family, and the healthcare team.

EXHIBIT 6-7 Planning Based on Outcomes

Patient 1
Outcomes this shift:

- _____
- _____
- _____

Long-term outcome:

_____
_____

Interventions to achieve the planned outcomes: Who will do:

- _____   • _____
- _____   • _____
- _____   • _____
- _____   • _____
- _____   • _____

Patient 2
Outcomes this shift:

- _____
- _____
- _____

Long-term outcome:

_____
_____

Interventions to achieve the planned outcomes: Who will do:

- _____   • _____
- _____   • _____
- _____   • _____
- _____   • _____
- _____   • _____

This works well with a mixed group of staff facilitated by a staff educator. Select appropriate patients for your area, and use the planning tool in Exhibit 6–7.

SHIFT YOUR FOCUS

Task Orientation to Outcomes-Based Clinical Management

Select from the following list the patients who would be on your unit during the day shift.

Plan your assignment, identifying your patient outcomes first! Determine which tasks you would delegate based on your team members and the planned outcomes.

- M/S: 65 yo total hip, day 2, has hyperal, is confused, family problem, very unhappy with care.

- M/S: 35 yo bowel resection, day 3, very happy that cancerous bowel was removed, ready to begin to learn home care.

- M/S: 82 yo cholecystitis, day 1, patient admitted by daughter because she wanted to go on vacation. Physician furious that ED physician admitted him. Patient is very stable and fun to take care of. Requires little care, will probably be sent home or to another place if tests okay. Doubt pain is cardiac.

- OB: 35 yo total hysterectomy, day 2, very stable, requires little care, ready to go home in a.m.

- OB: 40 yr para 1, gravida 1, delivered at 6 a.m., epidural in place, cramping and complaining of pain, wants to nurse baby, husband at bedside, upset at continuing pain and wanting to help his wife.

- ICU: 49 yo thoracotomy, new admit from OR, on vent with chest tube, pressure tubing to be assembled, needs lab drawn, Stat ABG, EKG, wife anxious and waiting.

- ICU: 57 yo MI, family at bedside, patient goes into Vtach and codes. ACLS initiated, attending needs to be called.

- IMCU: 74 yo TIA, day 1, CVA now evident, extending, family discussing code decision with physician, very unstable vital signs, on q 15" neuro checks.

- IMCU: 10 yo motor vehicle accident, day 1, multiple lacerations, bruises, dressings and wound care with saline/peroxide flush, takes about one hour to do wound care.

- ED: 14 yo female is vomiting and complains of abdominal pain. Workup has not been done yet to rule out possible etiology.

- ED: 2 yr old, fell 6 feet, with LOC 10 minutes immediately after fall, has vomited three times since arrival.

- PEDS: 12 yo insulin-dependent diabetic, blood glucose this a.m. of 50, mother insisting that daughter is okay, wants her to be able to eat anything and "act normal."

Samples of Patients by Clinical Area

ICU

1. 62 yo male, 6 hrs status postop Cabg x3. ETT in place, vent settings: FiO_2 40, IMV 2, Peep +5, Vt 850. Spontaneous RR 16. Has just met extubation parameters. CT x3 in place (2 pleural, 1 mediastinal) to Pleurevac @ –20 cm suction, no air leak, minimal hourly drainage 20–30 cc/hr. SG in place, CO 6.5, CI 2.1, PCWP 14. IVs infusing D51/4 20 Kcl@ 500/hr, Ntg @ 50 mcg/min., dopamine @ 2 mcg/kg/min. Pt awake and follows commands, cooperative. Spouse and daughter very anxious, asking a lot of questions. Cardiac monitor NS/ST 90–100s with rare pacs. A/V pacer wires in place with external pacer off @ present.
2. 57 yo female s/p AMI, s/p TPA given yesterday. HHD O_2 @ 2l/nc with SaO_2 93%—denies chest pain, SOB. VS stable. IVs: NTG 10 mcg/min, heparin 800 u/hr. Cardiac monitor NS 60s no ectopy. Up in cardiac chair @ bedside. Awaiting transfer orders to telemetry. Spouse in earlier, supportive—went to work.

Telemetry Team

1. 52 yo male, 2 days s/p IMI, just returned from heart cath procedure (needs A/V femoral sheaths removed) AAO x3, denies C/P—plan is medical management. O_2 @ 4l/nc, SaO_2 93%, HHD ordered, IV NS, INT. Needs cardiac rehab activity and discharge instructions. Cardiac monitor SB 58.
2. 56 yo male, 4 days s/p CABG. Cardiac monitor NS with rare PVC. O_2 @ 1 L/nc. Needs q shift incision care, ted hose application, ambulating 4 x day. Oral controlled diabetic taking oral hypoglycemic bid, 1800 cal ADA diet, INT. Routine VS, daily wts, plan discharge in am. Will need home O_2 arranged. Lives alone, one daughter lives in town.

Pediatric ICU

1. 30-week gestational male, now 2 days old, transferred from General Hospital yesterday. Intubated on a ventilator with a chest tube. Mom had an emergency C-section and has not seen the baby, Dad is really stressed and insisting that he needs to stay with the baby for all procedures, etc. He is not taking in any of the information from the hospital staff.
2. 2 yo baby girl s/p open heart surgery today. Intubated and not aerating. Needs to be reintubated and also needs multiple IV drips started ASAP. A chest tube also needs to be inserted.
3. 13 yo male gunshot wound to neck 2 weeks ago, transferred from downtown hospital. Trached with complex surgical site at neck. Conscious and angry, needs much assistance with daily activities. Gang friends trying to see patient at all hours.

Intermediate ICU

The day shift RN has these four patients and shares an NA with another RN:

1. 50 yo male, s/p CVA with neuro changes, scheduled by MD to go home today. Long-term IV needs to be inserted. Wife and patient very anxious. Discharge planner not aware of patient previously, not sure discharge is best idea.
2. 65 yo male, IDDM. DC planned, but MD calls in at 0800 that he is ill, patient will need more than 10 medications clarified prior to discharge. Pt has history of noncompliance with DM care but is now seeking instruction.
3. End-stage CHF patient, eligible for DC based on meeting activity criteria, four family members present, anxious to go home ASAP. History of poor compliance with CHF management.
4. 45 yo female, active bleeding GI hemorrhage. Patient anxious, scheduled for Stat nuclear med exam, needs RN escort. Anxious family.

OB

Six RNs are scheduled for the night shift. At the change of shift at 1900 hours, one RN had called in sick. There is no recovery nurse because coordinator was unable to find coverage for sick call. There is an on-call nurse for recovery all shift.

1. Room 1: in OR for delivery—fetal distress? C-section vs. vag delivery. Three day shift RNs in back for delivery; vag del @ 1913; neonatal concerns led to day shift recovery nurse staying over and pediatrician coming in to assess. IV started, labs run.
2. Room 3: stable primip needing maternal and neonatal assessments.
3. Room 4: 35 1/2 week PIH pt breech. Unsuccessful version.
4. Room 7: pt SROM 1240 breech, no contractions, 36 wko, FHT reassuring.
5. Room 8: pt pushing since 1730; maternal temp, thick meconium, fetal tachycardia, decreased variability with laxes. MD here, trial vac/forceps.
6. Room 10: vag delivery @ 1730. Pt out of recovery but nurse went back to help in OR.

Emergency Department

The following patients have presented in your emergency department. You will need to make assignments of tasks based on outcomes. What should the RN do? What should the ED tech do?

1. 2 yo, fell 6 feet, with loss of consciousness 10 minutes immediately after fall, has vomited 3 times since arrival.
2. 3 yo asthmatic has come in very SOB, wheezy, parents have been giving him an inhaler every 10 minutes since early am. No SVN used at home. HR tachy. Now 6 pm.
3. 27 yo vomiting and complaining of abdominal pain. Workup has not been done to rule out possible etiology.
4. 79 yo female with hx of IDDM, cardiomyopathy, now complaining of SOB, diminished breath sounds, 3+ edema both lower extremities.
5. 62 yo male, recent BKA (2 weeks ago). Complains of limb pain, unhappy with need to be here, wants to smoke a cigarette outside. Color poor, drainage noted at end of stump, temp 102.

Psychiatric Medical Services

1. 22 yo male, bipolar disorder, depressed at this time. Has increased suicidal ideation this past shift. Hx of ETOH abuse, no drinks for past 2 days.
2. 32 yo female, major depression. MHP hold, q 30 min checks, multiple OD. Cardiac arrhythmias secondary to OD. On telemetry, alert and oriented, has not signed goals. BP stable before transfer from CCU last night.
3. 66 yo male, ETOH dependence, COPD. On O2 2l per nasal cannula, restricted to unit, nebulizer treatments q 4 hours. On librium, agitated.

Ambulatory Care

You have the following personnel to complete this assignment: one medical assistant, one medical receptionist, MD, and yourself, an RN.

am scheduled appointments

9:00:   mother with sick kid (6 yo), sore throat, poor appetite for 2 days, no fever. You have had several phone conversations with mother over the last few months.

9:15:   second visit for a newly diagnosed diabetic (IDDM) scheduled for RN and MD.

9:45:   female for annual Pap/pelvic.

10:00:   female with recurrent UTIs.

10:30:   7-day visit for newborn.

10:45:   10 yo for ear checkback.

11:00:   65 yo female, posthospitalization for CHF.

In addition, you have the following:

Telephone calls

- mom calling for throat culture results on her child (8 yo) with sore throat. Fever continues.
- male calling for results of cholesterol/triglycerides.
- male calling for refill of Tolectin.
- 15 yo calling for results of pregnancy test.

Drop-ins:

9:00:   63 yo female with chest pain and hx of MI.

9:20:   female who needs Rx refilled.

10:00:   mom with child (3 yo) who fell and hit her head on coffee table.

CONCLUSION

There is so much to be done, and there are only a limited number of people to do the job. How do you best plan to delegate appropriately while ensuring efficiency and effectiveness? Remember to use the nursing process: assessing, planning, implementing, and evaluating your practice.

By realizing your part in the determination of what needs to be done, you are allowing yourself the time to practice the professional component of nursing—the implementation of the nursing process. Your extensive knowledge and sound judgment are the key ingredients to planning and delivering quality patient care.

Focus on outcomes and an awareness that evaluation of the achievement of those outcomes will increase nursing's visibility in all areas. Prioritize care, using the parameters of "life threatening," "safety," and "essential to the medical/nursing plan of care," and delegate by matching the correct individual to the job based on a simple job analysis.

By realizing your part in the determination of what needs to be done, you are allowing yourself the time to practice the professional component of nursing—the implementation of the nursing process. Your extensive knowledge and sound judgment are the key ingredients to planning and delivering quality patient care.

ANSWERS TO CHECKPOINTS

6–1.   a

6–2.

The PTA Model	Professional "The Whole Picture"	Technical "Expert Skill Level"	Amenity "The Extra Touch"
Example 1	discharge planning	passing medications	changing linen
Visible to	colleagues	physicians/patient	patient/family
How measured	length of stay	medication errors	patient surveys/ letters
Example 2	diabetic teaching in the home setting	giving insulin injections	fixing a snack for the patient's family
Visible to	patient, family, physician	patient, colleagues	family
How measured	patient behavior, follows Rx	# of attempts	patient survey, response
Example 3	medication instructions	changing a dressing	changing ice water
Visible to	patient, family, physician	physician, patient, colleagues	patient, family

The PTA Model	Professional "The Whole Picture"	Technical "Expert Skill Level"	Amenity "The Extra Touch"
How measured	patient behavior	healing status	patient/family comments
Example 4	your choice		
Visible to			
How measured			

6–4.

1. Life threatening

2. Essential to care plan

3. Essential to care plan

4. Nice

5. Safety

6. Safety

6–5.

1. Assessment of a.m. vital signs:

    a) knowledge—how to take pulse, temperature, respirations, and blood pressures

    b) skills—math, ability to work electronic or mercury thermometer, electronic or manual sphygmomanometer

    c) traits—conscientious, friendly, organized

    d) who—NA or any trained unlicensed assistive personnel would be best choice

2. Teaching insulin administration:

    a) knowledge—process of administration, side effects and desirable effects of insulin and the various types, sites for injection

    b) skills—ability to give a subcutaneous injection, psychomotor skill

    c)   traits—calm, confident, reassuring

    d)   who—LPN or RN. (In Washington state, in group homes or adult family homes in the community, legislation and rulemaking is underway at the writing of this book for specially trained and certified nursing assistants to administer routine insulin in those settings only and not to teach this task.)

6–6.

1. yes

2. no, maybe to an LPN

3. yes

4. no

5. yes

6. yes

REFERENCES

AACN. (2007, July). *White paper on the role of the clinical nurse leader.* Retrieved November 19, 2007, from http://www.aacn.nche.edu/Publications/WhitePapers/ClinicalNurseLeader.htm.

American Academy of Nursing. (2007). *Project improves nursing practice through technology.* Retrieved November 19, 2007, from http://www.ahanews.com/ahanews_app/jsp/display.jsp?dcrpath=AHANEWS/AHANewsNowArticle/data/ann_071107_AAN&domain=AHANEWS.

Bulechek, G., Butcher, C. & Dochterman, J. (2007) Nursing interventions classification (NIC). St. Louis, MO: Mosby.

Bulechek, G., & McCloskey, J.C. (2003). *Nursing interventions: Effective nursing treatments* (3rd ed.). St. Louis, MO: CV Mosby.

Clark, S., & Aiken, L. (2003). Failure to rescue: Needless deaths are prime examples of the need for more nurses at the bedside. *AJN, 103*(1).

Donahue, M.P. (1985). *Nursing: The finest art.* St. Louis, MO: CV Mosby.

Evans, S.A. (1991). Delegation: What do we fear? *Heart & Lung, 20*(1), 17A–20A.

Floyd, J. (2001, Spring). Envisioning new nursing roles and scopes of practice. *Reflections on Nursing Leadership.*

Lindeman, C. (1996). A vision for nursing education. *Creative Nursing, 2*(1), 5–8.

Manthey, M. (1991). A pragmatic concern. *Nursing Management, 22,* 27–28.

Mason, D.J., & Talbott, S.W. (1985). *Political action handbook for nurses.* Menlo Park, CA: Addison-Wesley.

Miller, K. (1995). Keeping the care in nursing care. *Journal of Nursing Administration,* 25(11), 29–32.

MNR. (1994). *244CMR 3.05 (6) Registered nurse and licensed practical nurse, section, 1996.* Retrieved November 19, 2007, from http://www.mass.gov/Eeohhs2/docs/dph/regs/244cmr003.pdf.

National Council of State Boards of Nursing. (1995). *Delegation: Concepts and decision-making issues.* Chicago:Author.

Needleman, J., & Buerhaus, P. (2007). Failure-to-rescue: Comparing definitions to measure quality of care. *Medical Care, 45*(10), 913–915.

The Joint Commission on Accreditation of Healthcare Organizations. (1994). *Accreditation manual for hospitals.* Oakbrook Terrace, IL: Author.

Urden, L., & Roode, J. (1997). Work sampling: A decision making tool for determining resources and work redesign. *Journal of Nursing Administration, 27*(9), 34–41.

Washburn, M. (1991, January). Delegation: The art of getting things done through others. *AZ Nurse Times,* 1.

Wolf, G. (2007). Blueprint for design: Creating models that direct change. *Journal of Nursing Administration, 37*(9), 381–387.

Know Your Delegate

Ruth I. Hansten and Marilynn Jackson

CHAPTER SKILLS

+ Identify the delegates in your workplace.
+ Compare official expectations of each role, practice acts and regulations, and actual workplace expectations.
+ Review standards of competency maintenance.
+ Prepare to assess the delegate's weaknesses and strengths.

RECOMMENDED RESOURCES

▶ Check the Web site for your specialty organization (such as the ENA, AACCN) and research any delegation recommendations that have been published.

▶ Research cultural implications for healthcare delivery in the major populations in your area.

▶ Call or go online to clarify your state regulatory board's rule for working with LPNs (LVNs).

▶ Go to your state board of nursing's (or state quality assurance association) website to get an update of rules for assisted living facilities and group homes such as adult family homes.

"Sometimes we are assigned a float nurse in our very specialized ophthalmology day surgery area. Some do okay, others are frightening to work with because they just don't know what they don't know! How can I feel comfortable working with these people? The way I understand the supervision clause in the state nurse practice act, I need to know the competencies of those to whom I delegate."

W e've put a bit of energy into examining ourselves. We've looked at what needs to be done and how the RN is accountable for leading the team to achieving outcomes. Now it's time to examine the other most pivotal person in the delegation process: the delegate. For those nurses who have been used to doing all their patient care without help, trusting some of the tasks to another person is difficult at best. But it is possible to know that delegate, just as we get to know those we serve.

As an example of how we get to know those to whom we delegate, think of the family. Whether you must hearken back to your family of origin or have a family now, think about how you've found out about the strengths, weaknesses, motivation, and preferences of those in your family. If you tell a 10-year-old to clean out the kitty litter box or fix dinner while you are at work, chances are the assignment will be incomplete or, worse yet, forgotten unless you supervise on a one-to-one basis. If you go to work and a parent or a responsible young adult son or daughter is at home during the day, chances are they won't even have to be told to do the breakfast dishes or get dinner in the oven. Within your work group, you might see variations in the need for supervision and also many different manifestations of strengths and weaknesses (more politically correct, "areas for improvement") in your staff, as well as how they fulfill the requirements of their job descriptions.

In this chapter, we'll briefly revisit the fundamental importance of state practice acts, explore job descriptions and competencies, and then identify strategies to clarify the personal expectations you might hold for your coworkers. Then we'll examine how we can best assess each delegate's strengths, weaknesses, motivation, and preferences and how these combine to give you the information you need to match the best delegate to the work at hand.

WHO ARE THE DELEGATES?

To whom do you delegate on a daily basis?

_____

_____

_____

_____

Here are some of the answers we've heard from nurses throughout the country:

- Student nurses
- New personnel (RNs)
- LPNs, LVNs
- Nursing assistants
- Orderlies
- Home health aides
- Respiratory therapists (or speech, occupational, or physical therapists)
- Multiskilled workers (combination of roles such as therapists, nursing assistants, phlebotomists)
- Pharmacy personnel
- Secretaries
- Volunteers
- Social workers
- Medical students
- Physicians (nurses report asking doctors, especially medical students, to do some of the care!)
- Psychologists
- Medical technologists
- Phlebotomists
- OR technicians

Whether we are delegating to all of these people in the strict sense of the nurse practice act or asking them to do things for our clients as we coordinate the care, the same principles apply. As we look into the future to identify potential team members, we might be supervising robots and evaluating the electronic data collected by telemedicine technology (Vastag 2007; Gandsas, Parekh, Bleech, & Tong, 2007). Those nurses who are attempting to find a workplace in which there is no delegation might need to think twice. How frequently do you find yourself in a supervisory role as a delegator?

CHECKPOINT 7-1

○ I have located the mission and/or a values statement for my organization.

○ I have also located recently revised job descriptions for those I work with, as well as my own job description.

○ I have called the state board of nursing and have obtained current copies of the regulations, rules, and administrative code for RNs, LPNs (LVNs), CNAs, medical assistants, or other healthcare workers in my facility.

Reviewing these documents now, I can answer the following questions:

1. I know what type of healthcare professional (which job description and practice act) is allowed to:

    a) pierce the skin to perform procedures

    b) start IVs

    c) monitor IVs

    d) perform the nursing process

    e) gather data for the nurse as he or she performs the assessment, nursing diagnosis, planning, intervention, and evaluation

    f) perform hygienic care

    g) deliver medications

    h) be "in charge" of coordinating patients' care in my healthcare setting

    i) educate the patient

2. I can locate several competencies in our job descriptions that reflect our mission and the values of the organization.

ASSESSING THE ROLE PLAYED BY EACH DELEGATE

What was it like in your family? Did your mom do the cleaning and the cooking and the yard work? Did dad or grandpa or uncle fix the car? Roles that were standard in the *Leave It to Beaver* or *The Simpsons* eras are no longer useful in the present lifestyle configurations, but no matter how your family or significant-other group is formulated, each person has certain roles. The analogy of the family situation might not fit for all of us as we compare it to work life, but the new flexibility and resiliency we find in family or social roles are characteristics that are also required of us in our organizations as we explore new methods and caregiver job descriptions.

What was your job description in your family of origin? It might not have been written, but it was certainly present. In our healthcare organizations, we must pay close attention to the written as well as the "unwritten" roles given to each worker.

OFFICIAL EXPECTATIONS OF EACH ROLE

Before we explore the underlying issues of what people really are expecting of each other in your workplace, let's take a closer look at the official documents. In Chapter 3, we asked you to examine the practice act for those with whom you work each day.

Do you know the job descriptions for all the workers in your facility and how your state's practice statutes are reflected in the organization's policies? Is it clear what each person is expected to do? How does each role reflect the values and mission of your organization?

With the practice statutes, your organization's mission and/or values statement, and your job descriptions by your side, let's examine how these documents determine the official expectations of each role.

PRACTICE ACTS AND REGULATIONS

As we discussed in Chapter 3, the fundamental expectations of each healthcare worker's job are based on state regulations and rules. In assessing your delegate, these statutes are the necessary framework on which you base your supervision and assignment of the delegate. For example, in New Hampshire there has been a decision to license nursing assistants. Other states (Ohio, for example) have developed specific rules for delegation to assistive personnel. These provide a basis for the tasks that are delegated.

One concern that we have voiced as we travel across the country has been the decision of some state boards of nursing to issue a task list for assistive personnel. Although these lists are often requested by the nurses within the state and seem to be helpful to organizations as they draw up job descriptions, we question any list that would seem to eliminate the licensed nurse's responsibility and accountability for delegating based on his or her assessment of the individual delegate's competency and of the situation and the patient at that specific time. This warning has been seconded by the National Council of State Boards of Nursing (NCSBN) (Simpkins, 1997, p. 1).

> By creating task lists for UAPs (unlicensed assistive personnel), an unofficial scope of practice is created. . . . Training of UAPs is not based upon the notion that such individuals will be performing

activities independently. . . . Task lists suggest no need for delegation, as the UAP already has a list of nursing activities he or she
may perform without waiting for the delegation process. But what
happens when the condition of a client changes? Is the UAP with
75 hours or more of training astute enough to recognize there has
been a change in the client's condition and alert the licensed nurse?

It's not condoned (or common!) for an organization or facility to assign
duties in job descriptions that are beyond the scope of legal practice as
determined by the practice acts of the state. More frequently, however,
facilities can interpret regulations differently or limit scope of legal practice within their organization, or individuals might attempt to practice
beyond the legal and official boundaries.

The NCSBN has responded to questions of competence resulting from
the work of the Pew Commission (see Chapter 2, "Know Your World")
and public concerns regarding continued competence of the nurse and
other healthcare workers due to the number of medical errors (Institute
of Medicine, 2003). Their interdisciplinary and multistate work on determining competency (in conjunction with other professional boards) has
been pivotal in determining the future direction of healthcare worker
competency evaluation and will be covered in detail later in this chapter.
(Don't miss it; these emerging trends will surely affect your practice!)

As you examined your state practice acts and your facility job descriptions, did you find any questions or inconsistencies? (If you are a student,
ask your clinical experience facilities for examples of their job descriptions.) If you found some discrepancies, take time now to answer your
questions by initiating a phone call to your state regulatory board or
discuss the issue with administrative personnel.

Many forces (in the form of official commissions, state boards, and the public) have converged to address this question of competency, a question we hear nurses voice on a daily basis. "How can I be sure the people I am working with are competent? How can I be sure they are still competent, even if they were once 'checked off' or tested?"

THE QUESTION OF COMPETENCY: EVALUATING AND MAINTAINING FROM A REGULATORY PERSPECTIVE

As referred to earlier in this chapter, the rapid changes
in healthcare roles have provided impetus for challenging the old methods used to initially assess the
competency of a new worker from a state licensing
perspective. Technology has moved forward very
quickly, new roles have developed, and delivery
systems have left both regulatory agencies and the

public concerned about the accountability of the individual practitioner, the employer, and regulatory boards in protecting the public. In 1994, the Nursing Practice and Education Committee of the NCSBN published the Model Nursing Practice Act and Model Nursing Administrative Rules to act as a guide to some standardization for national competency of licensed nurses (RNs, LPNs); they revised the document in 2002 (NCSBN, 2002). The Pew Health Professions Commission (1995) Taskforce on Health Care Workforce Regulation recommended that states should standardize practice entry requirements and that state regulatory boards should evaluate continuing competency requirements as well as continuing or improving their disciplinary processes. In a report published by the Citizen Advocacy Center, the concern was voiced that the public cannot be confident that healthcare professionals remain competent as they deliver care (NCSBN, 1997a). In response to the Institute of Medicine (2003) recommendations that evidence-based teaching methods and curricula in health professions education would be evaluated for outcomes, recent graduate RNs described discomfort with their competencies in the areas of direct care and medication administration to larger groups of patients than they handled as students, in delegation and supervising others, and in determining the point at which a physician should be consulted and how to communicate with the MD (NCSBN, 2006a).

Regulatory boards for all professions are required to provide assurance to the public that the practitioner (whether a physician, nursing assistant, or speech therapist) has met entry-level competency standards, that those who do not will be disciplined in a timely manner, and that this information is available to the public. To approach these responsibilities in a systematic manner, the regulatory boards must take the following steps:

1. Define competence.
2. Set standards of competence.
3. Evaluate the practitioners.
4. Identify measurable behaviors that demonstrate competence.
5. Implement a system to discipline those who fail to meet those standards (NCSBN, 1997a).

Defining Competence

The NCSBN further clarifies the process of demonstrating competence by establishing requirements for licensure at certain stages (see **Exhibit 7–1**): at entry level into practice,

> Competence is defined as "the application of knowledge and the interpersonal, decision-making, and psychomotor skills expected for the practice role, within the context of public health, safety, and welfare" (NCSBN, 1997a, p. 5).

at renewal of licensure, when reentering practice after extended time out of practice, and after disciplinary action (NCSBN, 1997a, p. 7). Three processes, including competence development, competence assessment, and competence conduct, are defined.

EXHIBIT 7-1 Licensure Competence Requirements

	Competence Development	Competence Assessment	Competence Conduct
Initial entry	Graduation from an approved program	NCLEX	Board review upon application; discipline check
Continuing authority to practice at renewal	Verified practice during authorization period	Subject to random/targeted group assessment; board-identified mechanism, e.g., peer review, professional certification, professional portfolio, testing, retesting	Board review upon application; discipline check
Reentry to practice after absence	Refresher education	Retest, e.g., NCLEX	Board review upon application; discipline check
After discipline	Board-identified mechanism, e.g., continuing education	Board-identified mechanism	Board review upon application; discipline check

Source: Used with permission of the National Council of State Boards of Nursing, Inc., Chicago, Illinois.

"Competence Development: the method by which a practitioner gains, maintains, or refines practice knowledge, skills, and abilities . . . through [a] formal education program, continuing education, clinical practice, and is expected to continue throughout the practitioner's career . . .

Competence Assessment can be accomplished through peer review, professional portfolio, professional certification, testing, re-testing. . . . Identified triggers could be used . . . a practitioner in independent or isolated practice, multiple jobs in a short period of time, prior discipline . . .

Competence Conduct refers to health and conduct expectations which may be evaluated through reports from the individual practitioner, employer reports, and discipline checks." (NCSBN, 1997a)

The Interprofessional Workgroup on Health Professions Regulation (IWHPR) Views on the Licensure and Regulation of Health Care Professionals (November 1996) defines competence similarly:

Professional competence is "the application of knowledge and skills in interpersonal relations, decision-making and physical performance consistent with the professional's practice role and public health, welfare and safety considerations." (IWHPR, 1996)

This workgroup recognizes that the standards or requirements for competence are changing over time as the practitioner specializes or as other factors (technology, overlap of scopes of practice) influence the roles. It has also indicated that uniformity throughout the states should be encouraged but not mandated and that there must be a distinction between initial, minimum practice standards and those of ongoing competence, and that each should be measured (IWHPR, 1996, p. 6). This group includes audiology, chiropractic, medical lab technology, dentistry, dietetics, medicine, nursing, nursing home administration, occupational therapy, optometry, pharmacy, physical therapy, physician assistants, respiratory care, social work, and speech-language pathology, adding up to over 4 million healthcare practitioners (IWHPR, 1996, p. 1).

Both the NCSBN and the IWHPR agree that the primary responsibility for remaining current and competent lies with the individual professional and that each person must ensure his or her own competence through choosing education or other means for maintenance and improvement of skills, as well as participating in peer review and by acting on any conduct by other practitioners that would indicate incompetent performance.

Setting Standards

The NCSBN has led the way in setting standards and in testing nurses by formulating and administering the NCLEX RN and NCLEX PN (LPN or LVN) examinations for entry into practice. It has based its work on research into job analysis of newly licensed nurses, both RNs and LPNs, and the input of educators and expert clinical practitioners across the United States. Model nurse aide administrative rules were published by the National League for Nursing in 1990, and a Nurse Aide Competency Evaluation Program (NACEP) was established in 1991. In 1997, development began on a national nurse aide assessment program, which includes the strengths of the Assessment Systems, Inc. National Nurse Aide Examination and the NACEP and is based on 1995 research into job analysis of the reality of nurse aide roles in the United States (Wiesmiller, 1997). The NCSBN analyzes nurse aide practice every 3 years to determine changes in the actual tasks that are performed by nursing assistants across the country (NCSBN, 1998). The Model Nursing Practice Act was also revised in 2004. Practice changes such as nursing assistants delivering medications in select settings such as assisted living are increasing (Reinhardt, Young, Kane, & Quinn, 2006).

In addition to state practice commissions and national boards, specialty nursing associations have made recommendations regarding RN and assistive personnel roles. The Society of Gastroenterology Nurses and Associates (SGNA) delineated the roles of assistive personnel in their practice arena. In a revision of their Position Statement (2006), they list competencies for UAPs and strongly encourage them to complete the GI Associate's skills validation test and achieve the title of GTS (GI Technical Specialist) (SGNA Practice Committee, 2006). The Emergency Nurses Association (ENA) had recommended in 1994 that triage and other processes using clinical judgment would not be delegated to UAPs (ENA, 1994). In reality, Zimmerman noted

2 years later that 85% of the RNs surveyed stated RN professional judgment in the emergency department was being performed by unlicensed assistive personnel (Zimmerman, 1996). However, the practice of triage by UAPs continues, and in 2004, a study by Paulson showed that a triage system using nurses (RNs and LPNs) rather than UAPs resulted in wait times being decreased by 73 minutes, and patients leaving without being seen were reduced by 85% (Paulson, 2004.) Evidence-based practice would seem to support clear delineation of assigned competencies related to educational preparation and clinical outcomes. (We also recommend that you consult your own nursing specialty organization to review the most recent guidelines.)

As we have previously discussed, the setting and circumstances are fundamental when determining possible skills to delegate. For example, assistive personnel administer medications (when certified) in assisted living, long-term care, and some home care settings in some states. LPNs often lead teams of rehabilitation aides in long-term care (Reinhardt, et al., 2006).

For RNs, three standards for competence have been developed:

+ Apply knowledge and skills at the level required for a particular situation.
+ Demonstrate responsibility and accountability for practice and decisions.
+ Restrict and/or accommodate practice if an RN cannot safely perform essential functions of the nursing practice role (NCSBN, 1997b).

The NCSBN's expected behaviors for individual nurses include the caveats that nurses must attain competence and must be responsible for evaluating and maintaining competence according to the current job requirements and any change in practice setting (NCSBN, 1997c). The expected behaviors for individual practitioners amplify the three general standards with specific and measurable performance, with the methods or sources for maintaining that competency included after each standard. (See **Exhibit 7–2.**) In 2007, the NCSBN continued to develop a plan for evaluating continued competence in nurses, with a collaboration of educators, employers, and other professional regulatory agencies, and has termed this Continued Competence Regulatory Model (NCSBN, 2007).

EXHIBIT 7–2   Individual Competence Evaluation

1. Apply knowledge and skills at the level required for a particular practice situation.
   a. Identify role expectations through
      - position descriptions
      - review of literature
      - networking
      - observe, shadow another nurse
   b. Determine individual level of knowledge and skills needed for the role.
      - skills inventory
      - assessment test
      - cognitive appraisal
      - peer review
   c. Identify strengths and learning needed.
      - cognitive comparison of role expectations and individual abilities
   d. Develop and implement a learning plan.
      - job or role orientation
      - formal or continuing education
      - independent study
      - refresher course
      - precepted learning experience
      - simulated learning experience
      - other experiential learning
   e. Evaluate the effectiveness of learning and its impact on the practice role.
      - reassessment (formal or informal)
      - testing
      - peer review
      - performance evaluation
2. Exercise sound nursing judgment.
   a. Synthesize knowledge and skills relevant to client needs in carrying out the nursing role.
   b. Delegate nursing activities appropriately.
   c. Identify cause and effect relationships.
   d. Recognize limits of knowledge and skill.
   e. Use resources appropriately.
   f. Monitor outcomes.
3. Employ personal principles reflective of professional, ethical, and legal standards of practice.
   a. Articulate an awareness of regulatory, professional, and ethical standards.

- Nursing Practice Act
- American Nurses Association Code of Ethics

4. Ensure that client welfare prevails.
   a. Articulate respect for the social, cultural, and spiritual diversity of clients.
   b. Maintain therapeutic boundaries.
   c. Ensure that clients' needs are articulated.

5. Enable client participation in healthcare decisions and outcomes.
   a. Facilitate client decision making by providing information.
   b. Facilitate the identification of choices and possible outcomes.
   c. Support client decisions.

6. Participate in professional activities that support the nursing knowledge and skills needed for safe and effective practice.
   a. Develop professional growth and development criteria recognizing individual level of experience.
   b. Conduct regular evaluation of professional development needs. (See standard 1.)
   c. Select professional development activities based upon identified needs.
   d. Review own professional development portfolio.

7. Collaborate with appropriate professionals to attain desired client healthcare outcomes.
   a. Differentiate nursing functions from functions of other providers.
   b. Communicate with the healthcare team.
   c. Assess the effectiveness of referrals.
   d. Monitor outcomes by assessment of the impact of collaboration on health promotion, maintenance, and illness prevention for the client.

8. Recognize the relationship of personal cognitive and functional abilities to safe and effective practice.
   a. Identify abilities necessary for the essential functions of a nursing practice role.
   b. Identify accommodations needed to ensure safe and effective practice.
   c. Limit practice based on abilities and accommodations.

9. Demonstrate responsibility and accountability for nursing practice decisions and actions.
   a. Identify the legal and ethical obligations of the profession.
   b. Answer for one's own actions and decisions.

Source: National Council of State Boards of Nursing, "Individual Competence Evaluation," Assuring Competence: Attachment One (Chicago: NCSBN, 1997), 1–6.

ACCOUNTABILITY FOR COMPETENCE

Although we have already established that each practitioner, no matter the role, is accountable for maintenance of his or her own competence, the NCSBN has offered some guidelines regarding the accountability of the regulatory boards, the employer, the individual, and the educator. **Figure 7–1** demonstrates the complexity of maintaining safe practice of myriad practitioners from entry into practice through the rapid changes in practice inherent in health care today. The model places the consumer of care in the center, emphasizing the real reason behind all this focus on competence.

JOB DESCRIPTIONS

As described in the previous discussion about accountabilities for the employer, organizations must incorporate state standards into institutional policies. These policies, coming in the form of job descriptions, have many structures and can be based on competencies or standards, performance criteria, the nursing process, or specific required behaviors or responsibilities. These documents can double as competency checklists or as performance review tools. Job descriptions can be considered a type of contract between the employee and the management team to perform a given role as specified within the written information, which will include such topics as the necessary qualifications, reporting relationships, scope of responsibilities, and a position summary discussing the overall role. In unionized environments, the union contract for each type of worker will also influence the roles played by each union employee and should be in agreement with the job description.

CHECKPOINT 7-2

Pat reviewed his state practice act for LPNs and found that there was nothing specified as to IV therapy. It also stated that the LPN acts as an assistant to the RN in completing the nursing process. However, he noted that LPNs were monitoring IVs and giving IV medications in his hospital. Many LPNs functioned just like RNs as primary caregivers. He wondered how this could be possible or legal.

What do you think might be occurring in this hospital? What should Pat do?

See the end of the chapter for the answers.

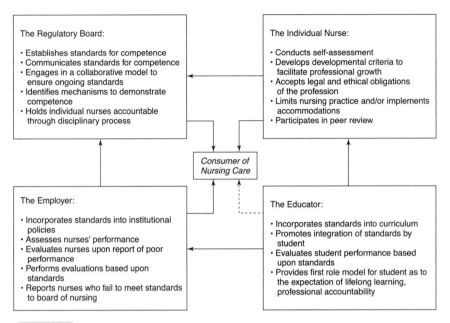

The Regulatory Board:

- Establishes standards for competence
- Communicates standards for competence
- Engages in a collaborative model to ensure ongoing standards
- Identifies mechanisms to demonstrate competence
- Holds individual nurses accountable through disciplinary process

The Individual Nurse:

- Conducts self-assessment
- Develops developmental criteria to facilitate professional growth
- Accepts legal and ethical obligations of the profession
- Limits nursing practice and/or implements accommodations
- Participates in peer review

Consumer of Nursing Care

The Employer:

- Incorporates standards into institutional policies
- Assesses nurses' performance
- Evaluates nurses upon report of poor performance
- Performs evaluations based upon standards
- Reports nurses who fail to meet standards to board of nursing

The Educator:

- Incorporates standards into curriculum
- Promotes integration of standards by student
- Evaluates student performance based upon standards
- Provides first role model for student as to the expectation of lifelong learning, professional accountability

FIGURE 7-1 Competence Accountability. *Source:* Used with permission of the National Council of State Boards of Nursing, Inc., Chicago, Illinois.

For our purposes here, turn now to the job summaries and lists of duties or responsibilities you've assembled from your clinical areas. Generally, RN job descriptions will contain such descriptors as:

- provides patient care, utilizing the nursing process
- assists in coordinating patient care activities
- acts as a communication liaison among departments and with physicians
- functions in a leadership role
- is accountable for the standards of nursing care
- assesses, plans, implements, evaluates, teaches

As organizations revise care delivery systems, job descriptions for the RN are beginning to include such statements as

- delegates appropriately and directs the activities of other team members
- effectively supervises team members
- evaluates care given by team members and gives feedback
- actively engages in solving problems in the organization

Job descriptions of assistive personnel reflect their dependence on the leadership of the RN:

+ works under the supervision of the RN and receives written and/or oral assignments and direction
+ gathers data for planning the care of the team's patients
+ reports appropriately and in a timely manner to the RN who is accountable for the care of those patients
+ performs various patient care and attendant activities under the direction of the RN
+ participates in planning, implementation, evaluation, and modification of the plan of care by sharing information and reviewing care administered

Duties or specific responsibilities are often outlined. These lists will help you determine what tasks can be assigned to a specific delegate when competency and understanding of the assignment are ascertained.

Examples of some of the duties listed for assistive personnel might be:

+ performs oral/nasal suctioning
+ assists with admission, transfer, or discharge as determined by the RN
+ measures and records intake, output, and vital signs
+ performs tasks such as bathing, feeding, and providing post-mortem care
+ assists in sponge count procedures as instituted by the RN
+ observes patient carefully for significant changes
+ maintains and orders equipment and supplies
+ performs CPR under supervision of an RN or MD
+ assists with bowel and bladder retraining

If the job descriptions in your organization do not reflect what is actually happening in your department or facility with your patients, ask some questions!

VALIDATED COMPETENCIES: THE ORGANIZATIONAL PERSPECTIVE

Many of you might have enjoyed the opportunity to supervise the completion of a competency checklist for a peer, an orienting employee, or assistive personnel. Often attached to the job description or as a part of the orientation packet, these checklists are based on what the state law says about scope of practice, how the organization interprets those rules within its system in the form of job descriptions, and the education or orientation attended by the employee. The portion of the state regulatory information that describes the subject matter for the educational program, as well as standards and competencies expected for the beginning graduate of an educational program, might provide a starting point for competency checklists for new employees.

For an example of what is commonly required in some assistive roles, let's review the State of Arizona's project in which the Arizona Department of Education (1985) published a validated competency list for nursing assistants, LPNs, and associate degree RNs. Fifty competencies were expected for the beginning nursing assistant, each divided into more specific behaviors. In this document, nursing assistants were expected to be competent in such skills as:

+ collecting sputum and stool specimens
+ testing urine using routine methods
+ applying protective restraints, Ace bandages, flexible abdominal binders
+ applying ostomy appliances and irrigating established colostomies
+ taking vital signs
+ giving a cleansing enema

These competencies are consistent with the Standards of Function for the Nurse Aide first published by the NCSBN in 1990. The NCSBN warns that enemas might be delegated to nursing assistants but that sterile procedures should not be delegated (NCSBN, 1990). These guidelines have been a basis for the adoption of rules by states. Although multistate licensure is being implemented on a state-by-state basis, (see Chapter 3, "Know Your Practice"), it appears as of the writing of this book that each state might continue to maintain overall responsibility for interpreting statute, issuing rules that explain the statute, and being accountable for granting licenses, dealing with complaints, and performing disciplinary acts.

Validated competencies (Arizona Department of Education, 1985) for LPNs numbered 72, and included such skills as:

+ sterile technique
+ administering medications and IVs, including calculation of infusing rate and regulation of gavages and irrigation using previously inserted GI tubes

- timing contractions and measuring and recording fetal heart tones
- performing normal newborn care
- recognizing substance abuse in the child and adolescent

At the current time, LPN and LVN (licensed vocational nurse) practice and APRN (advanced-practice RNs) regulations vary widely state by state (NCSBN, 2005, 2006b). Surveys that were assembled in the 2005 Business Book by the NCSBN showed that about half of the states allow LPNs to delegate, and 33 stated that assigning was considered to be within LPN practice (NCSBN, 2005). IVs, blood administration, and TPN (total parenteral nutrition) were limited based on requiring additional education, whether the medication was IV push or through a central line (NCSBN, 2005), and duties such as independent care planning are normally precluded (NCSBN, 2005). It is clear that in all states LPNs must be supervised and cannot practice independently. Advanced-practice RNs, such as clinical nurse specialists, midwives, nurse anesthetists, and nurse practitioners, lack uniformity from state to state in terms of prescriptive authority, the schedule of drugs that can be prescribed, and criteria and standards for certification. The vision of the NCSBN is increased regulatory consistency, with boards of nursing being the sole regulators of APRNs (NCSBN, 2006b).

Documenting Competencies

Seminar participants often ask us clarifying questions such as, "Since Mrs. Fujini's bowel was perforated when Sally gave her that enema, how can I support or document that I was correct in asking Sally to perform that procedure?" When you are familiar with the job descriptions of a nursing assistant in your organization and when you also know that Sally was "checked off" on giving a cleansing enema, the job descriptions and competency checklist are your documentation. If Sally had also been performing enemas without problems, and if in fact you recently observed Sally's technique when you happened to make a home visit while Sally was performing this skill, even better! When you assessed the patient and there were no potential problems, your decision to ask Sally to give Mrs. Fujini the enema followed the delegation process to the letter.

Some facilities ask new staff to keep their competency checklist with them, especially during orientation, as an aid to the delegating RN. Other organizations have developed so many new, multiskilled worker roles that they have created a laminated skills checklist for these cross-trained workers to keep in their pockets at work.

THE IMPACT OF THE MISSION ON JOB ROLES

We've spent a fair amount of time focusing on job responsibilities and the details of roles within your team. Earlier in the chapter, we asked you to determine how the mission was reflected in your job descriptions.

As discussed in Chapter 4, a mission statement can include such phrases as the following:

+ provide high-quality, cost-effective, integrated health services that support independence and are responsive to the needs of individuals, families, and the community
+ promote wellness, absence of disease, comfort, education, and independence by the collaborative healthcare team in an environment that is responsive to the needs of the public, as well as taking into consideration fiscal accountability and responsibility

Values statements can include such concepts as:

+ the respect and dignity afforded patients, the public, and employees, with an emphasis on communication skills
+ a culture of professional growth
+ proactive leadership in shaping change

Examine your facility's mission and/or values. Do you see an emphasis on collaboration, high quality, cost effectiveness? Is the quality of personal relationships among the interdisciplinary team inferred, if not directly stated? If so, you'll recognize the related performance criteria in the job descriptions translated as:

+ demonstrates positive interpersonal communication skills that enhance patient care and the functioning of the interdisciplinary team
+ uses assertive language in interpersonal relationships
+ participates actively in solving problems
+ maintains confidentiality
+ effectively utilizes human and material resources in planning and implementing care

Certainly, all of us seek some kind of personal fulfillment in our jobs. This fulfillment comes not from the actual jobs that we do (is it very fulfilling to fill out the paperwork or do mouth care?) but from why we are doing the work we do. The why is closely connected with our personal purpose and how that purpose complements the mission of our organization.

+ responds positively to guidance and feedback
+ performs assigned work without discrimination on the basis of age, sexual preference, national origin, race, economic position, religion, disability, or disease

Why are we spending time detailing these parts of the official roles? Because you, as the supervisory RN, must understand fully the impact of the job descriptions and other organizational policies as you match jobs to the delegates and evaluate their performance. This information is necessary not only for making assignments but for giving feedback to your team. We are also applauding steps that organizations are taking to reinforce the importance of emotional intelligence and the positive interpersonal behaviors of their employees. As an RN, it is your job to lead, and leading requires the ability to create a climate of motivation, clarity of expectations, vision, planning, and feedback so that the team can be successful. These positive interpersonal relationship and leadership skills are vital to you, your team, and your patients.

UNOFFICIAL EXPECTATIONS OF EACH ROLE

In addition to the official expectations based on the state laws or regulations are the real expectations within your facility. If there is a discrepancy between what the state regulations say, what the job descriptions explain, and what really happens, there is a serious problem. Workers should not be performing beyond their roles in any case. Keep in mind the supervisory and evaluative responsibilities that are present in your state nurse practice act and that were discussed in Chapter 3.

> As the supervisory RN, you must know whether the tasks your delegate agrees to complete are within the state practice act as well as the facility's job descriptions.

CHECKPOINT 7–3

You've been working with a new multiskilled worker in your neonatal ICU. This person is a respiratory therapist who has been cross trained as a phlebotomist and nursing assistant. He is in school for LPN licensure. He seems to be doing quite well clinically but has been avoiding performing the care of infants who are HIV positive or are the babies of "crack" mothers (cocaine abusers). How does this employee's performance reflect that he is not fulfilling his job description if he is working in your facility?

See the end of the chapter for the answers.

However, there are often other "gray areas" concerning what each individual can expect of his or her coworkers. For example, if you as an RN expect that the home health aide will telephone you immediately if the patient is complaining that the current pain control isn't effective, and

> Often, the "unmet expectations" that cause anger and uncomfortable team relationships stem from silent "unofficial expectations."

that doesn't happen, you will be justifiably angry. The operational definition of anger is "unmet expectations." (We covered this in detail when we talked about the grief process in Chapter 5.) If a nursing assistant in the long-term care facility expects that you as an RN will be physically involved in helping him or her with hygienic care on a regular basis and you aren't doing that, he or she will be angry also. In the acute care arena, unresolved issues such as those in the following list will continue to cause conflict:

- Who is responsible for answering the phone?
- Who is responsible for answering the call lights?
- Who is responsible for talking with the physician?
- Who is responsible for communicating with the family members about code status decisions?
- Who has the right to sit at the nursing station? For what reason?
- Whose patients are these, really?
- Who communicates what to whom, when?
- Who really has the authority to "make" you do what you are asked to do?
- Who should clean up the equipment or break rooms?

Understanding what each job entails, discussing your expectations within the group, and being realistic about what's reasonable to expect will go a long way to promoting better teamwork.

There is a practical strategy for resolving these issues of "unofficial expectations." Each group must define its expectations of the other groups and discuss them in an open forum. We suggest that this be done within a staff meeting. If you are unable to do this in a more public and less threatening way (such as in a team meeting), then you must clarify expectations on a personal basis. For example, consider the last few times you've been angry or frustrated with a coworker. What expectation wasn't met by that coworker? It's time to clear the air and clarify what you expect. For example, "When you left the unit today with three patients left on their bedpans and didn't tell anyone, I felt concerned about the patients' skin breakdown. Tell me about what happened today." (Listen to response.) "I was expecting that you would come to tell me before you left for break or ask someone else to help

If you feel someone is angry with you, clarify his or her expectations. For example, "I noticed a few minutes ago that you sighed loudly when I gave you the same assignment as yesterday. I am confused about whether you are unhappy with the assignment or if something else is wrong. Let's talk about it so we're all on the same wavelength."

those patients. Let's talk about how you can be certain that patients are not left without someone responsible for getting them off the bedpan." (See Chapter 8 on assertive communication.)

You might wish to use Checkpoint 7–4 in your staff meeting and share the responses. You'll find that some people focus on the very concrete tasks ("passes medications"), and some will discuss issues that relate to organizational values ("shows respect to the public and coworkers; calls me by name"). You might wish to ask the questions in Checkpoint 7-4 of each other within your work group on a personal basis.

CHECKPOINT 7–4

(Fill in the blanks now for your own information, and plan to do this exercise as a group.)

I expect RNs to _____

_____

I expect LPNs to _____

_____

I expect CNAs to _____

_____

I expect patient care assistants to _____

_____

I expect the secretary to _____

_____

I expect _____ (fill in the blank) to _____

_____

I expect our boss to _____

_____

On a person-to-person basis:

1. Have I been performing the way you expect me to?

2. Are there things I have or haven't been doing that sometimes bother you?

3. In what ways am I doing a great job?

4. In what ways could I improve the way I do my job?

5. How could I help you perform your job better by the way I do mine?

6. Have you been disappointed about anything in your job?

The following list shows some of the most common responses that have been given by RNs and certified nurses' aides (CNAs) concerning their expectations of RNs:

- Competence.
- Do your job.
- Be a troubleshooter.
- Be an advocate.
- Call workers by name.
- Respect team members.
- Communicate progress and inform team.
- Sit at the desk: this means the RN is doing charting, coordination of care, problem solving.
- Share plan for shift clearly.
- Instructions should be clear and complete.
- Answer lights.
- Be courteous.
- Teach other team members.
- Assess.
- Evaluate.
- Plan.
- Chart.
- Trust others.
- Organize care.
- Give feedback.
- Give clear, concise reports.

The following are some expectations of CNAs reported by CNAs and RNs:

- Respect each other.
- Attend report.

- Find out if you have questions.
- Communicate progress, changes.
- Take initiative but ask questions.
- Answer lights.
- Be an extra pair of hands.
- Be honest.
- Trust.
- Be motivated.
- Follow RN orders.
- Be positive and cooperative.
- Work as a team.
- Be part of problem solving.
- Organize work.
- Beds.
- Baths.
- Vital signs.
- Don't talk to patient about diagnosis or teach.
- Don't have to clean up after RNs in kitchen or break room.
- Okay to sit at desk if patient work is done or to chart.

Talking about these personal expectation issues might seem like a risky process. However, not much is gained without risk. Throughout this process, you will find yourself understanding each other more fully. You'll clarify what one another's jobs should be, and you'll find many fewer conflicts will get in the way of excellent care of your patients or clients. Change frustration and anger to relief as you deal with those trying situations that make your job more difficult than it has to be!

ASSESSING THE DELEGATE'S STRENGTHS

Think back to your family. Do you know the strengths of your family members? Who was best at doing the vacuuming? Certainly you had years to get to know each other, and this lengthy process is not always available in health care. In each case, as we look at assessing the qualities of the delegate, we'll focus on how to determine the competencies of those you work with daily and those who are short-term help.

Before we consider methods of assessing strengths, it's important to remember why we are doing this. Think now of one reason you'd like to know your delegate's best qualities.

_____

_____

_____

_____

Perhaps asking this basic question seems too obvious. When we ask nurses around the country this question, it's common for participants to consider the good of the patients but rare for them to consider the positive effects for themselves or their delegates. You might have come up with other reasons, but we think several are compelling for all of us who are engaged in treating or caring for patients.

> The first, most obvious reason to consider your delegate's strengths is that when people are using their strengths to perform their care duties, the outcomes for the clients are the most effective. The second reason is that people grow when their strengths are recognized and utilized for the good of patient care. The third reason is that your ability to lead is enhanced because there are fewer needless worries each day when people are working within their areas of competency.

Let's look at a couple of examples.

1. Do you remember the last time your supervisor gave you an evaluation or yearly performance review? What do you remember most about it? We are willing to bet you remember the competencies your supervisor checked as "needs improvement." Human beings tend to remember the critical before they remember the positive. Think back, though, about a well-earned compliment you were given. Perhaps your boss or colleague said, "I've noticed that in your caseload you are especially effective in working with families of those who are dying. All of us are impressed with your ability to communicate clearly with them and help them through the grief process." That feels pretty good, doesn't it? And the next time you take care of another similar case, you'll find that you redouble your efforts to do a fine job. You might even think more about the methods you use to be so effective and find that you are able to help others apply the same principles.

2. At Memorial Hospital, a nursing assistant had worked for years on the plastic surgery and burn floor. When she began to float, she was able to alert the RNs on the other floors to special proce-

dures and information she'd learned as "tricks of the trade" in her past clinical areas. Although many of these were less experienced nurses and could have been threatened by her knowledge, they were anxious to learn from the CNA. This sharing of information encouraged a climate of mutual respect in a situation that could have been difficult.

3. The Visiting Nurse Service employed a nurse who had been quite negative in her outlook for years. She had been married now for the third time to a person with a substance abuse problem. She finally realized there was a pattern to her life and joined Al-Anon (a program for the families of alcohol-dependent persons). She learned about her codependent tendencies and further delved into all the literature about alcoholism and the community support available. Because of her specialized knowledge, she became the group expert on alcoholism, from treatment of the delirium tremens to the best programs for aftercare in the area. As she found that her home life was improving and found herself to be a valued member of the team, her entire attitude changed. She was making lemonade out of the lemons she had collected during her life, and it helped her grow as she shared from her experience.

The Delegate's Strengths: Benefits and Warnings

We are clear on all the reasons why strengths are important. When you reflected on how you are utilizing your own strengths and those of your delegates, you might have wondered how to discover the "gems" under the rough-hewn exteriors of those with whom you work. How do we determine those sterling qualities? As we discussed in our family example, we determine them from what we observe and hear. You see that Bob is a good cook and enjoys doing the cooking. On your unit or within your work group, if you have not been able to observe strengths in action, then ask. You might first ask someone, "What do you like to do best?" This is often a good indication of what that person believes he or she does best. If you haven't received enough information yet, ask the delegate, "What do you feel the most comfortable doing? What are you best at doing?"

For short-term workers such as floats, agency people, or others you might work with only for a short period of time, remember to just come out with it. Ask them what they are good at. Most people know.

A caveat is necessary, however. We have spent time focusing on the strengths, and we have established that they certainly are important. However, if people always do what they feel comfortable doing, they will not grow. Be careful not to get into a rut and allow people to become apathetic from a lack of challenge. (We realize that health care is not a boring, slow job and is full of challenges daily, but we feel it is necessary to remind people of the potential hazards of becoming too comfortable in one way of doing things.)

A related issue is cross training. An excellent example of what can happen is the case of the hospital that provides multiskill training for some individuals who had been phlebotomists, nursing assistants, EKG technicians, and housekeepers. The training began in the fall, as RNs, LPNs, and the new patient care technicians learned to draw blood. The next summer the physicians began complaining because the patients' arms were all bruised again, just as they were when everyone was learning the skill. Further problem solving showed that when people were "checked off" as being competent, those who were best at drawing blood (those who had worked in the lab for years) began to take over that task primarily. When summer came, one patient care tech was on vacation, another was on leave, and another was off due to a back injury, and none of the remaining staff had maintained competence in phlebotomy!

Another warning: Some people perceive that they are skilled at tasks or processes, but you might observe that they aren't. The RN who is supervising the group cannot afford to take at face value a statement of "I'm good at doing brain surgery." You might also find yourself falling into the trap of the "halo or horn" effect. The person who seems to be an all-out super crackerjack cannot be perfect in all areas. The delegate whose personality rubs you the wrong way is not really the devil in disguise. He or she has at least one or two strengths also. All of the assessment data regarding the delegate, the patient situation, and the work that needs to be completed are essential for your decision making.

ASSESSING THE DELEGATE'S WEAKNESSES

The potential weaknesses of the delegates are the most frightening aspect for the RNs we've talked with across the United States. They are afraid that their license is on the line and that they will lose their licensure if a mistake is made by one of their delegates.

Remember that supervision means you will provide guidance for the accomplishment of a nursing task or activity, with initial direction and periodic inspection of the actual task or activity, and that the total nursing care of the individual

Keep in mind the need to vary assignments enough to sustain any cross training for long-term flexibility.

You are accountable for your decision to delegate. The delegate must decide whether to accept the delegation and then is accountable for his or her performance in carrying out your instructions.

remains the responsibility and accountability of the RN. The burden of determining the competency of the person who will perform the work and of evaluating the situation remains with the licensed nurse (NCSBN, 1990).

It is therefore very important to determine a delegate's competency, strengths, and weaknesses. We have already addressed the state regulations that limit practice, the job descriptions of your facility, and the competency checklists that can be used by your organization. These are all excellent guides for your decision making.

At this point, however, the RN must determine the competency of that one individual for a specific set of circumstances for one day, one shift, one caseload. There is no exact scientific formula for this. Once again, your decision rests on your nursing judgment.

CHECKPOINT 7-5

How are you now utilizing your own and your coworkers' strengths in the way you divide and apportion your work? Think about your last week of work and a few examples of how your delegates' strengths were used effectively.

If you were unable to come up with situations, spend a few moments thinking about the strengths of each of your coworkers and how they could be utilized for positive future impact.

There is not a profession on this earth that allows its practitioners to avoid making these kinds of decisions. An attorney's decision to plea bargain or to try for acquittal for his client based on his knowledge of the situation affects all involved. An accountant's decision to try a new tactic to use impending tax laws to the client's best advantage, drawing up a limited partnership agreement, is based on her best judgment of the future and her past education and experience. As a professional RN, you are called upon daily to make these types of decisions many times. You decide when to call the physician, when to approach the family for a code status, how to plan therapy for the newly diagnosed schizophrenic, how much IV pressor to administer to reduce the potential for renal insufficiency.

For the short-term worker within your organization, the person that you don't know well, you might ask the following questions: "What do you feel you are best at doing? Have you completed these kinds of procedures before at our facility? There is a new procedure written up for this task. I'll get it for you and we'll go over it. Do you have any questions now? Let me tell you about our patients in more detail. I'm on this beeper if you have any questions later on."

Some organizations that use floats or short-term help frequently have developed "float cards" or other evaluative tools for the agency or internal float pool. These allow the RN to give written information to the person's immediate boss for positive and negative feedback or to determine learning needs. They are not a substitute for verbal discussion with the delegate at that time, however. Feedback and communication will be covered in more detail in Chapters 10 and 11.

> Your nursing judgment is based on your assessment of the delegate, the situation, and your past experience and is one of the reasons you are being paid as a professional. "Judgment is a process of forming an opinion or evaluation of a situation arrived at by reasoning, discerning and comparing from premised or general principles" (NCSBN, 1986, p. 7).

For those colleagues who are within your workforce on a general basis, how have you assessed their weaknesses in the past? You might be aware of their weaknesses from several sources:

+ from personal observation as you have supervised them or followed them
+ from the competency checklist
+ from asking them for input as to what they feel uncomfortable doing or what they need to learn more about
+ from the "grapevine"

Let's look first at the "grapevine." The grapevine can be valuable in that you might be aware of a potential need for increased supervision if you have heard that someone is "a quart low on energy." However, beware of the grapevine. Most nurses have heard of situations in which a new staff member was branded by a person who didn't like students or didn't approve of some aspect of the staff member's personality, and a negative image was spread across the organization. Remember that an open but observant and listening attitude is the most useful.

This kind of communication will reap rewards in the future. For example, a new

> Asking the person for input is extremely important and can be the most simple way to uncover potential problems. An atmosphere that allows people to be imperfect, having some space for growth, is essential.

graduate might be frightened to death of patients with tracheotomies, but after being guided in caring for them, that staff member might be the most careful and the most well prepared to work with that type of client. Use your experience and judgment, and open your mouth and ask people if they are uncomfortable with any aspects of their assignments. For example, if you're working on a pediatric unit and there is a cerebral palsy patient who has a special feeding and needs to be fed, what will you ask the nursing assistant who is going to help with feedings today? "Have you ever worked with dysphagia feeding before? I'll show you today, and we'll do it together until you are comfortable with it. I'll have to check on the suction apparatus as well."

Use your competency checklists and job descriptions! Find a place for team members to keep them so they can be responsible for having them available for your discussions.

What about the problems that you've seen with delegates because you've followed them or observed or heard their actions? These short-comings generally fall into the following categories:

1. They don't understand what is expected of them.
2. They don't understand that their perception of their activities does not fit within your acceptable parameters for behavior.
3. They might have unmet educational needs.
4. They might need more supervision and guidance.
5. They might not care.

Let's look at each of these underlying reasons for performance weaknesses, often aptly called "areas for improvement and growth," and determine your course of action with each.

1. *They don't understand what is expected of them.* Understanding expectations is essential. We have covered this in detail previously in this chapter; when someone doesn't know that it isn't okay to sit at the desk and eat chocolates while others are performing CPR, he or she needs to be told. Some people truly need to be told things that we might suspect "should be" common knowledge. Remember, don't "should" on each other. Clear communication about your expectations is essential. "I expect you to be answering lights when you are not directly involved in the code situation."

2. *They don't understand that their perception of their activities and your assessment do not directly coincide.* As we discussed when we evaluated delegates' strengths, delegates might not recognize

that they are not doing their job the way you believe it should be done. When you find this is the problem, remember to focus on outcomes. Does it make any difference to the patient outcome that John does the bath in a different order or that Pat's charting on the intake and output chart is done after break? It may or may not be significant. Just realize that some of us tend to be a bit set in our ways and have difficulty seeing things done differently, even if it doesn't affect the outcome in any way. Be clear about what you expect and why it makes a difference.

If patient welfare or safety is involved, immediate action must be taken. If you see a CNA giving a medication to a patient (in most states this is not acceptable except in certain long-term care arenas with specially certified CNAs), you should immediately ask the CNA to step out of the room and talk about unlicensed practice, and bring this to the attention of the manager.

3. *They don't know, understand, or have sufficient information.* Some weaknesses might be educational needs. Perhaps the delegate doesn't want to care for AIDS patients because he or she is afraid. If the staff member understands more about the transmission of the disease and attends the mandatory education about HIV, there will be a change in the delegate's behavior and acceptance of the assignment.

4. *They need additional guidance and supervision.* As we discussed in our example of family roles, there are those in our family or social group who need more supervision than others. The spouse who goes to the grocery store and picks up the children at the soccer game might need exact directions and a specific list of items to buy at the supermarket. The roommate who pays the electricity bill might need a reminder when it is due, whereas other roommates might clean out the tub without being reminded. Some of your delegates will take more energy than others in terms of your time and observation.

Remember that there is a bell curve of performance. The majority of people are on the competent level. Some are overachieving "stars" as they go above and beyond the most highly competent and superior ratings in their job descriptions, but there are a few that waver at the marginal performance line. These individuals cause us the most consternation, but because we can't eliminate the possibility that we'll always have one or two (or more) within our staff, we must address how to deal with these marginal performers.

As we talk with nurses across the country, they often tell us that the most difficult part of their work life is dealing with this type of delegate. They often express anger at the managers: "Why doesn't the manager fire this person! She (he) should know that this person isn't performing well!" We then ask, "What have you done about the problem?" Part of your professional role is as patient advocate. You are required to report and to deal with any behavior that would adversely affect your charges: your patients. The nurse manager or other supervisory person must be given the exact data that will assist him or her in dealing effectively with the performance problem. As an RN who supervises others, you must confront any performance that does not fall within legal parameters or job descriptions or that could be detrimental to the patient. Changing the bed in a certain way might be just a personal preference issue, but leaving a confused patient in a bed in high position with the side rails down is unacceptable from a safety standpoint. Again focusing on potential outcomes, how will these behaviors affect the patient care or organizational goals?

As we'll discuss in more detail in Chapter 10, RNs must give their perceptions of the performance to the delegate and send on any information that will be necessary to the manager involved in formal performance counseling.

Let's discuss a difficult situation: that of the staff member who is wavering on the line of competent/incompetent while being assisted to either improve his or her performance or be counseled into another position (one perhaps that won't involve live human beings!). How does the RN supervise this delegate? Very carefully! This person will not be assigned tasks or processes that have been problematic in the past and will often be buddied with a competent person who understands the limitations. The RN must then be very careful to check on the progress of this delegate, observing, assessing, asking questions, and obtaining report information from the delegate more frequently. This type of staff member poses special problems when the staffing is low. Remember that there are other methods of care delivery. If this person can handle vital signs and other housekeeping tasks well, perhaps that is what he or she should be assigned. This situation, although rare, challenges RNs to use all their creativity and innovative approaches to encourage

Working effectively with marginal performers is one of the most challenging aspects of supervising others, but this offensive task is an essential accountability within the supervision process.

the marginal delegate to use all of his or her strengths for the best possible patient care and safety.

5. *They might not seem to care.* This brings us to another parameter we need to be aware of as we assess the delegates: What makes them tick? What motivates them to do their job? We'll explore the delegate's motivation next.

ASSESSING THE DELEGATE'S MOTIVATION

How often have you traveled home from your workplace, wondering why Sue or John ever showed up to work today at all? Why do some staff members bother to come to work when their apparent lack of commitment and energy forces us to push and pull them through the day?

CHECKPOINT 7-6

1. You have noted that Joy, a new LPN (LVN), telephoned a physician for orders yesterday. This is not recognized as the LPN's role in this organization. You realize that Joy:

   a) might not know the role expectations in this facility

   b) might have done this in past jobs and feels competent to do so, no matter what you say about this

   c) probably won't do this again, and you decide not to mention it to her

   d) will need to be told about the expectations and that you might need to give feedback to the nurse manager, depending on her response

2. Zachary, the secretary, has made several transcribing errors today as new residents are being admitted to your Alzheimer's unit. You, as supervisory nurse to Zachary, decide to:

   a) wait until the facility director of nurses hears about the problem

   b) tell the director of nurses

   c) find out if Zach's problem is an educational need

   d) recommend action to the director after first discussing it with Zach

3.   Patty, an experienced worker in your outpatient surgery area, has the combined job of nursing assistance and environmental services (housekeeping). She often interacts with the public, and you've noticed that she sighs loudly as she bends over, making groaning noises that disturb the families. She also seems to need constant direction. You decide to:

a)   let it go. She's not your problem.

b)   ask her about her behavior. Find out if she's having back trouble, and find out if she knows her job description.

c)   determine why she is having trouble finding things to do when there is so much work needing to be done, without accusing her or putting her down.

d)   discuss your findings with her and ask her for some ideas for solutions. Share your conversations with the supervisor.

4.   A float nurse has just come to work with you on your unit. Your nurse manager had given you the feedback that this person has made several errors and is being helped with her problems through the clinical nurse specialist. How will you assess what this person will be able to do today?

a)   Ask her for her competency checklist.

b)   Tell her you're having her work in a nursing assistant role and that's that.

c)   Question her carefully on what she's done before, what she feels comfortable doing. Arrange for someone to be available and for specific checkup times for assessing and assisting.

d)   Call the supervisor and demand a competent person to care for your patients.

See the end of the chapter for the answers.

The motivation of our coworkers becomes a significant issue for the quality of our work lives and certainly becomes essential for our ability to assess our delegates and match them with the work that needs to be done.

Return to your past knowledge of Maslow's hierarchy of needs (Maslow, 1970). In clinical situations, for example, we know that if a family needs food and shelter, these basic needs must be supplied before we educate them about their child's diabetes. In the work situation, we might all come to work for different reasons each day, and often these reasons are related to where we are currently functioning on the hierarchy of needs. **Exhibit 7–3** shows these different levels of need and your possible response, as a supervisor, to employees who function at these levels.

The first step of the hierarchy of needs is that of safety and security needs. Few of us are independently wealthy, and most of us certainly would notice if our paychecks were to disappear, but most of us have other reasons for working in the type of job we choose. Coworkers who are working only for their paycheck so that they can put food on the table and keep a roof over their heads will need to be supervised differently from those who chose health care because they feel an affinity for it. If the only thing that motivates people is getting that paycheck, they need to know that they must fulfill their job expectations for performance to remain employed. Although this might seem to be a "hard-nosed" point to emphasize, as an RN supervising others you must be prepared for such employees. They must know that if they do not fulfill the job requirements, they won't get their paycheck.

> Motivation comes from within the person. You can provide an environment that will encourage growth and excitement, but you can't force a person to be engaged and enthusiastic about the teamwork and the outcomes you are all achieving together.

EXHIBIT 7–3   Levels of Employee Needs and Supervisory Responses

Functioning Level	Your Response	Examples
Self-fulfillment	Encourage involvement in department functioning, variety, and new challenge Keep an eye on vision and purpose	Volunteering to head a new committee to discuss new care delivery design
Ego	Positive feedback (necessary) for all motivation stages	Saying thanks Detailed feedback
Social or belonging	Use social strengths for patients who need it, might need to observe progress closely	Potlucks, celebrations of the outcomes of a difficult case
Safety and security	Safe, secure climate; close supervision	Clear expectations Security guards in parking lot

When there have been severe personnel shortages, many staff members are concerned only about taking care of the safety and security needs. Few nurses will volunteer for a special committee or become excited about a quality management program when they are worried about having enough staff for their next shift. If it's impossible for your night shift workers to find enough warm, nutritious food at night when your diet kitchen is closed down, don't expect they'll have gone out of their way to get a start on the oncoming shift's work.

Keep in mind each person's individual reason for being at work, and use this to your best advantage for the best patient care. As staff members become more confident that their basic needs will be fulfilled, they might catch the excitement and climb to a higher level of motivation. We all waver in our motivational levels in a manner related to our personal life and how we perceive our impact on the world through work and other institutions.

The second level of motivation is that of social or affiliation needs. Many of us find fulfillment from the personal relationships we enjoy in health care, whether with one another or with those we serve. The staff members who are significantly motivated at this level might be those who love to talk and to organize the baby showers or social events. They might hold very dear the time that they have to interact with their clients on a one-to-one basis. This staff member might be the perfect person to assign to the elderly client who requires more interpersonal time. He or she can also be buddied with a coworker who is very goal directed but gives the affiliation-need partner much positive feedback.

The third level of motivation is that of ego needs for self-respect or status leading to self-esteem. Staff members who would like recognition and job growth might be motivated from this level. As RNs assign work or supervise staff at the ego level, the use of positive feedback, opportunities to be involved in task forces, recognition in the form of clinical ladders, and educational opportunities might be the most energizing. A CNA who functions primarily at this level might want to care for patients who have different diagnoses that he or she can research and use in their care.

A note of caution here: When nurses or other healthcare professionals identify themselves too closely with their job description, so that they themselves become interchangeable with what they do (i.e., what I do equals who I am and my value as a human being), and then their job roles change, they will be most disturbed. If asked who you are, how do you respond? Do you immediately think, "I'm John Jones, an oncology home health RN"? You as a human being have value beyond what you do for employment or as a profession. Be aware of this tendency when changes rock your workplace, and be especially good to yourself as you cope with the changes.

The fourth level of Maslow's hierarchy is that of self-fulfillment or self-actualization. We hope that, as professionals, many of you are doing your job because you are aware of how your role affects the lives of others and that you are aware of how you affect your own growth and the growth of those you serve by what you do. Staff members who are motivated at this stage are a joy to work with because they often help you, as supervising RN, look beyond the daily frustrations to the real reasons that you do your job.

YOUR RESPONSIBILITY FOR THE "GENERAL CLIMATE" OF MOTIVATION

Whether you are currently working in the role of a student nurse, staff RN, charge nurse, or nurse manager in any portion of the healthcare system, you have an influence on the environment in which you work. It is true that you can't be in control of others' behavior, but you can behave in a way that will affect others positively.

Multiple studies have been done—within health care, with nurses, and in business—about what motivates workers. Research has also proven a positive correlation between productivity, commitment to the organization, and job satisfaction. Specific leadership behaviors have been proven to directly influence productivity, commitment, and job satisfaction. The critical behaviors of "inspiring a shared vision, enabling others to act, modeling the way, challenging the process, and encouraging the heart are all positively related" (McNeese-Smith, 1992, p. 396) to the results you want to achieve in establishing a climate of motivation in your team. A positive climate of motivation also affects nurse retention when teams that work together, support one another, and resolve conflicts encourage the nurse to stay (Anthony, et al., 2005). Impacts have also been measured from the negative as research finds that lack of peer cohesion and poor working relationships have been noted as factors in nurse burnout (Garrett & McDaniel, 2001).

Your communication with others is fundamental to building relationships in your facility.

Most researchers would agree that the significance of the work being done, the degree of autonomy or decision making within the job, and the feedback given to workers affect job satisfaction and motivation. The types of relationships among workers also influence the climate of motivation within a group.

You might not be the CEO of the organization, and you might not sign the paychecks. However, pay raises are short-lived as motivators. Long-lasting motivation comes from being involved, feeling appreciated, and being clear about what you are to do and why. Each of you, every member of the team, is an integral part of establishing the climate of motivation in your facility.

When you tackle problems with a proactive, positive outlook, others want to be around you. (How many people follow leaders or want to be around colleagues who consistently express feelings of defeat, discouragement, and gloom?)

A climate of achievement is promoted when everyone understands what he or she is expected to do and where he or she is going. Reinforcing expectations, making goals clear, and encouraging everyone to participate in decision making as much as possible will provide a basis for clear and open communication. With that open communication, trust will develop. Reminding people why they are doing what they are doing (your mission) will energize them as they recognize how what they are doing contributes to the group's goals. Positive feedback (discussed in detail in Chapter 10) is one of the most powerful motivators in your formulary.

ASSESSING THE DELEGATE'S PREFERENCES

You might be surprised that it's taken us so long to get to the point of assessing the delegate's preferences. You will note that this is not the first of the criteria on the assessment list. This is because, all too often, the most aggressive delegate's preferences determine the assignments given to all the delegates. When it's possible, and it reflects your best judgment clinically, delegates appreciate doing the tasks they like best. However, again there might be an issue of whether the comfort zone is the best choice, and if it seems unfair that "Railroad Rita" has an easier assignment and avoids caring for Mr. Difficult Patient once again, it's important to analyze the other criteria for matching the delegate to the assignment more carefully.

Also remember our discussion about reliance on the strengths of an individual when many are cross trained. (Remember the hospital with the phlebotomy problem?) Keep in mind the long-term results of staff who all do only what they do best. None of them will remain competent in all the tasks they once learned, and flexibility will be lost for those times when staffing is marginal and all staff members must perform to the full extent of their potential.

EXHIBIT 7-4 **A Review: Know Your Delegate**

QUESTION ONE:

The vision of the National Council of State Boards of Nursing (Vision Paper 2006) includes:

a) Increased regulatory consistency among the states
b) Boards of nursing being the sole regulators of advanced practice nurses
c) LPNs practicing independently without RN supervision to help care for patients during the current nurse shortage
d) A and b but not c

Answer: d

QUESTION TWO:

Knowing your delegate and thereby improving teamwork could reap what benefits?

Answer:

A positive climate of motivation, resolution of conflicts, and team support affects nurse retention (Anthony et al., 2005)

Lack of peer cohesion and poor working relationships have been noted as factors in nurse burnout (Garrett and McDaniel, 2001)

Matching delegate skill level with tasks that need to be done will allow for better patient outcomes

QUESTION THREE:

In assisted-living settings, and in some states in long-term care and home settings, nursing assistants who have been certified as medication aides may administer medications. True or false?

Answer: true

QUESTION FOUR:

LPNs function as team leaders for rehabilitation aides in long-term care and assisted-living settings. True or false?

Answer: true. RNs in these settings, depending on the type of organizational licensure, are supervising and planning resident care while LPNS often function as team leaders. Additional regulations will likely emerge related to assisted-living and other care settings for the elderly and disabled. Check current state and federal regulations as this area of practice is a rapidly growing and dynamic field.

ASSESSING CULTURAL DIFFERENCES

As we work together to care for patients of diverse cultural backgrounds, we, the caregivers, are also influenced by our rainbow heritage of every hue of race, creed, color, gender, sexual preference, and age group. Even the community in which we grew up affects the way we communicate, prioritize and perform our work, and relate to one another.

A story illustrates the challenges we face as a multicultural team. A second-grade teacher announced to the class, "Boys and girls, there were four blackbirds on the limb of a tree. One was hit with a rock from a slingshot. How many were left?" One little boy immediately waved his hand and breathlessly shouted, "I know, teacher, I know! There were three blackbirds left!" A second boy interrupted. "No, there's not a chance any of those blackbirds would stick around! There were zero blackbirds left!" The first little boy placed a high priority on task, structure, and timely response to the teacher's question. The second little boy focused on reality and on relationships. Both were right.

This book is not a text on cultural diversity. However, we encourage readers to explore how their coworkers' backgrounds affect their understanding of the communications they give and receive each day. Even the body language and eye contact used by certain cultural groups can be misunderstood by coworkers. To you, is lack of eye contact a sign of respect or of dishonesty? It depends on your cultural heritage.

The first step to overcoming the possible hazards of miscommunication because of cultural differences comes from recognizing that these differences are a reality of who we are and consequently are not negotiable. The second step is to embrace the differences. The most important step is to communicate, communicate, communicate. Clarify questions and perceptions.

One could never find a totally homogeneous group with whom to work. Who would want to? Not only would it be boring, but there would be few variations to enrich the service we provide to our clients!

Ask questions of each other about backgrounds, such as "How did you handle conflict in your family?" Enjoy the attending special strengths that can be enjoyed with cultural diversity. A potluck with ethnic foods can be a tasty way to celebrate differences. For example, "When I told you that the vital signs in that room were a high priority, I didn't tell you that I meant within 5 minutes. Did you have another priority that came up?" (This situation can occur with a cultural background that looks at time in a different way.) "When you didn't look me in the eye when we were speaking together, I wondered if you were understanding me." (This type of clarification might assist you in learning that eye contact is not polite in the staff member's culture.)

As RNs understand more clearly their responsibility and accountability for supervision of the delegates, they will be less likely to choose the course of least resistance when delegating care.

Again, just as we must know our patients to care for them effectively, we must know our delegates.

CHECKPOINT 7-7

1. Knowing a delegate's motivation is important because:

    a) It is one of the assessment parameters that will allow me to make the correct decision about matching the delegate with the correct assignment.

    b) It will help me understand how to help him or her grow as we provide safe, effective patient care.

    c) I need to know how closely I will need to supervise this person.

    d) It's not important because no one could possibly take the time to know all this stuff about the people he or she works with.

    e) Understanding my coworkers better decreases the frustrations I might have to face each day.

2. I keep asking for feedback from Lew, but I can't seem to get an answer. She also asks someone else to do any personal care to any males. I can't decide if she's lazy or what!

    a) Both of these issues could be a cultural barrier we need to discuss.

    b) She might not be motivated to do the job.

    c) I will speak about this to her.

    d) I will just understand this is who she is and forget about straightening it out.

3. A student nurse will be caring for my patient who has a tracheotomy and a feeding tube. I will ask the following questions:

a) Nothing. The instructor should be there for all of the care. It's his problem.

b) I'll ask the student what parts of the care she is planning to do.

c) I'll ask whether she's done any of this care before.

d) I'll ask her detailed questions about positioning, suctioning, tube feedings, and tracheostomies and will be involved in the care of this patient all day.

4. Return to the questions we asked at the beginning of the chapter. Which type of healthcare professional in your organization can perform the following procedures?

a) Pierce the skin to perform procedures.

b) Start IVs.

c) Monitor IVs.

d) Perform the nursing process.

e) Gather data for the RN as he or she performs the assessment, nursing diagnosis, planning, intervention, and evaluation.

f) Perform hygienic care.

g) Deliver medications.

h) Be in charge of coordinating care in your healthcare setting.

i) Educate the patient.

See the end of the chapter for the answers.

CONCLUSION

Let's return to that pesky question that nurses ask, "What about my license?"

When you as the RN are following the supervision clause in your nurse practice act, when you are delegating appropriately, you

- know the job descriptions and official rules and regulations for yourself and delegates
- understand the concept of competency and how it affects your own performance and that of coworkers and your personal accountability for maintaining your competence

+ know delegates' strengths, weaknesses, motivation, and preferences
+ know the patients and clients based on your assessment, diagnosis, planning, intervention, and evaluation
+ use your professional judgment to match delegates to the work that needs to be done
+ continually supervise, evaluate, and give feedback to delegates

When you do these things, you are using your professional judgment and being responsible and accountable. The delegates themselves are accountable for their own actions as they perform their roles within their legal and organizational limitations. As much as you would like to control every one of their actions and protect patients from any mistakes, you cannot do that any more than you can prevent mistakes from happening within an all-RN staff. Delegates are accountable for their mistakes as they act within their job descriptions and practice limitations. You as an RN are accountable for the total care of the patient and for correcting the effects of the error. You must also address the cause of the delegate's error, be certain that charting and other paperwork (such as the Unusual Occurrence Report) are completed, and pass on the information to those who need to know (possibly the manager and the next shift). You have acted with excellent nursing judgment. Although you could not control every action of those you supervised, you followed professional standards to be accountable for your supervisory duties.

Getting to know delegates' qualities, just as you get to know qualities of family members, allows you to match delegates to the work that needs to be done for more effective patient care. In the next chapter, we'll discuss how to communicate your delegation decisions to the members of your team and how to keep the group from becoming a dysfunctional family!

ANSWERS TO CHECKPOINTS

7–2.   Pat needs to consult with an administrative person to determine what steps were taken as the hospital decided to introduce IV therapy into the LPN role. (Hopefully, they contacted the state board for an advisory opinion, which determined that LPNs could monitor IV therapy and administer some IV medications if educated in this area. Competency would have to be determined and "checked off" after the education program was completed.) As for LPNs as "primary nurses," the LPNs might be functioning nearly independently because RNs do not understand their own accountability by law. Pat needs to discuss his concerns about LPN supervision with his manager and help solve this problem. This hospital needs to determine the methods by which RNs will supervise LPN practice. RN's assessments and/or care planning involvement should be documented on the patient record as well.

7–3.   This multidisciplinary worker might be discriminating based on disease, or he might need some more education about HIV and how to treat crack babies. He might not be aware of the pattern of his behavior. (Read more about performance problems and giving feedback in Chapter 10.)

7–6.

1.   a, b, d

2.   c, d

3.   b, c, d

4.   a, c

7–7.

1.   a, b, c, e

2.   a, b (but probably not), c

3.   b, c, d

4.   We suspect that only RNs can perform d and h! Refer to your state practice act and organizational job descriptions to determine your answers.

REFERENCES

Anthony, M., Standing, T., Glick, J., Duffy, M., Paschall, F., et al. (2005). Leadership and nurse retention. *Journal of Nursing Administration, 35,* 146–155.

Arizona Department of Education. (1985). *Inventory of validated competencies and skills for nursing assistant, practical nurse, and associate degree nurse graduates.* Phoenix, AZ: Author.

Emergency Nurses Association. (1994). *Position statement: Role of delegation by the emergency nurse in clinical practice settings.* Retrieved July 20, 2007, from http://www.ena.org/about/position/pdfs/usenon-rn.pdf.

Gandsas, A., Parekh, M., Bleech, M., & Tong, D. (2007, July). Robotic telepresence: Profit analysis in reducing length of stay after laparoscopic gastric bypass. *Journal of the American College of Surgeons.*

Garrett, D., & McDaniel, A. (2001). A new look at nurse burnout. *Journal of Nursing Administration, 31,* 91–96.

Institute of Medicine. (2003). *Health professions education: A bridge to quality.* Washington, DC: National Academy Press.

Interprofessional Workgroup on Health Professions Regulation. (1996, November). *Views on the licensure and regulation of health care professionals.*

Maslow, A. H. (1970). *Motivation and personality* (2nd ed.). New York: Harper & Row.

McNeese-Smith, D. (1992). The impact of leadership on productivity. *Nursing Economic$, 10*(6), 396.

National Council of State Boards of Nursing. (1986). *National council position paper (1986): Statement on the nursing activities of unlicensed persons.* Chicago: Author. Retrieved from http://www.ncsbn.org/iwhpr/ipw/1196.html.

National Council of State Boards of Nursing. (1990). *Model nurse aide administrative rules by the subcommittee for model nurse aide language and the nursing practice and education committee.* Chicago: Author.

National Council of State Boards of Nursing. (1997a). *Assuring competence: A regulatory responsibility.* Chicago: Author. Retrieved from http://www.ncsbn.org/iwhpr/ipw/1196.html.

National Council of State Boards of Nursing. (1997b). *Definition of competence and standards for competence. Assuring competence: Attachment two.* Chicago: Author, 1–2.

National Council of State Boards of Nursing. (1997c). *Individual competence evaluation. Assuring competence: Attachment two.* Chicago: Author, 1–6.

National Council of State Boards of Nursing. (1998). *Job analysis of nurse aides, 1998.* Retrieved July 29, 2003, from http://www.ncsbn.org/public/testing/practice_analysis/naja98.htm.

National Council of State Boards of Nursing. (2002). Model nursing practice act. Retrieved July 29, 2003, from http://www.ncsbn.org/public/regulation/nursing_practice_model_practice_act.htm.

National Council of State Boards of Nursing. (2005). *Business book, NCSBN annual meeting. Mission possible: Building a safer nursing work force through regulatory excellence.* Retrieved August 12, 2005, from http://www.ncsbn.org/pdfs/V_Business_Book_Section 1_pdf.

National Council of State Boards of Nursing. (2006a). *NCSBN research brief, a national survey on elements of nursing education—Fall 2004.* Volume 24, July 2006.

National Council of State Boards of Nursing. (2006b). *Draft vision paper: The future regulation of advanced practice.* Retrieved July 20, 2007, from http://www.ncsbn.org/draft_APRN_Vision_paper.pdf.

National Council of State Boards of Nursing. (2007). *Continued competence.* Retrieved July 20, 2007, from http://www.ncsbn.org.919.htm.

Paulson, D. (2004). A comparison of wait times in patients leaving without being seen when unlicensed nurses, versus unlicensed assistive personnel perform triage. *Journal of Emergency Nursing, 30*(4), 307–311.

Pew Health Professions Commission. (1995). *Reforming health care workforce regulation: Policy considerations for the 21st century.* San Francisco: UCSF Center for the Health Professions.

Reinhardt, S., Young, H., Kane, R., & Quinn, W. (2006). Nurse delegation of medication administration for older adults in assisted-living. *Nursing Outlook, 54*(2), 74–80.

Simpkins, R. W. (1997). Using task lists with unlicensed assistive personnel. *Insight* 6(2), 1.

Society of Gastroenterology Nurses and Associates, SGNA Practice Committee. (2006). Role delineation position statement. *Gastroenterology Nursing, 29*(1), 64–65.

Vastag, B. (2007, June). Telemedicine's adolescent angst. *Hospital and Health Networks, 6,* 66–70.

Wiesmiller, W. (1997). Explaining the national nurse aide assessment program test development process. *Insight, 6*(2), 1–5. Retrieved from http://www.ncsbn.org/files/insight/vol62/nnaap.html.

Zimmerman, P. (1996). Delegating to assistive personnel. *Journal of Emergency Nursing,* 22: 206-12.

Know How to Communicate

Loretta O'Neill and Ruth I. Hansten

CHAPTER SKILLS

+ Select the most effective communication style for the situation.
+ Explore possible responses that could occur when you delegate to assistive personnel.
+ Use the 4 Cs of initial direction when delegating.
+ Practice the steps of assertive communication.

RECOMMENDED RESOURCES

▶ Review The Joint Commission's 2008 (or more current) Patient Safety Goals at http://www.jointcommission.org/PatientSafety/ NationalPatientSafetyGoals/08_hap_npsgs.htm.

▶ Discover what the Institute of Medicine says about quality in health care (www.IOM.edu) and what the Institute for Healthcare Improvement currently recommends for saving lives (www.IHI.org). Search on keyword "campaigns."

▶ Read another resource about emotional intelligence such as Daniel Feldman's book (1999). *The handbook of emotionally intelligent leadership: Inspiring others to achieve results.* Leadership Performance Press. www.leadershipperformance.com.

"Believe me, I'd love to delegate more of my routine care. I've tried in the past, but it hasn't been worth the effort. I get anxious about asking other people for help because I'm concerned that they will think I can't handle my assignment. Then when I'm really bogged down and do delegate something, I spend time worrying if it is getting done right or done at all, following up, finding out that it wasn't even done, and finally doing it myself. It seems I save a lot of energy by just doing it myself in the first place!"

S ound familiar? You can probably see the need for delegating in your workplace. You think it is important, but somehow in the thousands of details that make up your workday, learning the skill of delegation isn't at the top of your to-do list. When you delegate, you entrust another person to act in your place for that particular task or cluster of tasks. You are still responsible for the delivery of the task. How can you be sure it will be done satisfactorily and on time? Notice that the criteria for successful delegation are satisfactory accomplishment of the task (which includes important safety and patient interaction components) and on-time completion. Because the delegate is not you, he or she might not perform the task the exact way you would.

In addition to all those personal concerns about getting the work done, you have read that The Joint Commission has recognized team communication as the root cause for 65%–70% of sentinel events (JCAHO Sentinel Event Statistics, 2007), and the Institute for Healthcare Improvement (IHI) sees teamwork and communication as vital for saving lives (IHI 5 Million Lives Campaign, 2007). The National Patient Safety Goals (The Joint Commission, 2007) include the importance of hand-off communication. It's clear that the right communication is mandatory for patient safety and optimal clinical outcomes.

A key to successful delegation is in understanding, first, that delegation is an investment of time and energy that doesn't always have immediate returns, and second, that delegation is a skill, which implies that it has discrete steps or components, that it requires practice to improve, and that repeated practice of it will facilitate improvement.

CHECKPOINT 8-1

What percentage of sentinel events reported to The Joint Commission was related to inadequate communication among care providers?

COMMUNICATION AS A PART OF THE PLAN FOR THE DAY, SHIFT, OR CASE

In previous editions of this book, we left the manner in which initial direction and periodic follow-up communication was given up to the RN, dependent on the situation. However, as we are now older and wiser (perhaps), we have noted that many novice nurses are not afforded the opportunity to observe how experts incorporate the communication piece of team-work into their daily work. Put any assumptions to rest now: If the initial direction and ongoing supervisory connections with assistive staff are not planned as a part of your care delivery model or normal operating proce-dures, it will not occur. Or the interaction will be minimal, inconsistent, or less than stellar. For example, shift report is best offered at the bedside with oncoming assistive personnel present, and with patient involvement. Initial discussion with team members can occur there, so the patient and family understand the roles of each team member and the plan for the shift based on their intended outcomes. When the RN and NA discuss the schedule for the day, updates should optimally occur before and after breaks and meals. Meals and breaks should be planned for best coverage of the unit activities and knowledge of a group of patients. A planned short (5 minutes or less) meeting by midshift should transpire to discuss and/or adjust patient progress toward their priorities. Toward the end of the shift, a reciprocal feedback session is a best practice for improved teamwork and to encourage celebration of successful patient outcomes.

CHECKPOINT 8–2

Best practice would recommend that the registered nurse working on a medical surgical unit, for example, would plan for initial communication and ongoing checkpoints how frequently during the shift? Describe how an RN might plan the shift, engaging assistive personnel as a part of the team.

DELEGATE RESPONSES

Assuming that the task(s) delegated and the delegate selected were appropriate, your request might receive a number of responses, all of which are probably familiar to you. Here we assume that your communication instructions have been clear and complete.

The delegate's responses can fall into one of the following three categories: agreement, refusal, and absence.

Agreement Response

This represents the happy scenario of a delegated task that is willingly accepted. You delegate a task, and the delegate agrees to perform it. The response is basically, "Yes, I'll do it." You have delegated the authority to the delegate to complete the task. You have also indicated time frames for completion and situational boundaries for which you need to be notified.

Possible results of agreement responses are:

1. You monitor the delegate's progress and find out that the task(s) has been accomplished satisfactorily and on time.

2. The initial willingness of the delegate to perform the task leads to partially satisfactory results. The task might actually be completed but not satisfactorily, or it might be done correctly but not in the appropriate time frame. Many nurses habitually "fix it" when faced with this scenario. They complete the partially accomplished work or redo the incorrect work of their delegate. This has a number of negative effects. First, "plugging the gap" circumvents the accountability of the delegate to perform the agreed-upon task satisfactorily. The delegate needs feedback regarding what is and is not acceptable in the completion of the task. Without this feedback, the delegate is not likely to improve. Second, the delegating nurse becomes hypervigilant, checking, rechecking, and possibly redoing work that he or she thought was being done. This hypervigilance can lead to resentment toward the delegate, deterioration in the working relationship, and an unbearable workload for the nurse.

3. A frustrating variation on this scenario of initial agreement to perform the delegated task is the delegate who willingly and cheerfully agrees to do the task but does not actually perform it. When you follow up on the delegate's progress or lack thereof, you might hear, "I forgot," "I asked someone else to do that for me" (the delegate becomes a second delegator), "I got too busy with my patients," "I'm getting to it," or some other reason for nonperformance.

Once again, the delegating nurse will often reclaim the task and complete it him- or herself. Some of the rationales given by the nurse for this action include: 1) urgent need for patient data to be collected; 2) concern that the treatment or therapy needs to be done on schedule; and 3) concern that the delegate will be angry or upset with the nurse if confronted and will make a scene, take his or her feelings out on the patient, or make an error.

> If the nurse reclaims the task and does not offer corrective feedback, the nurse shares responsibility for the delegation problem.

In possible results 2 and 3, the delegating nurse shares responsibility for creating the delegation problem, usually by failing to monitor the delegate's progress until the deadline, then taking the task back.

In doing so, the nurse participates in setting up a frustrating cycle: delegation; unsatisfactory accomplishment of the task by the delegate; reclaiming of the task by the delegating nurse; resentment and/or anger for both parties; recommitment to "doing it all myself"; work overload for nurse; attempted delegation. This cycle fails to motivate or develop the skill level of the delegate in doing the task or of the delegating nurse in holding the delegate accountable. It can also frustrate and stress both the nurse and the delegate unnecessarily.

As we discussed in Chapter 3, "Know Your Practice," the delegate's accountability includes accepting the delegation as well as his or her actual performance in carrying out the task that was delegated.

Refusal Response

This represents the unhappy scenario when the nurse attempts to delegate a task and the delegate indicates verbally or nonverbally, "No, I won't/can't do it." This might be accompanied by a number of reasons for the refusal. The reasons offered might be rational and based on stated but conflicting goals. For example, the nurses' aide can't stay at the bedside of a confused and fall-prone patient while simultaneously helping to pass out meal trays. Or the refusal might be due to an inability or lack of knowledge about how to perform the requested task.

On the other hand, nonrational reasons based on hidden and unstated goals might be behind the refusal. The intended delegate's desire for personal power, prestige, or revenge might motivate the refusal response. For example, a delegating nurse, on her way to administer a pain medication to a patient, stops and requests another staff member to help one of the nurse's patients on the bedpan. The intended delegate places her hands on her hips, glares at the nurse, and states in a loud voice, "I am not your slave!" and walks away. This refusal of a delegated task is based on a desire to equalize a power imbalance in the relationship between the delegating nurse and the delegate. This response might also be based on past experiences within the team. For example, a nursing assistant who repeatedly asks for help from the RN but is not accommodated, or who observes an RN on the phone chatting with her relatives, might harbor resentment toward the other team member.

Absence Response

In addition to the responses of "Yes, I'll do it," "No, I won't/can't do it," and a nonrational attack, there is another scenario, that of the missing delegate. With the use of electronic supports such as pagers, cell phones,

Nurses, desirous of delegating routine and noncomplex tasks to others, note that some of their ancillary staff are "missing in action." It is indeed difficult to delegate to someone who is avoiding the additional work.

and other communication devices, the actual location of the UAP might be easily retrieved. However, these devices might also be "missing" or the delegate might be located tapping her foot at the time clock a half hour prior to the end of the assigned shift.

As in a bad game of Tag, you are forever "it" because you can't find the delegate who is off the unit, hiding in an empty room, or otherwise occupied and unavailable to be tagged with a delegated task.

CHECKPOINT 8-3

The Institute for Healthcare Improvement, National Patient Safety Goals, The Joint Commission, and other organizations committed to patient safety cite hand-off communication as fundamental to patient quality and protection from error. List several junctures in a patient's progress through the healthcare system when hand-off communication could occur.

COMMUNICATION STYLES: PASSIVE, AGGRESSIVE, ASSERTIVE

How do you, as the delegating nurse, deal appropriately with this wide scope of possible behaviors? How can you find the right words to communicate to the delegate, keep communication channels open, and resist the temptation to just do it all yourself? The words you choose and the way in which they are delivered to the delegate make the difference between a successful and a frustrating episode in delegation. Further, your words will make the difference in whether the workplace environment supports retention by providing the respect that is seen as a universal need among all of us. Authors DeLellis and Sauer (2004) suggest that there are many components of respectful communication including active listening, assertive speech, and avoidance of passive–aggressive communication. Disturbingly, they found that 79% of the respondents to their survey indicated that workplace respect was seriously lacking in the United States, and that if healthcare workers would respect each other as much as they respect their patients, the work setting would significantly improve. It seems there is a lot of potential here to make things better! So whether delegating or just working side by side, what approach are you using? Your communication choices fall into one of three general categories: passive, aggressive, or assertive. Let's take a look at each of the three possible styles, taking passive first.

Passive or Nonassertive

After listening to reports, you make out the shift assignments based on the acuity of the patients and the skill level of the staff available today. The LPN counts up each person's patient load and says, "I have all of the heaviest patients. I think this should be divided up evenly between the RNs and LPNs, since LPNs do everything but." You think the assignment is appropriate, based on the previous criteria, but this particular LPN can be quite difficult to work with and you don't want to start the shift with a scene, so you say, "Oh, here. I'll take one of your patients in 334. I have the other patient in that room and will be in there a lot anyway."

This is a typically passive or nonassertive response, also termed avoidance. Although it is not advisable or even possible to deal with every conflict situation, a habitually passive response stems from a number of feelings, including fear, anxiety, timidity, inhibition, hurt, self-denial, helplessness, and physical and emotional stress. If words are spoken they are often not reflective of the actual thoughts or feelings of the passive individual, adding an element of emotional dishonesty to the communication. Internally, an intense dialogue rages, with repeated replaying of the situation and various alternate responses that the passive person could have given.

The costs of habitually passive behavior include lowering of self-esteem and self-confidence, a negative self-image, avoidance of responsibility for the quality of one's relationships and life, and lost opportunities to develop skills in managing conflict and resolving issues. Problems are not faced or solved. Consequently they multiply at the feet of the passive communicator. Effective delegation becomes impossible, and the delegator ends up doing more and more work him- or herself. If the delegator's passivity is excessive, the delegates might become even less cooperative and control the amount and quality of work done. Consider the overtime costs for the organization as well as the RN's home life and physiological reactions.

Through constant acquiescence, the goals of others get accomplished, not the goals of the passive person. In addition, nonassertive behavior can engender feelings of pity, disgust, irritation, confusion, and anger in others.

Passivity, avoidance, and accommodation all go together to create overworked RNs and a poorly functioning team.

Why on earth would anyone choose this communication style when the results seem so negative? A passive response is based on the fear of rejection and retaliation caused by displeasing others. Conflict is avoided at the price of denying one's own feelings and needs. The reward is immediate avoidance of an unpleasant situation and the attendant feelings of tension. We will discuss these responses more in our next chapter about conflict.

Eventually this strategy of avoidance backfires because feelings stay suppressed only for a time. Like a toxic chemical solution buried in a rusty drum, feelings of anger and resentment begin to leak out. These negative feelings show up in subtle, hostile behaviors and quiet ways of punishing or manipulating others such as forgetting, unconscious sabotage, withdrawal, sulking, or crying.

The helpless, withdrawn, silent martyr actually has a method of communicating, though it is indirect and manipulative.

Aggressive

You and two nursing assistants are working the night shift. One assistant on the Alzheimer's unit is off the unit on an errand. You are already behind schedule in giving medications when you find that a patient, Mr. Smith, has untied his restraints, been incontinent of urine, and slipped and fallen on the floor. You go to the desk and see the remaining aide reading a magazine with his feet up on the desk. When you request his help, he replies, "This is not my side of the hall," and returns to his reading. You lose your cool and in no uncertain terms tell him, through clenched teeth, in a low and angry voice, "I don't really care whose side of the hall it is, you worthless, lazy bum. This patient needs help, and you are going to help me get him back to bed and cleaned up right now. I'm tired of seeing you sit around here when these people need help. You do this every night. Get out of that chair now and don't let me catch you sitting down the rest of the night!" You stomp off to Mr. Smith's room.

In this scenario, the nurse has no problem expressing her thoughts, feelings, and wants. She is expressive, and her words honestly reflect the feelings she experiences. You can see that she is annoyed, stressed, impatient, and angry.

However, her direct communication comes at the expense of the other. Her words carry a tone of righteous superiority and "loaded" terms such as "worthless," "lazy," and "bum." Such phrases have not been known to engender cheerful acceptance of delegated tasks! The communication she uses in this aggressive response is riddled with "you" messages of blame and labeling. How do you imagine the nurses' aide feels about himself? Probably hurt and humiliated. His feelings about the nurse are likely to be angry and vengeful. She even throws in a general condemnation about how he has used his time previously. These characteristics of aggressive communication typify the verbal attack.

> Aggressive behavior is an encroachment or attack upon another and is almost always hostile in intent. The communication flows from the aggressive person outward. Little listening takes place while he or she talks at, not with, others. This style, long on criticism and short on praise, successfully suppresses ideas and feedback from others. Such a tension-filled relationship evokes passive–aggressive behavior on the part of others, which perpetuates the cycle of overbearing authoritarianism and indirect aggression.

In another setting you might have witnessed aggressive behavior without actual speech. The pediatric clinical specialist who has just lost a neonate after a long fight might enter the nurses' station area with a flourish and then begin to throw charts or slam the telephone down on the hook when the lab doesn't respond immediately to his call.

The will of the aggressive person often prevails in the conflict situation. The goal is to dominate and hurt the other. The price of winning is the animosity of the recipients. During the verbal storm, the aggressive person speaks as if he or she has no mental filter but says whatever is on his or her mind. This brutal directness fosters fear and resistance, sabotage, and resentment in the listener. Delegating with an aggressive manner of communication often has the same ultimate result as a passive style because real problems don't get solved, and the delegator is avoided and ends up doing more work him- or herself.

Assertive

You assign a staff member to take postoperative vital signs on a C-section patient. When you go back to check on the readings, the last two sets are

No one approach will be best for handling every delegation situation, but knowing how to express yourself assertively can help you with the people-related problems of delegation.

not on the flowsheet. The last set of vital signs charted is over an hour old. You find the staff member and say, "I was in Mrs. Miller's room and noticed that the last set of vital signs charted is from an hour ago. I am concerned about her blood pressure. Do you have a more recent set?" The staff member gives you vital signs written on a scrap paper in her pocket. You say, "These look fine. In the future, please chart them all on the bedside flowsheet. It will save us both time."

Assertive communicators are confident and positive and lay claim to their own right to speak up for themselves. In the example above, the nurse is direct and expresses what she has observed, thinks, feels, and wants in this situation. The message is congruent with what she feels, so it is emotionally honest. She clearly addresses the problem without belittling herself or the other person. She knows what she wants and asks for it without apology. Assertive people feel good about themselves at the time they communicate and later. They are not ambushed by feelings of anger, resentment, or guilt. Because this style of communication addresses the problem in the situation, real problems get solved and stay solved.

Other people generally respect the assertive person because they themselves are treated with respect, not with deference, as in passivity, or with dominance, as in aggressiveness. Because the assertive person communicates directly when there is a problem, others can trust that problems will be shared with them and not inappropriately with others. This leads to the development of trust, an essential component of effective delegation.

At the heart of delegation is the skill of clear, effective, assertive communication. Improving your ability to express yourself can have a number of positive effects on your mental health and work life. Some benefits for you include increased feelings of self-confidence, improved communication with coworkers, resolution of problems, nonmanipulative negotiation for behavior changes, and the ability to act as an advocate for patients. A key strategy is to begin assertiveness practice in small nonemotional situations and build upon your success. The most difficult, negative staff member on the unit is not the ideal recipient of your first efforts. Start out small and practice. Assertive communication will become easier and more natural to you. Please complete Checkpoint 8–4 (page 283) before reading on.

CHECKPOINT 8-4

Determine what type of communication style is being used by the following personnel.

1. Rashad attended the team meeting with all the rest. When the topic of role clarification for assistive personnel came up, he stated that he thought part of his role was to anticipate the needs of the patients for toileting and personal hygienic care. Robin, one of the staff RNs in their psychiatric care group home, raised her voice as she firmly stated, "You are only an aide. That is in the RN role. We don't expect you to think, just to do what we tell you to when we tell you." Rashad sat quietly without responding because he needed to keep his job but began his plan on how he'd make Robin pay for her statement. Maybe he wouldn't do anything without being told.

2. Pamela, one of the school nurses in a rural county, was following up on some vision and hearing testing done by one of the volunteers, Brigite. She was concerned about the accuracy of the work due to the way these readings compared to previous readings. Instead of discussing this with Brigite, she decided to do it all herself and retest everyone.

3. Rosa managed the ambulatory care surgical center for a large healthcare conglomerate. Mabel, one of the surgical technicians, told her that she would not consider scrubbing in any orthopedic cases. Her rationale was that they were too physically stressful. When Rosa mentioned that, although she wanted the staff to work together as a team, with everyone using his or her strengths to bring the best care for the patients, and that being involved in orthopedic cases was a part of Mabel's job description, Mabel told her menacingly that she was the granddaughter of the chairman of the board and that she'd "get Rosa's head on a platter."

See the end of the chapter for the answers.

EFFECTIVE ASSIGNING

The first step in effective communication related to delegation is to be clear in your own mind about what you need to have done by the delegate, based on the outcomes you and the patient and family have determined are the priorities for this shift. A handy mental checklist can be borrowed

Sharing why, who, what, when, where, and how with the team member will help the communication be clear and complete.

from journalists, who routinely use the why, who, what, when, where, and how format in getting the details of their stories. By taking the time to share each of these aspects of the assignment with the delegate, you are communicating your specific expectations regarding the performance of the task.

Let's look at each of these in turn, starting with why.

Why

In giving feedback to others, you'll find that when goals and feedback are combined, performance effort is more than doubled (see Chapter 10). What would it be like to be a robot, each day going from patient to patient, doing the usual "beds, baths, and vital signs" without a clear understanding of why you are doing those tasks? In Chapter 6, "Know What Needs to Be Done," we emphasized the importance of first determining patient outcomes in partnership with the patient. Now you, as the team leader, must communicate the priority outcomes to the team members. For example, if you've noted that a high priority for Ms. Jones for this shift is to be able to breathe more comfortably, relieve her pain, and begin to build up her nutrition, then communicate that to others who will be assisting you.

> Imagine the difference in performance effort if you told Alicia (patient care assistant) to "Be sure Ms. Jones is fed this shake every two hours and let me know about her oximeter readings and pain," versus saying, "Alicia, for Ms. Jones to be able to stay off the ventilator and out of ICU, we have to be able to build up her nutrition quickly. We also must keep careful watch on her oximeter readings since I have given her pain medication and that can slow her breathing. Please be certain she eats at least 100 ccs of the shake at 10 a.m., and let me know how much she takes in at noon too. Also, tell me immediately if she complains of pain or you hear her oximeter alarms go off."

When people understand why they are doing their jobs, the difference might be critical, ranging from a melting nutritional shake left at the nurses' station for several days and a trip to ICU to the positive effects of celebrating Ms. Jones's return to the previous care facility!

Who

Usually at least two people are involved in any patient care delegation situation: the intended delegate and the patient. Who is the delegate for this particular task? In Chapter 7, the process of identifying and assessing a delegate was discussed at length. The delegate might be a nurses' aide, patient care technician, LPN/LVN, another RN, or someone outside the work group, such as a member of the patient's family. Be sure to specify the person who is your intended delegate.

> It is much clearer and more effective to say, "Mary, would you take this specimen to the lab?" than to generally announce, "Who has time to take this to the lab?"

The second "who" is the patient or receiver of the task. This seems incredibly simple and obvious, but avoidance of patient care errors begins with correct identification of the patient. An example of being clear about who is to receive the service or task is as follows: "Tracy, would you please take Mrs. Miller [who] into exam room #2?"

What

What is the job or task to be done? Be clear and specific regarding the task or assignment that you are delegating. Unless you already know that the delegate understands the task, you need to take the time to explain the task thoroughly. Without adequate information, the chance that the task will be completed to your expectations is slim. What exactly do you want done?

Here are some examples of being specific about the delegated task.

+ "Sandy, could you go [what] to the diet kitchen and pick up [what] a late tray for Mr. Sams? Please check [what] that it is an 1800 ADA diet."

+ "James, I've noticed that your documentation of patient teaching on eye surgery patients is clear and thorough. Would you be willing to review [what] the patient teaching sections of these ophthalmic surgery patients' standardized care plans for completeness and update [what] the references to reflect current practice?"

+ "Patricia, will you please go [what] to Mrs. Paulson's home today instead of tomorrow to do her [what] hygienic care?"

> Clarity means that you have not clouded the issue with too much information. Being concise will help. If you ask someone to chart an intake and output for you, it's not necessary to go into detail about how the diuretics work on the kidney and those pressure gradients! Confusion will ensue as the delegate wonders what you were asking him or her to do.

> Even experienced staff members have gaps in their knowledge and might appreciate being shown exactly what needs to be done, saving them from admitting they do not know how to perform a task.

At this point, many nurses feel and respond to their own overcrowded schedules. "I don't have time to explain what he (she) needs to do. It's easier and quicker for me to do it myself." This is probably accurate. Unfortunately it also ensures that you, and only you, are the one spending precious time on tasks that could be delegated. On the other hand, if you work with the same staff members often and begin to invest a little time in clearly delegating one new task at a time, you will develop the delegates' repertoire of skills and expand the pool of competent persons.

Nurses not being complete in their communication to others is often a cause of incomplete work or unmet expectations. As we work with assistive personnel across the nation, they continually state, "Please tell the nurses to just tell me what to do and what they expect, and I will do it. I can't read their minds!" As an attorney friend once told us, "The trouble starts when people stop talking."

A quick reminder as we discuss the "what" of communicating assignments to delegates: The task must fit within their scope of practice and job description and must be something they are competent at completing. Consistent with chapter six's discussion of the Rights of Delegation, the 4 Cs of communication (clear, concise, correct, and complete as a helpful memory device will be discussed in more detail later in this chapter. The task you delegate must be correct, that is, legitimately within their capabilities and scope.

Another method to communicate the "what" of the task to delegates is to show (teach) them rather than tell. Take the delegate with you the next time you'd like to delegate a task. Use this opportunity to show him or her what is to be done the next time.

When

When, meaning what time or by when, do you want the task completed? And when, or under what circumstances, should the delegate notify you? Your communication of the time frame for completion of a delegated task is crucial to on-time completion. Only when you specify the time parameters will the delegate share your prioritization of the task. Examples of communicating the "when" follow.

- "Audrey, Mr. Pong needs to have his a.m. care done by 0730 because he is scheduled for an arteriogram this morning."

+ "Angela, Mr. Phillips is back from surgery. I took the first set of vitals, so he gets three more q 15 minutes, starting now [when to do the task], then the rest of the routine schedule. Let me know if he has significant changes in BP or pulse or any bleeding on the dressing [when or how often to notify you]."
+ "If you receive a call on the answering machine about a poison control question, please notify me as soon [when] as I walk in the door."

The 4 Cs of Initial Direction

Another method of remembering what should be communicated during the initial direction portion of delegation is the 4 Cs: clear, correct, concise, and complete.

+ Clear—Is the information muddled, or would anyone else walking by understand what you are attempting to convey? Have you included some type of written communication as well as a plan for ongoing checkpoints with the delegate so that any emerging questions can be answered? Vague, passing comments such as, "It's the same assignment as yesterday," would probably not be construed as initial direction in a court of law.
+ Correct—Is the right patient/family, room number, and task being described? Is this a task the assistant is able and/or willing to perform? Is this task consistent with the patient's and family's preferred outcomes and long-term goals?
+ Concise—Don't add so much information that any original simplicity or precision is lost. Describing the purpose of the task is essential for encouraging motivation. "We are checking his blood glucose every 2 hours today because he is on such high dose steroids that he could run into problems like last admission."
+ Complete—"Complete" communication is judged by the ear of the listener. Asking "What else will you need to know to be able to be successful at this plan?" will help the delegate consider what else he needs to know. The comprehensive nature of initial and ongoing direction will be based on the needs and expertise of your team member. For a novice, complete direction might include him observing you performing a task; to another trusted teammate, ample communication takes place best during the first rounds of the day when you introduce yourselves to your patients. "Rose, today you and Mrs. Peters can plan to ambulate twice before lunch and before

afternoon PT. Since you (Mrs. Peters) want to get back home to that puppy, getting ready for admission to rehab a will mean being up four times. You and Rose make quite a team, and Rose will let me know if there are any blood pressure or pain issues, okay?"

Where

Communicating where you want a task done could mean either an anatomical location on the patient or a geographic location. For example:

+ "Susan, when you take the TED hose off Mr. Johnson, please clean the graft incision on the calf [where—anatomical location] with warm water."
+ "Mary Ellen, please ambulate Mrs. Darcy from her room to the patient dining area and back [where—geographic location or distance] twice this shift."
+ "Liz, would you go to Materials Management and pick up a replacement sterile instrument kit? The department is on the first floor behind the cafeteria [where—location]."

How

How do you want the task to be done? There is a large range or scope of possibilities in answer to this question. Essentially, ask yourself if you have any assumptions about how the task will be completed. If you do, it is important to communicate these specifics to the delegate. Two examples of communicating "how" follow.

+ "Beth, Mr. Barnes is coming up from the ED. He has a rebreathing mask on, so when you do his admitting vital signs, he needs a tympanic temp taken [how]."
+ "Judy, please stay at the bedside with Mrs. Murphy and take her vital signs before and after dangling [how]. She has a history of fainting and subsequent fractures."

Combining the Elements

It might seem that these components (why, who, what, when, where, and how) would be a lot to remember and take ages to communicate, but such is not the case. It is actually a quick, clear, and thorough method to delegate successfully. For example, "Martha [who—delegate], do you have 10–15 minutes to ambulate [what] Mr. Parker [who—patient] before lunch [when] please? Good, thanks. He is slightly weak on his right side, so please walk on his left side [how] to give him support on his unaffected side [why].

See if you can get him to walk the length of the hall [where]. Thanks."

When you are giving those instructions, ask yourself quickly, "Have I discussed the why, who, what, when, where, and how, and am I being clear, concise, correct, and complete in what I have told them?" This is a good time to ask the delegate, "Have I given you enough (or too much) information?"

In four short sentences, you have explained exactly the why, who, what, when, where, and how of a delegated task! Although it might seem obvious, note that a liberal sprinkling of "pleases" and "thank yous" really makes a difference to your coworkers!

In communicating assignments to the delegate: remember the 4 Cs:

Clear—Am I saying what I want to say, and is the delegate hearing it?

Concise—Am I confusing him or her with too much information?

Correct—Is this a task I can comfortably delegate to a competent individual, within his or her scope of practice?

Complete—(This is where we most ofter err.) Am I stating the outcome we want to achieve (why this is being done)? Have I given times and parameters for reporting? Does the delegate have enough information to do the job accurately?

ASSERTIVE FOLLOW-UP

You have now clearly delegated a task. On the follow-up, you find that it has been done satisfactorily and on time, that it has been done partially satisfactorily, or that it has not been done. How can you respond in an assertive way, mindful of your needs and those of the delegate? How can you communicate assertively in all these situations? How can you think of the appropriate words when you are pressured for time and have strong feelings about the situation?

CHECKPOINT 8–5

Decide how you would clearly communicate the following tasks to be completed:

1. You want Geraldine, a medical assistant in your office, to check the axillary temperature of all the babies under 3 years of age when they come in for a well-child checkup.

2. Linnea, your secretary, must still complete the Medicare forms, or your rehab center will not receive reimbursement.

3. You'd like Antonia to pick up the psychiatrist's evaluation and referral from the homeless shelter on her way back from home visits.

See the end of the chapter for the answers.

Step 1. Determine an Outcome

Before you begin, think about what outcome you'd like to achieve from your talk with this individual. Determining the outcome (what you want to have happen in the future) will create time to allow you to decompress, think clearly, and plan what you will say. This first step is the most essential!

Step 2. "I Noticed That . . ." or "When You . . ."

Here you describe the actual observable, verifiable behaviors that you have seen, heard, or noticed. Be specific and give as many concrete, specific details as you can recall, such as time, place, and frequency of action.

For example, "Melissa, I asked you to go to Admitting to pick up Mr. French 15 minutes ago. Since then I noticed that you have been on the phone discussing your plans for the evening. I am anxious to get the patient admitted. Please go to Admitting now and pick him up." Notice that this is a description of the events, not an assumption about Melissa's motivation or character flaws.

If you give others feedback about their behavior now, take note of your language choices. Do you use "you" messages, such as "You are late!" or "You forgot to ambulate Mr. Smith"? A "you" message sounds like an accusation and others might feel defensive and resistant to hearing your message. An important principle of assertive communication is the use of "I" messages, such as "I've noticed that . . ." or "I would like you to bathe Mrs. Dove."

Step 3. "I Feel . . ."

Here you describe an emotion. You communicate a great deal to others when you share the impact of their behavior on you. They can get a clearer picture of the effect on others. An example is, "When I asked you to float off the unit just now, you slammed the chart down on the desk and said, 'No way! I am not going to float up there.' I feel angry. Every staff nurse has taken a turn floating off the unit, and now it's your turn."

> "I noticed that . . ."
> or . . . "when you . . .,"
> "I feel. . . .,"
> "I want . . ." (the desired outcome). This is the recipe for assertive communication.

Use this step judiciously. If you are confronted with an angry physician who is throwing charts, you might not wish to share that "I feel intimidated by your behavior." That physician might be so angry as to state, "Well, I hope you are intimidated! That was my intent, to get someone to react to get something done around here!" You may, however, want to share your concern that "I am concerned that the patients and families will hear you, and that one of those charts will hit someone."

Step 4. "I Want . . ."

This is where you are able to use that outcome that you determined in the first step. Here you specify what action you want the person to take or what behavior you want him or her to change. Your best bet is to start by requesting small changes of behavior and only one or two changes at a time. But let's face it, by the time you have noticed a behavior significant enough for you to spend time, effort, and adrenaline to ask for a behavior change, you really want more than a small change. In your heart of hearts, you secretly wish for a complete conversion experience that totally reforms both the offending behavior and the accompanying attitude! When you point out the problem, you want the person to say, "You are absolutely right! I am so grateful to you for showing me the light. I can't believe I didn't see this about myself. Believe me, from now on I'm going to be different. Thank you again." This is an entertaining but unlikely fantasy.

> Remember, it can take years to change an attitude. Focus on a small change in behavior related to your goal. Remember that you cannot control another person's behavior, but you can best influence them by your good communication and example!

An illustration is, "Jeff, you are later than I expected getting back to the unit. I expected you 20 minutes ago. The next time you get tied up in another department, I would appreciate it if you would call me [small behavior change] and let me know you are going to be late so I can plan for it."

CHECKPOINT 8-6

Use the outcomes-based communication formula to address a problem with the manager of your unit. You have noted that she is "off at meetings all the time," and although you're sure there must be some reason for those meetings, you've perceived that quality has dropped since she quit making rounds on the floor.

NONVERBAL BEHAVIORS

Research on human communication has shown repeatedly that the majority of the message we communicate comes from the nonverbal components.

What you say is very important, but how you say it carries even more weight. Nonverbal behaviors can either enhance or conflict with the verbal message. When confronted with such a mixed message, most listeners choose to believe the nonverbal message is the "real" one, so paying attention to your nonverbal behaviors can strengthen your verbal message.

Voice

The assertive delegator uses a level, conversational tone of voice and audible volume appropriate to the situation. Words are enunciated firmly and confidently. The assertive delegator is also comfortable with silence and pauses after key points to allow others to process the information. These behaviors communicate that the speaker has the legitimate authority to delegate and that the delegator is respectful of the delegate.

Eye Contact

An assertive delegator has a relaxed, steady gaze into another person's eyes. Looking away or down while speaking is usually suggestive of lack of self-esteem or confidence, although there are cultural variations on this interpretation. Avoid staring, blinking, squinting, or excessive eye movements.

Body Posture

How you hold your body while speaking says a great deal about you and your message. Face the person you are speaking with and place yourself at the same level, sitting or standing appropriately close. Hold your head erect and avoid slumping. Lean forward slightly. If you are standing, avoid shifting your weight from one foot to another. These are attending behaviors that say you are paying attention to what is being said.

Gestures

While speaking assertively, maintain a relaxed use of your hands and arms. Use gestures for emphasis, but avoid gestures such as arms folded across the chest (defensive), making a clenched fist (threatening), or finger shaking (aggressive/shaming). Also avoid the myriad other distracting nonassertive behaviors, such as excessive head movement; covering your mouth with your hand while speaking; and playing with jewelry, coins, keys, hair, beard, clothing, and so on. This fidgeting distracts from your message.

Facial Expression

Your facial expression should be relaxed with a pleasant to neutral expression. Most importantly, be consistent with the verbal message. If you are angry or upset, do not smile because this nullifies your words. Relax the muscles in your face and maintain a neutral expression. Avoid a drawn, tight-lipped mouth, wrinkled forehead, repeated swallowing, or other nervous habits such as excessive throat clearing or lip licking.

Personal Space

Maintain an appropriate distance, not crowding or invading the personal space "bubble" of the other. Avoid wandering and pacing.

CHECKPOINT 8-7

First determine the outcome or intended result.

"When you . . ." or "I notice that. . . ,"

"I feel . . . ," and "I want. . . ."

Use the steps above to respond to the following situations:

1. The jail chaplain has once again intruded into a counseling session when you are discussing problems with one of the assistive workers from the clinic.

2. The roster for your family planning class was finally located; it had been placed in the wrong public health nurse's mailbox by the agency secretary.

3. The rehabilitation aide has not charted the range of motion exercises for the last 2 days.

4. Patient call lights are blazing, but Joan is sitting at the desk eating chocolates.

See the end of the chapter for the answers.

CONCLUSION

Nurses have tremendous responsibilities and need to be able to delegate effectively through clear, assertive communication. Assertiveness is a learnable skill that improves with successful practice. Start out in small, low-emotion situations and gain skill and confidence.

Whether the response to your delegation is agreement, refusal, or absence, you can develop an assertive dialogue with your delegate that addresses the real problem and begins the process of resolution. What is in it for you? Just increased feelings of self-confidence and self-respect, improved communication with coworkers, resolution of actual problems, above-board negotiation for behavior changes, and the ability to act as an advocate for yourself and your patients.

ANSWERS TO CHECKPOINTS

8-1

    1. 65-70%

8-2.   Best practice for initial direction: initial instructions and description of the plan for the day is recommended to occur at the patient's bedside with the off going RN and the oncoming RN. Time is saved if the RN is able to describe the plan for the day with the patient and assistive personnel present, including the patient in the discussion. The plan for the day should include at the minimum:

    •   The RN will update the nursing assistant with any differences in assessment data or preferred patient/family outcomes after the RN performs assessment and patient focused interview at the bedside.

    •   The RN and team members engage in discussions before and after breaks and all meals.

    •   Anyone leaving the unit for any other reason would perform an update and handoff so that care can continue.

    •   Toward the end of the shift, the registered nurse and team members will plan a short period of time to discuss the outcomes that patients have achieved, celebrate the impact of the work that they have done, and give each other feedback. This celebration checkpoint is essential for team growth and development, job satisfaction, and critical thinking as revisions of care are planned for the next shift.

8-3

    1. On transfer from areas of care, such as in home care to the emergency department, emergency department to surgery,

surgery to post anesthesia care, to the surgical unit, to the ICU, to long-term care

2.   Shift reports

3.   Case hand-offs for weekends or holidays (such as between physician partners, between home health nurses, or care managers)

4.   RN initial direction and ongoing communication throughout a shift with assistive personnel

5.   When a care provider leaves a care area for breaks or meals.

8–4.

1.   The psychiatric nurse was being aggressive. Rashad responded by being passive but planned to be passive–aggressive in the future.

2.   This school nurse was being nonassertive.

3.   Mabel was aggressive. Her boss was being assertive.

8–5.

1.   Geraldine, will you please take axillary temperatures on all patients who are under 3 years of age when you do their admission work for the next 2 weeks? Please let me know verbally before I go in to their physical assessment if any are over 100°F. I think we've had some problems recently with the accuracy of the tympanic electronic thermometer, and I'm sending it off to get it fixed. Any questions? Great! Thanks, I think we'll avoid giving sick kids their immunizations this way!

2.   Linnea, I am concerned about this new Medicare paper-work. If we don't get it right and send it in before 2 days have elapsed postdischarge, we won't be paid the full amount we have coming. Let's go over how to fill it out. Is there any reason you can't get these sent off the day they leave, or at least the day after? Great! I appreciate your help in keeping this place open!

3.   Will you possibly have time to go by the Midtown Home-less Shelter before you come back to the office today after

visits? Good! Mrs. Burns' psychiatric evaluation is waiting there at the front desk to be picked up. I'll call Sammy, the secretary there, and let her know you'll come about 3:30 to pick it up today. Thanks! We need this evaluation to do her team planning tomorrow morning.

8-6.   First determine the intended outcome: The manager (or someone) would make rounds to observe for those quality issues (to see if your perception is correct) and make sure that quality is improved if it needs to be.

"Susan, I have observed more skin redness and breakdown the last several weeks, and I'm not sure if that is an increase in incidence or not. I am concerned about some other quality issues, and I'm wondering if staff have quit paying attention to some of these details of care since you have been so busy with those budget meetings. I feel nervous that our quality of care could be less than optimum without close observation and rounding from someone in management! I would like to know your thoughts on this concern." "Yes I would be willing to be involved in some observations and chart review to help out."

8–7.

1.   When you come into my office when I'm involved in a private conversation, I feel concerned about maintaining confidentiality, and I'd appreciate it if you'd knock before you come in.

2.   I noticed that the class roster was in the wrong mailbox today. I felt panicked when I couldn't find it. Would you please put it in my in-box the next time? Thanks!

3.   I noted that the charting on range of motion has not been completed the last few days, and I feel particularly frustrated by this because the state health department is visiting tomorrow. Please chart them now and plan to get them in the charts as soon as you can after completion. I appreciate it!

4.   Joan, when there are patients who have put on their call lights for assistance and you are sitting at the desk eating chocolates, I feel angry and concerned about patient safety. I want you to get up and help answer the call lights. (Please note: This is not all you might say in these circumstances. We will add to this kind of communication when we discuss conflict resolution and giving feedback in the next chapters.)

REFERENCES

DeLellis, A., & Sauer, R. (2004). Respect as ethical foundation for communication in employee relations. *Laboratory Medicine, 35,* 262–266.

Institute for Healthcare Improvement. (2007). *Protecting 5 million lives campaign, getting started kit: Reduce surgical complications.*

The Joint Commission's 2008 Patient Safety Goals. (2007). Retrieved July 6, 2007, from http://www.jointcommission.org/PatientSafety/NationalPatientSafety-Goals/08_hap_npsgs.htm.

The Joint Commission's Sentinel Event Statistics: Causes. Retrieved July 6, 2007, from http://www.jointcommission.org/NR/rdonlyres/FA465646-5F5F-4543-AC8F-E8AF6571E372/0/root_cause_se.jpg.

Recommended Reading

Anderson, K. (1993). *Getting what you want.* New York: Dutton Publishing.

Burley-Allen, M. (1983). *Managing assertively: How to improve your people skills.* New York: John Wiley & Sons.

Cohen, Shelley. (2004, October). Delegating vs. dumping: Teach the difference. *Nursing Management, 35*(10), 14–18.

Feldman, Daniel. (1999). *The handbook of emotionally intelligent leadership: Inspiring others to achieve results.* Paonia, CO: Leadership Performance Press. http://www.leadershipperformance.com.

Genua, R. (1992). *Managing your mouth.* New York: American Management Association.

Goleman, Daniel, Boyatzis, R., & McKee, A. (2002). *Primal leadership: Realizing the power of emotional intelligence.* Boston: Harvard Business Press.

Walzak, B., & Absolon, P. (2001). Essentials for effective communication in oncology nursing: Assertiveness, conflict management, delegation, and motivation. *Journal for Nurses in Staff Development, 17*(2), 67–70.

Know How to Resolve Conflict: Getting Coworkers to Work Together as a Team

Ruth I. Hansten and Marilynn Jackson

CHAPTER SKILLS

+ Identify the major sources and costs of conflict in your workplace.
+ Reflect on the origins of your own preferred strategies for handling conflict.
+ Apply the best option for resolving conflicts to select situations.
+ Use an outcomes-based conflict resolution model to resolve a work conflict.

RECOMMENDED RESOURCES

▶ Read Patterson, K., Grenny, J., McMillan, R., Switzler, A., & Covey, S. (2002). *Crucial conversations: Tools for talking when the stakes are high*. New York: McGraw-Hill Publishers.
▶ Attend any workshop in your area on how to resolve conflict, get along with others, handle difficult people, etc. It does not have to be nursing specific!

"You may tell me to do this assignment, but that doesn't mean I'm going to do it. In fact, there's no way that I am going to care for Mrs. Smith or work with Jerry!"

CONFLICT AS A CONCEPT

In the last chapter, we discussed how to communicate clearly and assertively and began to look at situations in which delegation can precipitate some uncomfortable interpersonal situations.

Conflict! It is definitely something most of us fear or avoid. However, when working with people, conflict of some kind is inevitable. Our attitude toward the possibility of conflict often influences the manner in which we delegate. "But if I tell staff to do something or give them feedback, there's a chance they will disagree, and then there will be conflict!"

Conflict, although uncomfortable, must be accepted as a part of living and working together. Consider the whole concept for a few moments, and think about what life would be like without any conflict at all. (Those of you who are breathing a sigh of relief and envisioning a world with prancing Bambis and fluttering butterflies, read on!)

There would be no new ideas or inventions. Most of these arise from conflicts over which idea is better.

Some of us would not put in the required effort to improve our performance. If negative feedback is given to us, even though we might disagree and begin a discussion about our own perceptions, we will be more aware of our supervisor's perceptions and focus on those problem areas.

More open relationships and better communication occur when colleagues are not afraid to disagree. Each person's point of view can be considered, and patient care improves from sharing varying perspectives.

Procedures and systems can improve through conflict. When a member of the team argues that things need improvement and that his or her way is better, it offers a window for changing things that need to be changed.

Conflict can be constructive, depending on the way it is handled. As the energy from the conflict is channeled to make things better for all, staff performance and better patient care can result.

Unless you work totally alone, we know you probably have ample opportunity to experience conflict. You might have developed your own philosophy of the origins of conflict. To make certain that you've covered all the bases when you steam away in frustration at those difficult situations in your work setting, let's take a look at the more common sources of conflict.

SOURCES OF CONFLICT

Why bother to look at sources of conflict? As nurses, you know there are at least 100 horrible physiological events that begin to take place in the human body when a patient is immobile, and you've learned to expect them and take measures to avoid the negative sequelae of such conditions as constipation, pneumonia, or deep vein thrombosis. Similarly, if you understand the usual sources of conflict, you'll be able to anticipate them as normal, even healthy, phenomena. This mind-set will make dealing with those issues much less stressful, and you might even be able to take steps to plan for them.

Ambiguous Jurisdiction

Not knowing who should be doing what and how roles and duties overlap is a common cause of conflict. This is often a problem when new roles are undertaken and systems of care delivery change. Inherent in these conflicts are questions of responsibility and authority. Instead of wasting energy on unnecessary disagreement, clarify job descriptions, state practice acts, and role expectations to reduce this source of conflict.

Conflicts of Interest

Where do you see these types of conflicts occurring in your healthcare setting? Everywhere! Whether an administration is perceived by staff to be solely interested in the bottom line or whether staff seem to define quality of patient care by the numbers of patients they care for, we see conflict of interest each day. In your specific setting, you'll see delegates experiencing conflict about care methods or about priorities based on their own personal values. Recognizing conflicts of interest will help you begin the conflict resolution process by identifying what each party really wants. (This will be covered later in the chapter.)

Communication Barriers

Physical and time barriers abound in health care. The very nature of our work in acute and long-term care facilities requires shift work. The pharmacist who works in the third-level underground in the medical center might not have as clear a concept of the needs of the nursing department on the oncology floor as the pharmacist who works in a satellite on the 12th story. The inpatient care coordinator might find that conflicts occur regularly with the outlying ambulatory care clinics. The French have a wonderful saying that translates as "He who understands all, forgives all." Our communication barriers prevent us from understanding each other, and conflict results.

Dependence of One Party on the Other Party

Delegation, from the physician to the nurse, the nurse to the assistive personnel, or the nursing care team to other departments, creates potential for disagreement and anger. When one party doesn't complete the job on time or correctly, righteous indignation blooms as the delegator sputters, "But I was counting on you! The patients were counting on you!" When one party is dependent on another and the process doesn't progress

"He who understands all, forgives all."

well, expect this kind of reaction. Anticipating it allows you to take steps to rectify the problem and will encourage the necessary communication and supervision to be certain the work is completed as planned.

Association of the Parties

The dictator type of management, in which the supervisor does not request participation and input, is uncomfortable for staff and stifles creativity and job growth. However, as interaction increases among workers, the potential for disagreement also grows. We've stated previously that disagreement can be positive, and a climate that encourages participation is excellent for improving staff motivation and the overall products we produce. Increased association of the parties becomes a source of conflict when the parties are unable to tolerate disagreement, do not have the communication skills to deal with the disagreement positively, and are working in a pressure-cooker environment. Expect that you'll need to help resolve conflicts when all have been under particular stress and when some members of the team do not employ assertive communication skills.

Behavior Regulations

Standardized policies, procedures, and rules seem to do two things at once. These regulating mechanisms are intended to reduce conflict by providing guidelines for performance. In some circumstances, however, the individual who wants more autonomy and less structure will chafe under the organization's regulations. For example, if your state's nurse practice act allows an LPN (LVN) to perform many procedures that are prohibited by your organization's job description for LPNs, expect some annoyance from some of the LPN staff. This discomfort will certainly surface as conflict.

Unresolved Prior Conflicts

The most common cause of conflict is unresolved prior conflicts. Consider those people of whom you aren't extremely fond, and time how quickly a list of past insults or negative incidents arises in your memory. Human beings often store up data that reinforce their viewpoint of a given individual. This data storage has been called "gunny sacking," a process that promotes an aching back and head. When the offending person once again commits his or her "crime," the gunny sacker finally dumps the overflowing bag onto the unprepared recipient. "You never listen to your assignments! You always act like a lazy bum!" The ability to deal with conflicts effectively as they arise allows both parties to feel better about themselves and their work, unencumbered by the weight of past unresolved problems.

Conflicts Unique to Health Care

While these are broad, somewhat generic categories of sources of conflict, it's also important to note some very specific areas of conflict unique to health care. Consider the following:

- Physicians versus nurses—An age-old battle still goes on in some settings due to many factors, including a gender bias, "curing versus caring," the interdependence of the roles, and the impact of healthcare revisions on both professions.
- Nurses versus the rest of the world—Nursing service, the largest part of any acute care facility, often feels unfairly targeted in terms of costs, need to change, restructuring demands, and staffing limitations. Nurses will often cite examples of how "pharmacy did not have to consider delivery of PRNs and stat meds as part of their jobs, and now nursing has to pick up the slack!"
- Nurses versus assistive personnel—If a change in care delivery models is imposed on nurses, rather than being of their own design, conflict often results. A difference in values and accountability is perceived. Nurses have been heard to say, "Assistants don't care about the patients as much as I do!" and "I'm the one who is accountable here; they will never be as accountable as me!"
- Healthcare payors—Like a steamroller running over all of us, changes in reimbursement practices have had a tremendous impact on healthcare providers. Physicians feel their opportunities for independent practice are restricted, patients feel their choices are being limited, and nurses are in the middle advocating for patient care and resisting the limits imposed by managed care plans.

Review statements 1–5 in Checkpoint 9–1. Think about how the norm for handling conflict in your family has affected the way you deal with, or avoid, conflict at work. Those of us who learned that any kind of disagreement was very painful might find it more difficult to respond to conflict in a positive, open manner. If significant others in our past modeled ineffective communication skills, which culminated in rearrangement or destruction of our family unit (whatever our definition might have been), we might be baffled and confused by those who enjoy a good argument and don't feel threatened when confronted by conflict. People who learned to keep quiet and passive, then fly into a rage, might find it more difficult to bring out issues that might trigger conflict until the situation becomes unbearable.

CHECKPOINT 9-1

Consider the conflicts you've encountered in the past 2 weeks in your work setting. Which source of conflict was responsible for each situation? In what ways could positive resolution of those conflicts be constructive for your team and your clients?

Let's take a look at how your past might be influencing your attitude toward conflict. Answer the following as true or false.

____ 1. I am afraid of conflict. In my family, conflict meant people yelling and fighting, which always translated into heartache for someone.

____ 2. In our family, we argued for fun. The neighbors often thought we were really fighting, but it was our way of showing we cared about each other.

____ 3. My parents never raised their voices to each other. I never knew things weren't going well until they were ready to get a divorce.

____ 4. The people in our family didn't ever disagree until someone was really very angry. Then one little thing would put Dad (or Mom) into a screaming rage.

____ 5. I grew up in the only nondysfunctional family in our town. We all discussed any issues that bothered us openly and freely, and calm, insightful, respectful discussion was the norm.

COST OF CONFLICT

We've discussed the potential benefits of a willingness to recognize and resolve conflict, and we have identified the sources. What about the cost? When teamwork fails, when people are unhappy with each other or themselves, when staff members feel overburdened or taken advantage of or, worse yet, powerless, a price is paid. We all know nurses who think of the work setting as an adversarial "us against them" type of environ-

ment. These people usually do not have a positive outlook, feel powerless and victimized by
the system ("I have no choice"), and will either
withdraw or leave the organization. If they stay
around, it is with detachment and a sense of
"just putting in my time." The impact on others
is significant because this attitude is contagious.
Morale goes down, and staff members are less
likely to be actively involved in working for the
improvement and advancement of their department. (Administrators then consider themselves
lucky if the staff is just getting the work done!)

> The impact on others is significant, as this attitude of a helpless withdrawal is contagious. Morale goes down, and staff members are less likely to be actively involved in working for the improvement and advancement of their department.

The organizational cost of conflict might be financial, as reflected
in lengthening of patient stays due to missed treatments or care; lack
of collaboration among the team members, leading to disputes over
approaches to care; staff calling in sick when they do not want to face
a continuing negative environment; and so on. A survey of over 1100
new nurses (practicing less than 1 year) in New Zealand reported that
because of conflict at work there were high levels of absenteeism, many
considered leaving the profession, and the majority of those who experienced a significant "distressing event with a coworker" declined to report
it to management, fearing retribution or other consequences (McKenna,
Smith, Poole, & Coverdale, 2003).

The impact can be felt on a personal level as well. The unhappy staff
member might internalize the conflict between herself and another staff
member by misusing avoidance, a poor resolution that affects her physically (stress ulcers, high blood pressure, maladaptive coping through
substance abuse, etc.). Yet the fear of confrontation or the feeling of helplessness can be so powerful that the personal price is paid, and the situation is endured and not resolved. A study of 141 nurses working on 13
inpatient units validates these effects of conflict, concluding that intrapersonal and intragroup conflict are directly associated with lower levels
of work satisfaction and low perceptions of team performance effectiveness (Cox, 2003).

We have seen many efforts fail due to the inability of the staff to satisfactorily resolve the conflicts that arise when developing a team. Differences in personal values, role confusion, unclear goals, and a need for
control (usually on the part of the nurse) are contributing factors to team
dysfunction. Conversely, we have witnessed many success stories where
staff members were willing to take the personal risk, were supported,

> "Unchecked, conflict has the potential to divide alliances and departments. Conversely, providing an ongoing forum for differences of opinion to be voiced and understood creates an environment where expectations can be shared and ideas are more likely to be expressed openly."

and were able to resolve the inevitable disagreements that result when people work together. "Unchecked, conflict has the potential to divide alliances and departments. Conversely, providing an ongoing forum for differences of opinion to be voiced and understood creates an environment where expectations can be shared and ideas are more likely to be expressed openly" (Forte, 1997, p. 121). Our assessments of nursing departments around the country continue to demonstrate that the opposite is more often the case, and more likely conflict will go "underground" or be discussed behind the backs of the people most involved.

STRATEGIES FOR CONFLICT RESOLUTION

Now that you have some idea of how you react to conflict, let's review how effective your preferred coping mechanism becomes in different situations. This section's adaptations of the Thomas-Kilmann Conflict Resolution Inventory (TKI) grid show how attitudes toward conflict reflect our intensity toward our own interest and the self-interest of the other viewpoints. **Exhibit 9–2** also summarizes the cost and benefit of each of the choices.

CHECKPOINT 9–2

Evaluate your attitude toward conflict and your strategic response repertoire by answering the questionnaire in Exhibit 9–1. Most people use different coping mechanisms in conflict situations depending on the setting and the future implications, but use your first reaction for the questionnaire.

EXHIBIT 9-1 Conflict Questionnaire

	Very Unlikely	Unlikely	Likely	Very Likely
1. I am usually firm in pursuing my goals.				
2. I try to win my position.				
3. I give up some points in exchange for others.				
4. I feel that differences are not always worth worrying about.				
5. I try to find a position that is between the other person's and mine.				
6. In approaching negotiation, I try to consider the other person's wishes.				
7. I try to show the logic and benefits of my position.				
8. I always lean toward a direct discussion of a problem.				
9. I try to find a fair combination of gains and losses for both of us.				
10. I attempt to work through our differences immediately.				
11. I try to avoid creating unpleasantness for myself.				
12. I might try to soothe the other's feelings and preserve our relationship.				
13. I attempt to get all concerns and issues immediately out.				
14. I sometimes avoid taking positions that create controversy.				
15. I try not to hurt the other's feelings.				

SCORING: Very unlikely = 1, Unlikely = 2, Likely = 3, Very Likely = 4.

	ITEM	ITEM	ITEM	
COMPETING	1	2	7	TOTAL
COLLABORATING	8	10	13	TOTAL
COMPROMISING	3	5	9	TOTAL
AVOIDING	4	11	14	TOTAL
ACCOMMODATING	6	12	15	TOTAL

Source: Reprinted from Thomas, K.W., Toward Multi-dimensional Values in Teaching: The Example of Conflict Behaviors, Academy of Management Review, Vol. 2, p. 487, with permission of the Academy of Management, © 1977.

EXHIBIT 9–2 Five Choices for Resolving Conflict Among the Team

#1 Avoidance: "There's no problem"

Used as a short-term solution to calm down and to buy time.
Cost: It does not solve the problem.
Benefit: It allows time for cooling off and thinking.

#2 Accommodation: "You win, I lose"

Sacrificing own interests to please the other member of the team. Okay if the issue is not important to you or the resolution is short term and will be problem solved later.
Cost: It does not achieve your own interests.
Benefit: It allows for immediate solution.

#3 Competition: "I win, you lose"

For quick, decisive action on vital matters.
Cost: Other party might not be satisfied and might be resistive.
Benefit: Your goals are achieved.

#4 Compromise: "I win and lose some, you win and lose some too"

Temporary solutions to complex problems, with resolution by mutual consent.
Cost: It takes time; you might have to give up optimum goal.
Benefit: Both parties feel successful and part of solution.

#5 Collaboration: "I win, you win"

Process that evolves over time, working through feelings that have interfered with the relationship and finding an integrative solution.
Cost: It takes strong commitment from both parties.
Benefit: It is a long-lasting solution with mutual satisfaction.

Avoidance

The first common strategy to resolving conflict is that of avoidance. Those who answered "True" on Question 1 in Checkpoint 9–1 might find avoidance to be an overused tool. It can be evidenced by the statements "I don't want to talk about it," "Let well enough alone," and "Don't rock the boat." Although avoidance works well in situations when you need more time to reflect, calm down, or get more information or input, it won't work for those situations that require your action and involvement.

A study of nurses' conflict resolution styles at three hospitals (Fowler, et al., 1993) noted that nurses use withdrawal, or avoidance, as their most common coping mechanism when confronted with conflict. The authors stated that this indicated a willingness to remove themselves from relationships and possibly a lack of interest in the outcomes of the conflicts as well. Additional research studies reveal that intensive care nurses generally prefer avoidance as a strategy to preserve relationships, provide a better example for student nurses, and reduce open confrontation (Kelly, 2006). Researchers used the TKI to survey nurses and other healthcare personnel at a large healthcare organization and found that avoidance was also the ideal approach to conflict for these participants (Reich, Wagner-Westbrook, & Kressel, 2007).

How do we decide whether to get involved? Certainly in health care it is easy for us to either brush conflict situations under the rug, leave it for the next shift or the next nurse, pass it off to a manager to take care of, or run in and save the day. It's certainly easy for us to put ourselves in a rescuer role when we don't need to be.

When making a decision about whether to get involved, focus on the intended outcomes. For example, what will happen if I do something about this issue? What will happen if I don't get involved? Examine the potential costs and potential benefits, and make your decision.

> A study of nurses' conflict resolution styles at three hospitals noted that nurses use withdrawal, or avoidance, as their most common coping mechanism when confronted with conflict.

Source: Adapted from the Thomas-Kilmann Conflict Mode Instrument. © 1974, Xicom, Inc., Tuxedo, New York.

Further, think about whether this situation affects your own safety, security, or goals. Does it affect the safety or welfare of those committed to your care? Does this conflict get in the way of achieving your group goals? If the answer to any of these questions is yes, then your strategy of avoidance had better remain an interim tactic only. You'll need to deal with this conflict.

Competition

Competition as a method of resolving conflicts shows a great amount of self-interest and low interest in whether the other party's viewpoints are considered. We see competition as an integral part of our society,

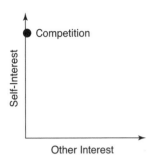

Source: Adapted from the Thomas-Kilmann Conflict Mode Instrument. © 1974, Xicom, Inc., Tuxedo, New York.

of our business world, and of the games we play in the Western hemisphere. In the past, boys were taught how to compete through the games and sports they played. Girls were encouraged to cooperate and be "nice" to everyone, and therefore women might not feel as comfortable with win–lose situations. The win–lose mentality works very well in some situations but is not satisfactory for making certain that everyone's positions are considered and for promoting a long-term supervisory relationship.

For example, if a school nurse and a school secretary have had repeated discussions about the necessity of instructing the asthmatic children how to use their metered dose inhaler properly, but the secretary refuses to do it and the nurse observes a child in real distress being merely handed the inhaler by the secretary as she glares at the RN, an "I win, you lose" or autocratic approach to resolving the conflict might be necessary for the short term. The nurse will want to intervene immediately to be certain the child's health is not at risk and will have to overrule the secretary's actions with her own, discussing the problem later with the secretary in a private place. Certainly when a client's health is at risk, time is not wasted to ascertain the other party's position on the matter.

Partially as a result of the serious nature of health care and nursing, rules or policies are considered to be important guides for practice. Some rules are based on reason and excellent rationales. However, in some organizations the culture (or "the way things are done here") might encourage forced compliance when conflicts occur. This becomes a kind of "corporate competition" when rules are enforced without reasoning why the policy was written in the first place. When situations like this occur, the agency itself is the "we win, you lose" competitor. For example, it's necessary for the safety of all concerned when a hospital enforces a rule that no one (except security or police) will be allowed to carry concealed weapons when visiting patients, and in a case when a visitor brandishes an AK-47 assault rifle and is carried bodily from the ICU, the "we win, you lose" method of solving a conflict might be best. But when the rule against bringing pets into an acute care institution is considered to be written in stone and is adhered to, even though nurses advocate for a short visit from a dying patient's dog, the competitive method of resolving a conflict might not be the most effective method for all concerned.

Just as we discussed the necessity of using your nursing judgment when delegating care, choosing the correct method of solving problems rests on your assessment of the situation and what tactics would be the most effective.

Accommodation

This style of resolving conflict develops when a person is much more interested in the other person's needs or desires than in maintaining his or her own point of view. Those whose answers scored high in accommodation might use this as a comfortable method of relating to others when there is some disagreement. Accommodation is effective in a situation that doesn't matter much to you. For example, if a delegate (a home health aide, for example) states in a challenging manner that she is planning to rearrange her schedule of home visits, and this does not present a problem to you or

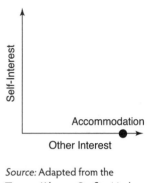

Source: Adapted from the Thomas-Kilmann Conflict Mode Instrument. © 1974, Xicom, Inc., Tuxedo, New York.

to your clients, it's fine to be accommodating. (The nurse in charge might also want to explore the situation more extensively and find out why the home health aide seems angry and challenging today.) If, however, a scrub technician in your outpatient surgical center states that she doesn't think she'll provide the correct instruments for Dr. Jones' orthopedic patients today, it's not time to accommodate her wishes.

The message of accommodation is this: Accommodate when it's truly okay with you. Use another method of conflict resolution if you feel uncomfortable or unhappy with the situation. (For those with codependent tendencies who tend to accommodate others, we recommend the classic *I'm Dying to Take Care of You* [Snow & Willard, 1989].)

Compromise

"I win some and lose some; you win some and lose some" is commonly used for conflict resolution in our society. The political process often uses compromise to come up with a reasonable middle ground as terribly complex issues are discussed by highly polarized groups. Each of these groups has principles or values that are ingrained to the core of each individual's personality and are at complete odds with one another. What is right and good and ethical will be very different for different individuals; therefore it is sometimes difficult to come up with a conflict

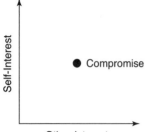

Source: Adapted from the Thomas-Kilmann Conflict Mode Instrument. © 1974, Xicom, Inc., Tuxedo, New York.

resolution in which all people are completely satisfied. If you discovered in your conflict questionnaire that you compromise frequently, you might be aware of the very common human tendency to avoid flexibility and understanding the opposite viewpoint when your opponent is so obviously wrong and you are so obviously on the side of "good and all that is right."

Compromise allows us to move ahead in situations that are terribly complex or polarized. When changes must be made in the admissions processes for an acute care medical center, conflicting ideas and positions will occur because literally scores of departments and hundreds of people are affected. Even if all departments are involved in creating the changes in procedure, not all of the personnel might agree wholeheartedly with the end product and might need to "give" a bit on their original position. Mutual consent that when the decision is made, all will implement it for the good of the whole will allow the medical center to continue to function as smoothly as possible during the admission process.

You might experience compromise frequently in your work setting. For example, if a new admission is coming to your area but all staff are overloaded, the admission process could be divided up into parts and shared, with one RN coordinating the process. If a dialysis RN asked for Christmas Eve off for the last year but ended up having to take call, perhaps the dialysis tech would share call and get the work done more quickly.

Collaboration

The "win–win" approach to conflict resolution, or collaboration, is founded on the ability of each party to focus on what each wants or needs, as well as their mutual goals. In collaboration, each party contributes to the problem-solving process so that views can be integrated. All relevant issues are discussed in an open and honest manner, with mutual respect for each individual's thoughts, feelings, and ideas. Both parties win because they have been heard and their ideas and needs have been considered and discussed. The final resolution should be acceptable, if not preferable, to all involved. This win–win approach will be discussed in more detail in the Hansten and

Collaboration requires trust, a clear understanding and appreciation of each other's position, and a willingness to reframe the goal to one of mutual concern.

Washburn Outcomes-Based Collaborative Resolution Process later in this chapter.

As you reviewed your organization's mission, we suspect you found some statements about treating those you serve with dignity and respect. These same precepts or values are necessary to work within a situation of conflict. Although all the methods can be used effectively within an appropriate problem situation, compromise and collaboration reflect a thorough consideration of each party's needs, emotions, and issues.

Collaboration is a time-consuming approach and should be used for those problems that require participative involvement for the success of a program, those where emotions are deep, and those where there is significant need for the relationship between the parties to grow and mature. Changing care delivery systems, adding new personnel, and redefining roles require a true collaborative effort.

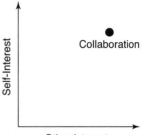

Source: Adapted from the Thomas-Kilmann Conflict Mode Instrument. © 1974, Xicom, Inc., Tuxedo, New York.

Changing care delivery systems, adding new personnel, and redefining roles require a true collaborative effort.

Conflict Evaluation Quiz

Let's look at a few issues and determine what method would be best to use.

1Q: There is a conflict between the RN who supervises the oncology program in this ambulatory care setting and the medical assistant who schedules the chemotherapy appointments and often gives the prechemotherapy nausea medication. The issue here is the timing of the medication and the administration of the chemotherapy.

Conflict resolution method of choice_____
Why? _____

1A: Collaboration should be attempted first because there are significant reasons to invest in this relationship: Its quality will affect both individuals, the team, and the patients. Both individuals are driven by the mutual goal of the most appropriate and effective patient treatment. It's possible that other personal needs are involved, and compromise might be necessary.

2Q: The rehabilitation team has worked extensively with a family regarding the home care plan for a paraplegic patient, Fred. However, one of the family members strongly believes, from a religious stand-point, that Fred should not be completing his own self-catheteriza-tion. Although this viewpoint is difficult for the healthcare team, there has been no change of attitude on the part of the caregiver despite many reasoned discussions.

Conflict resolution method of choice_____
Why? _____

2A: Compromise might be necessary in this situation. Reality dictates that if a procedure will not be completed due to pressure of a family member, another method might be needed. Perhaps the religious standpoint could be further explored and the exact nature or ratio-nale of the prohibition could be discussed so that creative solu-tions could be applied. Perhaps the family member will not have to be involved in this procedure. When deep values, such as religious teachings, are involved, it's difficult for everyone to be totally satis-fied with solutions.

3Q: Sally was brought up by an abusive, alcoholic mother. When making visits to the home of an alcoholic diabetic patient, she finds herself unable to listen carefully to the concerns of this patient. When she allows herself to be honest, she figures that he's killing himself anyway and that her time is wasted when she tells him to eat right and to take his insulin and medications as ordered. It's a constant argument, with Sally telling him what to do and the patient ignoring her.

Conflict resolution method of choice_____
Why? _____

3A: Unless Sally has already embarked on an effective personal coun-seling journey, it might be best for her to use avoidance and ask someone else to take over his care. Awareness of her inability to deal with the inevitable conflict successfully shows respect for herself and for her patient.

4Q: Pablo, a case manager for total hip patients throughout the healthcare continuum in a large healthcare conglomerate, notices that one of the subacute care facilities frequently sends total hip patients back to the ICU on the weekends and holidays. When he attempts to discuss this with the director of that department, she begins to shout about the level of staffing that is available during those periods.

Conflict resolution method of choice_____
Why? _____

4A: This situation calls for collaboration on the part of Pablo, who has legitimate concerns, and the department director, who seems frustrated at her staffing situation. A win–win solution will creatively address both individuals' concerns. Their mutual ground at this point is their need to assure patients' welfare.

5Q: Pat, an AIDS patient in a combined long-term care and hospice facility, has been very angry about the corporate visiting rules. She wishes to be married to her significant other, Kim, and wants to invite at least 50 friends. Her condition is declining. She is angry and shouts at you, the charge nurse for this shift, about the "inhumane corporate policies."

Conflict resolution method of choice_____

Why? _____

5A: The charge nurse has every reason to accommodate Pat's need to go around the rules. The nurse might need to ask Pat to compromise some on the number of guests, but, if possible, she can accommodate Pat's wishes. The charge nurse has very little invested in the corporate rules in this situation and will be even more satisfied if Pat wins.

6Q: The Medic One ambulance has patched in a serious arrhythmia on the monitor. The patient is about 10 minutes away from your emergency department in the middle of a traffic jam on the highway. You have instructed the medic to give a bolus of epinephrine. He states that he's just been to an update on arrhythmia treatment, and he thinks another choice of medication would be better. You have recently been through an advanced cardiac life support course and do not wish to argue as the patient's pressure drops.

Conflict resolution method of choice_____

Why? _____

6A: "I win, you lose" is the method of choice in this situation. The patient also wins if some antiarrhythmia treatment is given and is effective. You can be clear that you'll discuss the new treatment protocols later, but for now, "Give the drug!"

7Q: The materials management and environmental services departments have made a change in the location of the sharps containers for contaminated needles and other disposable instruments. These have been placed in the rooms of the patients and within the areas that nurses might need them. It is the evening shift, you are in charge, and you've been told that the containers will be moved during your shift to a central location on the unit. The materials management worker states sourly, "It's going to save $400 per day to have fewer containers to empty." Your obvious concern is safety.

Conflict resolution method of choice _____

Why? _____

7A: This situation calls for a collaborative approach in the long run. In the short run, the charge nurse can try competition ("I can't let you change them now because I am very concerned about patient, nurse, and environmental services workers' safety") or avoidance and compromise ("If you'll wait just one day, I'll get in touch with the department managers and we'll start a discussion about this change in procedure").

Before we move on to the Hansten and Washburn Outcomes-Based Collaborative Resolution Process, let's review the sources of conflict, the beneficial and destructive consequences, and the advantages to dealing with conflict appropriately to the given situation. Please review the flowchart in **Figure 9–1**.

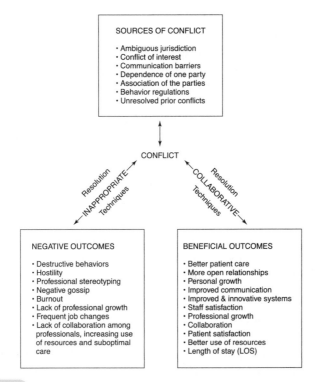

FIGURE 9–1 Conflict Flowchart. *Source:* **Dennis Burnside**

INNOVATIVE ISSUE RESOLUTION PROCESS: A COLLABORATIVE METHOD

Exhibit 9–3 outlines the collaborative resolution method. Quickly review the process steps and then proceed to the discussion. We'll ask you to apply the process in some clinical situations that you might have encountered.

EXHIBIT 9–3 Hansten and Jackson Outcomes-Based Collaborative Resolution Process

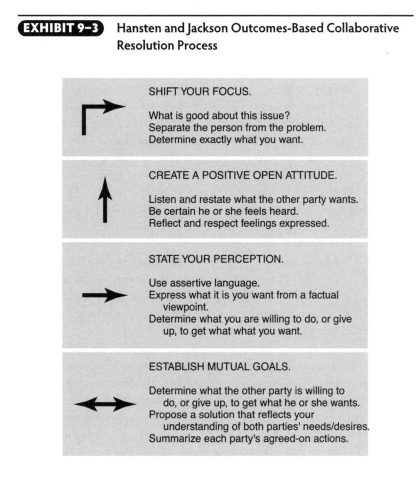

SHIFT YOUR FOCUS.

What is good about this issue?
Separate the person from the problem.
Determine exactly what you want.

CREATE A POSITIVE OPEN ATTITUDE.

Listen and restate what the other party wants.
Be certain he or she feels heard.
Reflect and respect feelings expressed.

STATE YOUR PERCEPTION.

Use assertive language.
Express what it is you want from a factual viewpoint.
Determine what you are willing to do, or give up, to get what what you want.

ESTABLISH MUTUAL GOALS.

Determine what the other party is willing to do, or give up, to get what he or she wants.
Propose a solution that reflects your understanding of both parties' needs/desires.
Summarize each party's agreed-on actions.

The first step in resolving issues or conflicts is to be aware of your state of mind. If you are angry and upset, your mind will be closed to creativity. If you feel threatened, your "fight or flight" response will be operant, and things will not proceed as effectively. In health care, we don't have the luxury of wasting time and money on uncontrolled, unexamined emotions.

1. *Shift your focus.* Instead of thinking of how you're being wronged or the negative characteristics of the Neanderthal person you're dealing with, blow out the flame of anger instead of adding fuel to it. There are several methods of remaining calm and logical as you attempt to resolve an issue.

   Stimulate your right brain and creativity by thinking about what is good about the problem. For example, in problem 7Q, the sharps containers being moved away from where sharps are used, consider what could be positive about this issue arising.

   Perhaps you are glad that this has happened on your shift because you feel so strongly about safety issues. Perhaps you are anxious to be more involved in interdepartmental planning and in "fixing" the system by which decisions affecting many departments are made. Perhaps this will allow you to get to know the support people better. This might sound like a Pollyanna part to collaboration, but it is essential to shift to a positive way of thinking so that the creativity necessary for problem solving can be used.

   Separate the person from the problem. This time-honored phrase has been used as fundamental to conflict resolution since people began to think about the process. Remember that the person who is removing the sharps container is not the problem; a decision that was made about the sharps containers is the problem. This allows you to view the person dispassionately, more as a pawn to circumstance than as someone who is personally plotting against your happiness.

   Determine exactly what you want. To do this, you must be calm enough by this time to take the energy produced by those emotions and harness it to think logically about what you'd like to reap from the time you'll spend on this issue. What is the bottom-line result you'd like to see? Basing this model on outcomes allows our brains to do the work for us in terms of creating the fastest paths to attain the predetermined goals we have in mind. In this case, you probably want the sharps containers to be where they can be used most safely and efficiently by all personnel.

   If you are still not calm enough to think about this problem logically, then take some time to relax and calm down. Deep breaths, counting to 10, prayer, and taking a short bathroom or coffee break are useful to

Identifying what's good about the problem allows you to stop the negative downward spiral of "ain't it awful" and begin to think of creative and positive options.

some. Nurses have also told us that they use such techniques as creative visualization and directive self-talk. These are not auditory or visual hallucinations. In creative visualization, you think of yourself in a safe, calm place, whether it is by a rushing stream in the mountains, fly fishing, or on your couch at home in front of a crackling fire with a cup of herbal tea. Others visualize themselves or someone that they admire dealing with the issue in an effective manner. Some visualize the offending opposing person(s) with his or her pajamas on, with a clown nose, or in other less threatening attire. Many people direct their self-talk, that continuous running commentary in your brain, to be positive: "I know I can handle this, I will be calm, and besides, no one will remember this day 100 years from now!"

> Determine exactly what you want (results). Most people fail to successfully resolve a conflict because they are reacting on an emotional level and have not clearly identified the outcome they would like to achieve.

2. ***Create a positive open attitude.*** Listen closely to what the other party is saying. By continuing to keep your focus shifted from your anger to what the other party's needs might be and trying to fully understand his or her position, you are influencing the potential for a positive outcome to the discussion.

    Listen carefully to what is being said. The materials worker who has stated that "it's going to save $400 per day to empty fewer containers" is probably discussing the rationale that he's heard for the change in procedure. As you restate what you've heard, you're clarifying and asking for more information. "So the idea here is to cut the material and personnel costs as a part of our money-saving plan? What else have you heard about why this decision was made?"

    Be certain that the other party feels he or she has been fully heard and that his or her position has been understood. "If I hear you correctly, your department is doing this as a cost-savings idea, but you're also afraid that a few more of these ideas, and you won't have a job left to do?"

    Reflect the feelings that have been expressed. In our example discussion, the worker has shared his concern about being laid off if he doesn't have enough

> Respect all feelings that are expressed. Judging whether a feeling is right, wrong, or justified is not helpful and only serves to further isolate the two parties.

to do. In many cases, people will not express their feelings clearly, and you might need to put yourself in their place, empathize, and then ask for confirmation. "You seem nervous and angry about this. I can certainly see where this would be of concern to you. Am I on target with how I think you are feeling about this?" Naming their emotions, fears, or concerns often allows people to be less guarded, discuss the issues without hidden agendas, and solve problems more effectively. If the other party is very angry or upset, stating that you've received that message will help take the wind out of their sails. "I can see this is upsetting for you and you seem to be feeling quite concerned. We understand that this was an order given to you and that you didn't make the rule yourself. Let's talk about what we can do together to solve it."

Respect all feelings that are expressed. Nurses are great empathizers; we might know how we would feel in the same circumstance. However, the range of human emotions and thoughts is varied, and whatever feelings are expressed must be respected as such. Judging whether a feeling is right, wrong, or justified is not helpful and only serves to further isolate the two parties. (Behaviors, however, are subject to feedback and comment. A discussion of methods of giving feedback will be provided in Chapter 10.)

3. *State your perception.* In this step, you are again sharing your viewpoint and what you'd like to accomplish by your discussion. Think back to our last chapter on assertiveness and use your "I noticed that, I feel, I want" recipe as needed. For example, you might state, "When one department makes a decision that affects another, such as changing the location of the sharps containers, the other department feels left out and devalued, and I'd like all of us to work together to determine a better system for interdepartmental decision making." This statement focuses on the long-term results and the reason you are feeling distressed. "For now, however, it seems that you've been given an order by your department that isn't one you like, either. I will talk with your supervisor so that you don't get into trouble, but I am asking you not to move those containers until we can find a better solution. The safety of the nurses, other healthcare personnel, and the patients might be adversely affected by moving those disposal bins."

In the preceding discussion, the nurse in charge has looked at the problem in two ways: one a short-term resolution (don't move the containers) and the other a long-term one (how can we find a better system to avoid these problems?). The nurse has used assertive language to express feelings and expressed what he or she wants from a factual viewpoint. The nurse has also determined that he or she is willing to do at least one thing to resolve it: Take on the responsibility of calling the materials supervisor about these concerns and thus providing some assistance to assuage the materials worker's anxieties.

What else might the RN plan to do to get started on resolving the long-term issue? Certainly he or she would be willing to alert the manager to the issue so that follow-up can continue. Perhaps he or she would be willing to be on a task force for determining the safest and most cost-effective manner to dispose of sharps. Perhaps the materials worker would want to join that committee as well. The RN might also want to research current methods of discussing and resolving interdepartmental issues and help solve this recurring problem within the organization.

4. *Establish mutual goals.* In any area of health care, the patient or client's service or care must be the mutual, bottom-line objective of all parties involved. When people are reminded of their shared goals, it is much less difficult to obtain participation. "Since all of us are here for safe, quality patient care, we all have to think about safety along with the costs."

    Determine what the other party is willing to do or give up to be a part of the solution. "Will you be willing to stop the process of changing the containers if I call your supervisor to explain?"
    Propose a solution that reflects your understanding of the needs and desires of the other party as well as your own, and then review what each party has agreed to do.

    "So you'll leave the sharps bins where they are, and please explain our discussion and our concerns with your supervisor also. You're also willing to be on a committee to solve these interdepartmental problems, and at the same time, you can think of ways to keep your job through added responsibilities, if necessary. I'll call your supervisor for tonight to explain why we don't want this done right now, and I'll discuss ways in which we can solve the short-term problem of the sharps disposal as well as what each of us can do to keep these interdepartmental issues from cropping up due to lack of understanding. We each have a couple of things to do, but it's worth it to keep us all safe and employed! Is this all okay with you? Great!"

This step allows us to clarify whether each party has remained clear and whether the parties are currently in agreement on a course of action. Each party has "won" and will be invested in the solutions.

Although the process of collaborative resolution seems intricate and involved, there are really four main issues:

1. Shift your focus to what's possible and away from the negative feelings.

2. Create a positive open attitude by listening and respecting the other party's position.

3. State your perception and position assertively, clearly, and factually.

4. Establish mutual goals and actions based on input and participation from both parties. Use the imagery of the arrows in Exhibit 9–3 to help you remember.

CASE STUDY ANALYSIS OF COLLABORATIVE RESOLUTION

Jamal is a jail nurse for a men's work release center. He has had some concerns about some nagging coughs that he's heard, particularly during the night and early morning hours. Although most of his clients have been smokers, some also had positive TB skin tests in the past without preventive drug therapy. He's read about the growing prevalence of a multidrug-resistant tuberculosis and wonders whether all of the prisoners would be infected with the current ventilation system. He's brought his concerns and a plan for follow-up TB skin tests or QFT-G tests (QuantiFERON TB Gold Test as recommended by the CDC), chest films, and sputum samples to the physician advisor, Dr. Richards. Dr. Richards, who is also responsible for the budget of the facility, reacts angrily: "Jamal, you are just like a mother hen! I am tired of hearing about all the real or imagined ills of 'your' patients! These people are heavy smokers, have been drug abusers, and are in horrible health all around. They are going to cough in the morning, for heaven's sake! Don't you have enough to do? We can't afford to do all those tests on these people!"

Follow the process to help Jamal respond to Dr. Richards. Write down your thoughts as well as your dialogue in this situation.

1. Shift your focus. _____

_____

_____

_____

_____

_____

2. Create a positive open attitude. _____

_____

_____

_____

_____

_____

3. State your perception. _____

_____

_____

_____

_____

_____

4. Establish mutual goals. _____

_____

_____

_____

_____

_____

CHECKPOINT 9-3

To feel competent in dealing with the Collaborative Resolution Process, it's necessary to practice it continually. As often as we've taught these communication skills, it is still difficult for us to use them in every situation. We recommend that you think about a recent issue or conflict and role play resolving it with a friend. If you feel uncomfortable doing that, make yourself a "skill card" with the process, and keep it in your backpack, purse, or pocket to use before you are planning to solve an interpersonal problem. After a conflict situation, use the process to evaluate how well you have done and where you might have needed to concentrate. Many nurses have found it effective to teach the process to their children or spouses and learn it better from teaching it.

Here are a few situations you can use to test your understanding. For further practice, look over the conflict issues listed earlier in this chapter.

1. You've assigned a nursing assistant to complete a task. She retorts, angrily, that you've been of no support or help to her, she's been working like a demon all day, and she is just too tired to consider taking on another assignment.

2. You return from a break and you notice that one of your psychiatric patients is having a serious problem because you see a code cart and several security guards by the door. One of your coworkers is on the telephone, talking about a date that is being planned for this evening. You motion for her to get off the phone and help with the other patients, and she glares and turns her back, continuing her conversation.

3. You and your supervisor have had a disagreement about your caseload and the home health aides and rehabilitation aides working with your patients. You feel overwhelmed and unable to take on more work, and you aren't happy with the performance of your assistants. Your supervisor is adamant, and the entire agency is under terrible financial stress.

4. You are an ambulatory care nurse working with several physicians. One of the physicians you work with has displayed some erratic behavior that might indicate he is being affected by a chemical dependency or some other intense personal problem. It has affected his work with the patients. You approach the senior physician, and she reacts angrily that you should keep quiet about this and that she is sure the other physician has "everything under control."

See the end of the chapter for the answers.

1. In shifting your focus, you wonder what is good about this problem. Perhaps this gives Jamal a chance to prove his clinical expertise and judgment or an opportunity to clarify his role expectations with Dr. Richards because they seem to be in conflict. It's

certainly good that Dr. Richards is reacting at all because he rarely seems to have an opinion on anything. Besides, it's necessary to get him involved in this potentially serious situation. In separating the person from the problem, you've identified that the real problem is the health of these coughing patients. What you want is an opportunity to further assess the etiology of these coughs and rule out TB or other infectious disease agents.

2. What is Dr. Richards saying here? Is he afraid that he can't really affect the wellness of the inmates without it costing too much? Does he feel out of control of their health due to the myriad other risk factors? He's obviously irritated. Jamal might respond, "Dr. Richards, I can see this is a frustration for you as it is for me. These people have just about destroyed their bodies before they got to us, and certainly we don't have enough money to give them all bionic parts! It's hard for us, me especially, to determine where I can best be of help to them all. Do you ever feel that way?"

3. Dr. Richards has verified this feeling of helplessness; now it's time for Jamal to share his position. "As frustrating as it may be, I am even more concerned when I hear the increasingly loud racket of productive coughs during the night and early morning hours. Some of the inmates are complaining of night sweats also and were never followed up on their positive skin tests. When I am confronted with all of these symptoms, I feel increasingly frightened for their safety as well as ours, and I want your help in deciding what kind of follow-up should be done with respect to efficacy as well as cost. The cost would be astronomical, both in terms of treatment and in terms of public outrage, if we had a TB problem and did nothing about it. I am willing to do overtime or whatever it takes, including getting the advice of the public health department experts."

4. Because Dr. Richards seems to be responding well to the facts now that Jamal has outlined them effectively, as well as being cognizant of the risks involved with not acting, it's time to remind him of the mutual goals. "After all, our jobs here, as I see it, are to ensure the optimal health of these clients, given the cost constraints and the material we are given to work with! We are certainly working together for the same goals, right?"

After Jamal asks Dr. Richards for suggestions, Dr. Richards determines he'll call an old friend at the health department for some input. He'd like Jamal to call the TB nurse specialist and find out how they could

> Conflict, and our response to it, will always determine whether we move ahead as a profession or become paralyzed victims of circumstance, unwilling to take the risk that conflict demands.

help. As the conversation continues, Jamal wants to restate the plan. "So I will call the TB nurse specialist for assistance, and you'll talk with your friend who's been involved in the program, and we'll get together to discuss this on Friday at noon? Great! I feel better checking this out. There are just too many indications to avoid exploring the cough problem!" Jamal also knows there is a long-term problem left to solve. How can he determine whether he is fulfilling Dr. Richards's expectations or if there is a problem? Is he really a "mother hen," or was that response a result of Dr. Richards's frustration? "You know, I am wondering if we could also discuss how you feel I am doing in my job. I'm not sure how to interpret the comments you made earlier in the conversation, so could you think about this and we'll discuss it on Friday? I want to be able to present my concerns to you and to do my job overall in the most effective manner, and I'd like some feedback." The physician may or may not respond now, but Jamal potentially will find out how he can better get his attention without having to resolve a conflict.

CONCLUSION

Conflict, and our response to it, will always determine whether we move ahead as a profession or become paralyzed victims of circumstance, unwilling to take the risk that conflict demands. We have seen countless nurses literally stopped in their tracks, victims at the mercy of everyone else's control, as they perceive the potential for conflict too great to take the chance. We have also observed many nurses who see conflict as a process of life and who have developed their skills in dealing with disagreement, just as they have mastered numerous clinical skills.

Nursing is in the people business. And people don't always agree. Appreciating the benefits of that disagreement and being confident in your ability to resolve conflict will position you for the most satisfying career you can imagine. Secure in your understanding of the basic four-step process of conflict resolution as outlined in this chapter, you will find yourself taking control of both your personal and professional growth. Isn't that the best outcome of all?

ANSWERS TO CHECKPOINT

9–3.   Scenarios: suggested dialogue:

1.   In shifting your focus, you realize that the real problem is
not this nursing assistant but the fact that there is a task to be
done and no one agreeing to do it. You consider what is good
about this problem: Perhaps you are glad to have the chance
to interact with this CNA, who has expressed her concerns
about overwork before. Perhaps you are rested today and feel
energetic about using your new conflict resolution method!
What you want is to find someone to take over the task assignment and to find out what's wrong with this CNA. To create a
positive open attitude, you'll respond, "Wow, Mei, I can see
that you are really overwhelmed! And I am sorry that I haven't
been as available as I'd like to have been to help you. We've
had a pretty rough day." In stating your perception, you might
say, "But Mei, when I come to ask you for help, and you react
by throwing the linens on the floor, I feel hurt. I'd like us to look
at the assignments and figure out what ideas you have for who
can do this work. Someone has to complete it, and I know three
of us will be on overtime already." Mei might discuss with you
that she needs to have foot surgery and that she isn't feeling
well. (You should certainly respond to this with a few caring
comments.) You might also express that you've looked at the
assignments and are unable to find anyone with time on her
hands and that you can't take on any more work yourself with
Mr. Smith being so critical. In establishing mutual goals, you
might also state, "Mei, I know we all want the patients to get
quality care and we also all want to get home and put up our
feet. Would you be willing to assist with this task if I ask the next
shift to finish whatever else you have to do at 3:45? I'll get 15
minutes of overtime authorized for all of us." Mei agrees. The
next day, when time allows, discuss the long-term problem of
Mei's feet and how you and she could interact more positively
regarding her assignments and supporting her as charge nurse.
Clarification of expectations, another concept covered earlier,
will be helpful.

2.   In shifting your focus, you take a few deep breaths. (If you
have a split second of time, you might consider that what is

good about the problem is that you finally have some objective evidence that this coworker is not performing. Usually she just disappears!) You know the real problem at hand is getting adequate assistance in the code and with the other patients, who will be very upset. This is time for using "competition" as a mode of resolution until you can work out a long-term solution. You might lightly touch your coworker and state, "Sue, I am going to help with the code. You must check on the other patients. Now." Or, after you ascertain that the code situation is under control, you can return to Sue. You can use your assertive language and say, "I understand that it's important for you to have some time on the phone with your friends, but when I come back to the unit after break and you are on the phone talking about a date while an emergency is going on, and you ignore me, I feel angry and frightened about the safety of the patients." You've determined what you really want: that Sue will participate in the emergencies on the unit. You've determined that what you are willing to do is to make a point of resolving the issue and discussing it with Sue. Your mutual goal in this situation is safe patient care. Sue might have the additional goal of getting break time or free time to resolve personal issues. If that is the case, you can discuss how she can also get those needs taken care of during breaks. A solution will certainly include all individuals being involved in caring for the patients during emergencies.

3.   You begin by shifting your focus. What is good about this problem is that it has finally come to a head and that you'll be dealing with it for the good of all involved. You determine that what you want is to be able to do the work as required but to have some impact on the way you supervise and evaluate the assistive personnel. You begin by discussing with the supervisor, "I know it's very tough financially here and we all want to do our best and keep the agency open and keep our jobs. You've got your hands full helping us to maintain productivity. But when I'm asked to do more than I'm sure I can do well, without having adequately trained assistants, I feel absolutely overwhelmed, and frankly, I am afraid. I'm not sure my patients are getting the care they need unless I have more time to supervise and teach these new assistants. I'm willing to take any suggestions you may have." As your supervisor under-

stands that you are trying to work things out, she'll be able to interact with you more positively. "What I'd really like from you are some ideas on how to make certain I can supervise, train, and evaluate them and still do the necessary caseload." As the discussion continues, your supervisor might give you many worthwhile ideas, assist in training or supervising your assistive personnel, or modify your assignment. Remember to summarize each other's agreed-upon actions.

4.   What's good about this problem? You've used your excellent powers of observation as a patient advocate. The problem here is the potential for unsafe care due to a physician's behavior. What you want is for someone to find out what is going on with him and to take action to protect the patients. You have another meeting with the senior physician, Maria Menendez. You begin by saying, "Maria, I know you are good friends with Dr. Putz, and it's tough to think there could be a problem. It's scary for all of us. But we all want to protect the patients if my concerns are valid. When you seemed to dismiss my objective examples of his erratic behavior yesterday, I felt even more concerned. I've lost sleep over this situation. This is definitely a matter that could go to the state board if you find there is a problem. In fact, this is our professional duty. I am willing to be involved in the discussion with him, if you'd like, or be of support to you when you talk with him. Are you willing to discuss it with him? Good. Will you let me know when you've talked with him, then?" Although we haven't added the responses of Dr. Menendez, she is aware that she must deal with the situation and determine what needs to be done. She also knows you aren't going to let the problem simmer when patient safety is involved. Good job!

REFERENCES

Cox, K. (2003). The effects of intrapersonal, intragroup and intergroup conflict on team performance effectiveness and work satisfaction. *Nursing Administration Quarterly, 27*(2).

Forte, P. (1997). The high cost of conflict. *Nursing Economic$, 15*(3), 119–123.

Fowler, A.R. Jr., et al. (1993). *Health Progress, 74*(5), 25–29.

Kelly, J. (2006). An overview of conflict. *Dimensions of Critical Care Nursing, 25*(1), 22–28.

McKenna, B., Smith, N., Poole, S., & Coverdale, J. (2003). Horizontal violence: Experience of registered nurses in their first year of practice. *Journal of Advanced Nursing, 42*(1), 90–96.

Reich, W., Wagner-Westbrook, B., & Kressel, K. (2007). Actual and ideal conflict styles and job distress in a health care organization. *Journal of Psychology, 14*(1), 5–15.

Snow, C., & Willard, D. (1989). *I'm dying to take care of you: Nurses and codependence and breaking the cycles.* Redmond, WA: Professional Counselor Books.

Recommended Reading

Hansten, R., & Washburn, M. (1993). *The nurse manager's answer book.* Gaithersburg, MD: Aspen Publishers.

Patterson, K., Grenny, J., McMillan, R., Switzler, A., & Covey, S. (2002). *Crucial conversations: Tools for talking when the stakes are high.* New York: McGraw-Hill Publishers.

Ramos, M. (2006). Eliminate destructive behaviors through example and evidence. *Nursing Management, 37*(9), 34–41.

Know How to Give Feedback

Ruth I. Hansten and Marilynn Jackson

CHAPTER SKILLS

+ Identify the benefits of giving and receiving feedback.
+ Apply the feedback model to delegation and supervision in your practice.
+ Practice giving feedback in specific delegation situations.

RECOMMENDED RESOURCES

▶ Read the Silence Kills report online at www.silencekills.com.
▶ Attempt to give someone feedback using our step-by-step method.
▶ Read a book about accountability such as Samuel, M. (2006). *Creating the Accountable Organization.* Katonah, NY: Xephor Press, or any of the Oz books by Connors, R., & Smith, T., such as *Journey to the Emerald City.* Paramus, NJ: Prentice-Hall Press or *The Oz Principle: Getting Results Through Individual and Organizational Accountability.*

"What? What do you mean, the nursing assistant has already left the building? I don't see any intake and output results being charted, and I never heard from her about the vital signs on that patient who is receiving blood, or the one who fell earlier today. Someone should talk to her about being more responsible!"

I n Chapter 7 we discussed the need to know your delegates in terms of their strengths, weaknesses, motivation, cultural differences, and preferences. Communication is an essential skill in assessing your delegates in these areas, and the specific process of feedback will allow you to maintain a continuous cycle of effective communication that will not only assess the progress of the delegate but motivate that performance as well.

Feedback is the final note in the circular process of delegation. Foregoing feedback is similar to singing the notes of the scale: do, re, mi, fa, sol, la, ti. . . . Everyone is waiting to hear "do," the last note, your words that will complete the cycle and will set the tone for the next time you work together. If they are left unspoken, you have failed to close the loop and to provide a solid foundation for the working relationship with your delegate. Lacking your feedback, the delegate might be making assumptions, filling in his or her own note.

The next time you work together, the delegate will be functioning with an unknown evaluation, and performance will be adversely affected by his or her unanswered questions. "Did I do okay? Does she think I'm a good worker? Does she even notice what I do?" Or the delegate will have formed an opinion of YOU: "She never notices, doesn't even say thank you after I've worked like a demon for her." "He never seems that busy, always sitting at the desk, talking to docs while I'm running around like crazy. I hate to work with him." Or, worse yet, "I hope I don't do anything wrong, but who knows? I never get any feedback, so what does it matter?"

In a 2004 survey of 1,700 nurses, physicians and other healthcare providers and administrators, VitalSmarts and the critical care nurses association (AACN) found that 62% of nurses and other clinical workers witnessed shortcuts being taken in care that was being provided, 48% of nurses were concerned about the clinical judgment of a coworker, and 53% of nurses were concerned about a peer's competence. Only 12% had spoken with their peer and shared their full concerns. Seventy-five percent of nurses and other clinical care providers were concerned about a peer's poor teamwork, but only 16% had spoken with this peer and shared their full concerns (Maxfield, Grenny, McMillan, Patterson, & Switzler, 2005). When the concern is the competence of a nurse or other care provider, only 3% of nonsupervisory employees confront an issue, and only 16% of the supervisors confront an issue (Maxfield, et al., p. 11). This information is frightening when we know that about 65% of sentinel events categorized by The Joint Commission from 1995 to 2006 were caused by team communication problems (The Joint Commission, 2007a). The Joint Commission has added two points to the 2008 Patient Safety Goals that would

Closing the communication loop by sharing some honest feedback during and at the end of the shift can go a long way in preventing a negative working relationship from developing. Isn't it worth the time?

address the issue of giving accurate and timely feedback (The Joint Commission, 2007b):

- Goal 2E—Under improving communication among caregivers, "Implement a standardized approach to 'hand off' communications, including an opportunity to ask and respond to questions."
- Goal 16—"Improve recognition and response to changes in a patient's condition."

CHECKPOINT 10-1

1. When 1,700 nurses, physicians, and other healthcare workers were surveyed about their feedback practices, what percentage shared concerns about a peer's competence?

2. In the same study, what percentage of supervisors confronted a concern about competence of a nurse or other care provider? What are the implications for nurses offering feedback to delegates?

Although these goals were not designed specifically for delegation and supervision issues among RNs and assistive personnel, certainly the nurses' handing off of communications to team members, which offer accurate instructions and ongoing supervision in feedback, would allow for better recognition and response to changes in the patient's condition. The ANA and the National Council of State Boards of Nursing issued a joint statement on delegation in 2006 that reiterated both organizations' stance regarding communication as a central issue and that feedback is the often forgotten, essential step in delegation. They ask the nurse to consider, "Were there any learning moments for the assistant and/or the nurse?" and "Was the assistant acknowledged for accomplishing the task/ activities/function?" (NCSBN, 2006, pp. 8–9).

In our quest for patient safety, we have consulted with airline pilots about what works in that industry where errors are infrequent. A shared planning of outcomes is standard practice. High reliability teams not only agree upon goals and a plan, but they use team debriefings to improve safety and process improvement. Questions about clarity of communication, whether mistakes were avoided, workload, what went well, and what could be improved are used in feedback sessions as best practice (Powell, 2007). We have advocated for planned feedback sessions for decades, and the best teams with world-class outcomes use this technique without fail.

CHECKPOINT 10–2

Think about the benefits you will realize from learning a process for giving effective feedback to your delegates. Jot down a few thoughts.

If delegates felt comfortable giving you some constructive feedback on your communication skills, leadership, or performance, how would that benefit you and your performance?

Even though giving feedback and communicating appropriately is supported by evidence to be essential to patient safety, giving and receiving feedback takes courage. It's difficult to tell people what's going wrong and easier to talk about what is going well. It might be harder still to ask your delegate for an appraisal of your performance, and you might feel that this is unnecessary in your role. When it seems that giving and receiving feedback is the absolute last thing you want to do, it's helpful to think about the possible benefits to you and the delegate.

BENEFITS OF GIVING AND RECEIVING FEEDBACK

Some of the following responses are most commonly given to us by nurses. We hope that you identified similar benefits as well as some that are particular to you.

- You learn how to better lead the team.
- Personal growth for both the RN and the delegate provides improved job opportunities for the future.
- The delegate learns and grows and is thus motivated to a more energetic effort.
- Positive performance is reinforced.
- Individual and team performance improves.
- Open communication helps overall teamwork.
- Patients receive better care.
- Patients are safe.
- We follow national patient safety recommendations.
- We apply the principles of the ANA and NCSBN joint statement on delegation and supervision.
- Besides, haven't you always wondered what your delegates and coworkers think about your performance?

THE POWER OF FEEDBACK

The value and benefit of feedback as a motivator cannot be stressed enough. Research studies repeatedly show that recognition, feedback, and constructive criticism are high-ranking factors in enhancing productivity and performance. When asked to rank work factors in terms of importance, the majority of those surveyed will list "appreciation of work" and "a feeling of being in on things" as more important factors than the amount of pay, the loyalty from the supervisor, or the physical conditions of the job (Jenks & Kelly, 1985). Now considered to be a classic in motivational literature, **Figure 10–1** illustrates the importance of feedback when considering multiple factors in job satisfaction and motivation.

Ninety-two percent of nurses ranked recognition as important to job satisfaction, but 28% perceived this recognition to be seldom or never given.

Feedback in the form of recognition is a significant factor to most of us. In a survey of nurses in the Midwest, 92% ranked recognition as important to job satisfaction, but 28% perceived this recognition to be seldom or never given. Verbal feedback was described

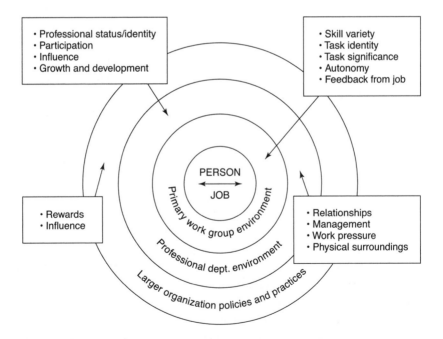

FIGURE 10–1 Factors That Affect Job Status and Motivation. *Source:* Reprinted from Henderson and Williams, The People Side of Patient Care Redesign, *Healthcare Forum Journal,* July–August 1991, p. 46, with permission of Healthcare Forum, © 1991.

> Discussing patient outcomes with team members and giving them both positive and negative feedback along the way can result in more than double the performance effort!

as the most significant form of recognition, and many looked to their head nurse, nurse executive, patient, coworker, physician, and hospital department heads for this feedback (Goode, et al., 1993). Unfortunately, studies show that nurse managers often do not see the process of motivating staff (giving positive feedback) as one of their tasks (O'Neil & Gajdostik, 1989). Press Ganey's 2007 Hospital Check-Up Report reviewed the perceptions of 193,163 nurses and other employees at 373 U.S. hospitals. The priorities identified included top leaders listening to employees' concerns, compensation, recognition for work, participation in decision making and staffing levels (Press Ganey, 2007). Even in the midst of a healthcare personnel shortage, when retention of qualified staff correlates with organizational success, there continues to be a gap in meeting employees' needs for recognition. What an opportunity you have as a colleague, knowing that a simple "thank you" or "good job" can take so little time to say and yet can have such a tremendous impact!

A study of how both goals and feedback affect performance levels and motivation was published in 1983 by Bandura and Cervone (Kouzes & Posner, 1993), and its message has not changed. They found that when an individual has a challenging goal and detailed feedback (both positive and negative) is given, there is a nearly 60% improvement in performance effort. This underlines the need to discuss the preferred patient outcomes with team members when assignments are given and to evaluate progress along the way. Connors, Smith, and Hickman, in their books about the Oz Principle, describe the power of feedback in becoming accountable as persons and as an organization. Both giving and asking for feedback help individuals to improve performance and think critically in their problem-solving process (Connors, Smith, & Hickman, 1994; Connors & Smith, 1999). A study regarding improving team relationships and care delivery models in a psychiatric unit showed that effort related to better communication and role definition improved job satisfaction by 14% (Allen & Vitale-Nolen, 2005). When reviewing the "10 Deadly Sins That Prevent Us from Attaining Results," Samuel lists two of the sins as related to lack of feedback. Sin number 8 is avoiding holding people accountable, and sin number 10 is failing to recognize success (Samuel, 2006). The effect of recognition is that it allows all staff to celebrate the results in partnerships with patients and families.

CHECKPOINT 10-3

Recall the last time someone recognized your efforts on the job or at home. How did you feel?

THE PROCESS

Many nurses would like to leave the process of feedback to the manager, believing perhaps that it is out of their realm of responsibilities and that the manager has more time to devote to evaluating and supervising employees. However, regarding the process of delegation, the National Council of State Boards of Nursing (NCSBN) states:

> The delegating nurse is accountable for assessing the situation and is responsible for the decision to delegate. Monitoring, outcome evaluation and follow-up are necessary supervisory activities that follow delegation. . . . The delegator would be expected to provide supervisory follow-up such as intervention on the behalf of the client and corrective action. (NCSBN, 1990, p. 3)

As stated earlier, the ANA, NCSBN, and other nursing organizations recognize the need for ongoing evaluation and feedback (NCSBN, 2006).

Consider whether your care delivery system or model includes built-in times for offering feedback. If the plan for the day or shift in your department does not include specific opportunities for giving initial direction and ongoing checkpoints for touching base and exchanging reciprocal feedback, the supervisory functions that are essential to patient safety might not occur. In every type of care delivery, there should be an expectation that feedback will be given not only throughout the shift or episode of care but also toward the end of the shift. We recommend that feedback be given at checkpoints before and after breaks and meals at prearranged flexible times. Merely saying that "we will see each other as we pass in the hallway" is not sufficient for actual review of care and coordination of the team. The value of the last reciprocal feedback checkpoint (or time for celebration of success) cannot be underestimated.

Repeatedly, when we work with assistive personnel, they say, "Please tell the RNs to let us know why we are to do the tasks they ask us to do (what are our goals?), let us know what they expect, and tell us how we are doing!"

These 2 to 5 minutes that are set aside for clearing up communications and role expectations, making the next episode of care more successful, will also strengthen teamwork and efficiency of care along with job satisfaction. Asking "What could we do differently tomorrow if we were given the same assignment?" is essential. Celebrate the outcomes the patient was able to achieve today with your assistance. Don't miss this opportunity!

CHECKPOINT 10-4

A 2006 joint statement on delegation by the NCSBN and the ANA emphasized that feedback is often a forgotten step of the delegation/ supervision process. What two questions do these sages ask nurses to consider using when performing feedback?

The feedback that you are required to give as a delegator involves some preparation in terms of assessment and analysis. The following basic questions will be helpful in preparing you to follow up with your delegate:

+ What do I see? Is the delegate having difficulty with the task? Is the information not where I expected it to be (e.g., daily weight not on the graphic sheet)?
+ How does it affect me? Is it making my job easier or more difficult?
+ What can I do about it? Can I offer additional training for the task he seems to be unable to do? Can I encourage her to share this skill with other members of the team?

When you provide feedback to your delegates, the information shared will usually be one of the following four types (Hersey & Duldt, 1989):

1. Clarifying—This will involve restating your instructions, making certain that any confusion regarding the assignment is cleared up so that you both are in agreement regarding parameters for reporting and the expectations of performance that you both have. "Please get the vital signs from the new postop in room 101 and report them to me immediately."

2. Interpretive—This particular type of feedback involves making an observation of the delegate's behavior and making assumptions about the meaning. "When I could not find you on the

unit, I thought you were out on the deck smoking as usual." Be careful about this type of feedback—check your assumptions first!

> Feedback is generally one of four types: clarifying, interpretive, judgmental, or personal reaction.

3. Judgmental—Similar to interpretive feedback, this form also involves drawing conclusions, this time in the form of a value judgment regarding behavior. "You're such a slob! How can we get any work done when you never clean up the treatment room?"

4. Personal reaction—When you provide the delegate with information about your personal feelings, you are giving a strong message of how he or she is coming across. "I feel relieved when you are working with me because you do such a good job, and I can count on you."

CHECKPOINT 10–5

Can you recall times when you have given feedback to coworkers that was: 1) clarifying? 2) interpreting? 3) judgmental? 4) a personal reaction? How did you feel on each of these occasions? Which type was most effective for you?

GIVING FEEDBACK TO THE DELEGATE

It is easy to see by reviewing the types of feedback that one can potentially do more harm than good. You can increase the defensiveness of the delegate and further alienate the members of the team if a few simple criteria are not followed. In further preparing your feedback message, consider the following criteria (LaMonica, 1983):

- ✦ It is specific rather than general.
- ✦ It is directed toward behavior the receiver can do something about.
- ✦ It considers the needs of both the receiver and the giver of the feedback.
- ✦ It is solicited rather than imposed.
- ✦ It is well timed.
- ✦ It is checked to ensure clear communication by asking the receiver to rephrase the message to make certain he or she understands.

Keeping these criteria in mind, let's look at a method for giving feedback. Our proposed recipe can be used for both positive and negative feedback. For our example, let's use the situation of a new student nurse who has been working with you. You've noticed that Brenda does an excellent job in working with patients who have been diagnosed with cancer and are in the beginning stages of the grief process. You'd like to comment on how wonderful it has been to work with Brenda.

Who needs to be told this information? Brenda certainly needs to know how you feel. It would be helpful for Brenda if your evaluation of her expertise was shared with her instructor as well. When you have positive feedback to share, feel free to shout it from the rooftops and tell everyone. Letting others know about Brenda's performance is certainly positive to the general atmosphere of the work setting. Just be certain to let the person most involved hear it first! However, if the feedback is negative, then only Brenda should hear the news. It might, of course, be necessary for the manager and the instructor to hear about problems. (Be sure to tell any delegate that you'll share the information with the manager or supervisory person prior to doing so.) Resist telling stories to others about the errors individuals have made. Adlai Stevenson said, "If you throw mud, you get dirty." Confidentiality in performance feedback of a negative nature is essential, and betraying confidences will cause the speaker to look bad as well.

When the feedback discussion takes place is also essential. As soon as you are aware that feedback needs to be shared, time should be planned to make certain it occurs. If emergency circumstances dictate that feedback will need to wait, then tell the person as soon as possible that you'll need to talk with him or her and set up a time. It is human nature to avoid the unpleasant, but in health care we do not have the luxury of avoiding giving performance feedback of a negative nature because human lives are at stake. (Think of late feedback you've been given about a circumstance that took place several months ago. It isn't effective for learning or for motivational purposes either.)

Where the feedback session occurs is also important for the success of the discussion. Obviously, negative feedback is never given in public, whereas praise is wonderful to hear in any setting. Negative feedback given without discretion to the time and place will belittle the importance of the message and be ineffective because the receiver will generally react defensively due to the shame of being repri-

> Adlai Stevenson said, "If you throw mud, you get dirty." Stick to the facts in a respectful, confidential manner.

manded in public. Instead of being useful, this is destructive to the results intended.

THE FEEDBACK MODEL

1. Get the delegate's input before proceeding.
2. Give credit for the delegate's efforts.
3. Share your perception of what you have observed, read, assessed.
4. Explore the situation more fully with the delegate: Discuss gaps in perceptions and causes of the problem.
5. Get the delegate's input or solution to the problem.
6. Agree on an action plan.
7. Set a time to check on progress.

APPLICATION TO THE DELEGATION PROCESS

As Susan, an RN, plans to give feedback to Brenda, she will first decide when and where it would be appropriate to discuss this with Brenda. She'll also plan how she'll share this with the instructor. She has chosen the setting of the coffee room, in private, when they go together on break.

1. Getting the delegate's input is essential, and it is the step that people often miss. In this case, Brenda responded that she felt she wasn't getting enough direction from Susan, and sometimes she felt that she might not be doing as well as she wanted to in understanding and explaining the effects of chemotherapy. If Susan had charged in with her positive feedback and glowing assessment, she might not have known that Brenda had these concerns about her supervision. The two were able to discuss that Susan had gained trust in her, that Brenda had always asked questions appropriately, and that Susan was assessing the patients' understanding of their chemotherapy herself.

2. There is no substitute for giving credit for others' efforts. When nurses work as hard as they do every day, it's frustrating when everything accomplished is overlooked, but a small detail is criticized. "I realize several patients have expired today and you've had three codes, but your charting is behind!" Avoid the negative consequences of focusing only on the negative. Some experts

> How information is shared will make a huge difference in how the discussion is perceived and acted upon. Being tactful and providing thoughtful, objective feedback without being judgmental is essential if the feedback is to achieve your desired goal.

recommend the sandwich principle: When giving negative feedback, be certain to give positive feedback before and after the negative. It makes the news somewhat easier to swallow, although most people will only hear the negative feedback. In this case, Susan tells Brenda how much she appreciates how well she is prepared each day before coming to clinical, not because she is trying to sweeten the message, but because she really believes that to be true. Honesty is always the best policy, and people do appreciate being appreciated.

3. It's now time to share the perceptions Susan has had. She tells Brenda that she has been very impressed with how well she has been communicating with the newly diagnosed cancer patients and their families. They seem to be pretty upbeat and are retaining treatment information well.

CHECKPOINT 10-6

Fill in the blanks below with your proposed responses.

1. Get the delegate's input before proceeding.	"Brenda, how do you feel things have been going?"
2. Give credit for the delegate's efforts.	
3. Share your perception of what you have observed, read, assessed.	
4. Explore the situation more fully with the delegate: discuss gaps in perceptions, causes of the problem.	
5. Get the delegate's input or solution to the problem.	
6. Agree on an action plan.	
7. Set a time to check on progress.	

Now, using the steps of the feedback model, refer to the suggested dialogue in the sample conversations in the text.

Maintain and preserve the self-respect of delegates by being respectful in your manner and speech. Asking yourself what you want delegates to remember from the conversation will help you to set the correct tone. Do you want them to remember how angry and upset you were? If so, be prepared for the situation to repeat itself because a display of anger will allow delegates to focus on your behavior, not theirs. It's a fact of human behavior that we tend to remember process, how something was said, much more readily than what was said. A calm, objective manner will overcome that tendency and keep the focus on the message, not your emotions.

4. As the situation is explored, Susan shares her assessment of Brenda's performance, stating that she has observed Brenda's patients to be much more knowledgeable about their treatment and better prepared for discharge. Brenda appreciates this appraisal but still feels that she is not giving adequate information to the patients.

5. Getting input and discussion from the delegate, Brenda responds that she didn't know her patients had been responding better than most, but she thought it had to do with the statistics she gave them and the discussion she had with them about their own participation in treatment. She states she has read a lot about the difference that attitude makes in treatment and gives Susan the names of several books.

As input is received from the delegate in a negative performance conversation, remember that performance problems are generally due to a combination of several factors. Delegates might not understand their role or your expectations. They might not know that the way they are performing their role does not correlate with what you desire or that it doesn't measure up. There might be barriers present in the environment (those systems problems), or they might not understand how to do their job or why it is supposed to be done the way you want it to be done. They might need further education or closer supervision, or they might lack the necessary motivation to do the job right.

6. Susan asks Brenda if she'd feel comfortable sharing her ideas with the regular staff. Brenda agrees to bring it all up at report and see if anyone is interested in having an inservice on what she's learned.

> Encouraging the delegate to be involved by offering input early in the process will help the individual experience accountability for his or her own performance and will set the stage for better results.

She might even be able to get extra credit for it! This action plan will begin on the next clinical day.

7. After setting a time to check progress, Susan states that she will facilitate the discussion during the next report and check with Brenda as the plan emerges to share Brenda's success with others.

Let's now use the feedback model process to give negative feedback.

Grant is in charge of the postanesthesia care unit today. The unit has been very busy, and they are short a secretary. Several patients have had rocky recoveries, and two were sent back to the OR. Pat, the OR supervisor, stops in and sees order sheets stacked up and the phone ringing without being answered. Pat is normally a very perceptive and caring individual, but today she walks by Grant and tells him, "Get your act together, The Joint Commission surveyors are on their way!" Without waiting for a response, she walks briskly from the room.

Grant knows he must give feedback to Pat about this incident. However, he knows that he'll have to wait to do this until after the emergencies are taken care of and after the staffing supervisor calls in the secretary she's been promising to reach.

When Grant talks with Pat the next day, this is the way the conversation proceeds.

Grant:	Pat, can we talk over here in private for a few moments? Good. Well, I was wondering how The Joint Commission survey went yesterday. How did your day go, considering all that stress?
Pat:	Well, I haven't consumed that many antacids for a long time. I was very worried that they'd come in here and see the chaos.
Grant:	How do you think we do here, overall, in keeping our act together?
Pat:	Well, generally things seem to be very organized, and the transfer of patients is excellently orchestrated. You do a wonderful job in keeping all these people alive and caring for the most critically ill. There haven't been many problems at all. Why do you ask?
Grant:	Pat, I know you have worked very hard to make this unit the success it is. You were here long before I came to work in this area. The reason I ask is that yesterday I was concerned about your conversation with me prior to the survey. When

you saw the situation and said, "Get your act together" without asking me what was going on, I knew you were very busy and under stress, but I felt invisible. I wanted to tell you that we were short a secretary, how busy things had been, and that I'd taken care of the situation by getting help to come in. I felt pretty awful about your response, even though I understood your pressure.

Pat: Well, I guess I didn't realize how I came across! I knew that you would have taken care of the tight staffing as best you could and that you had things under control—you always do! I was reacting to my own concerns, I guess. I probably don't tell you enough how much I do rely on your excellent leadership and judgment.

Grant: Thanks! I'm glad to know that. You are right, we need to figure out a method to give each other feedback more frequently so that these types of exchanges don't cause problems or concerns in our relationship. We have enough other concerns just keeping this place going!

Pat: Let's use our monthly meeting together for that purpose. I'll try to let you know when I'm stressed out, and if you'll let me know right away if I say something that's confusing, I'll be sure to let you know right away if I have any concerns. If I don't say anything, be sure to know I'm still extremely happy with your performance.

Grant: Thanks, Pat, I feel better knowing that you're not harboring some secret worries about how I am doing and how well this place runs during my period in charge.

Now give feedback to your secretary, Joe. His job description states that he will organize the clothing room of your residential psychiatric facility. Although he has been told repeatedly in the last 2 weeks that this task needs to be done, he has not completed the job. You've noted that he seems to have time on his hands because he's been playing cards with the residents.

Follow the process or role-play a feedback session. Describe the setting. Then follow the steps of the feedback process.

A possible conversation would proceed as follows:

Marion: Joe, how have things been going for you here with respect to your role and work?

Joe:	Pretty well, Marion, but I feel a bit like my skills are being underutilized. You know I want to become a mental health professional instead of a secretary. Otherwise, I think the job is okay.
Marion:	I'm glad to know you want to keep working in psychiatry, Joe, and I have very much appreciated how well you interact with the patients. You have a gift for talking with even the most disturbed without being afraid of them. I'd like to talk to you more about your plans to become a mental health professional. Since you feel underemployed, I can see why you aren't too excited about cleaning the clothing room. It doesn't seem like a priority, but it really does need to be done. When I ask you to do something several times, and then I see you playing cards with a resident, I feel frustrated. Unfortunately, this is something within your job description, and as much as it is not the most fun job, it doesn't make sense for the other members of the team to be doing that type of work either. They are also concerned because clothes have been lost and they have had to spend time searching for things for the residents or their families. How do you think this should be resolved?
Joe:	Marion, as much as I hate to clean, I guess I have been procrastinating. I can see how it would be frustrating for you all. Maybe this is like starting at the bottom and working up?
Marion:	Yes, Joe, I think it would work best if you did the job. I'd like it done once every week. You can determine when will work out best, but please be certain it is done. In fact, it may be best if you mark it on the sheet that we use to record the inventory in that room. Then the others will know it is being done regularly.
Joe:	Plus you can tell if I am getting it done, right?
Marion:	Right! Let's plan to talk more about your career plans when we evaluate the clothing room issue too. I'll get some information together for you at our next monthly meeting, okay?

CHECKPOINT 10-7

Review Grant and Pat's conversation and match the steps of the performance feedback process on the following chart:

1. Get the delegate's input before proceeding.	"How did your day go? How do you think we do here?"
2. Give credit for the delegate's efforts.	"You've worked very hard to make this unit the success it is."
3. Share your perception of what you have observed, read, assessed.	
4. Explore the situation more fully with the delegate: Discuss gaps in perceptions and causes of the problem.	
5. Get the delegate's solution or input.	
6. Agree on an action plan.	
7. Set a time to check on progress.	

Practice Feedback Scenarios

Below you'll find a few situations you may encounter in your work life. Use these problems to experiment with the feedback process. You may want to ask a fellow student or family member to role play with you and critique your communication style. Ask them for feedback regarding how you could improve in the next feedback opportunity.

1. In your family planning clinic, one of the assistants who also performs secretarial work has decided to telephone the patients with their HIV test results before consulting with you, the RN who generally counsels patients about these issues.

2. You have observed a new colleague drawing blood without using gloves. Someone needs to talk with her.

3. A medical assistant has been discussing confidential information about patients in the coffee room.

4. The psychiatric case worker talked with a patient's family to plan aftercare. After the case worker left, the family complained about the "condescending attitude" that was displayed.

5. A physician, who is the consultant for the school nurses' immunization clinic, met with some of the community leaders at an evening holiday open house. He had evidently had something alcoholic to drink because his breath smelled quite strong, although his behavior didn't seem altered. One of the community leaders asked, "Is this clinic run by someone with a drinking problem? I think that drinking alcohol is a bad example for the people of this community, where substance abuse is very high. You need to tell the doctor we don't want to smell alcohol on his breath again!" Margaret, one of the school nurses, has to decide whether to give this feedback to the physician, but she is afraid of the impact to the clinic if she doesn't.

6. Maria, the nursing assistant on the night shift at the long-term care center, routinely complains about having to turn patients who are "just going to die anyway."

7. Greta has come in to work late several times in the last week.

REQUESTING AND RECEIVING FEEDBACK

As you can see from our model, feedback requires an exchange of information to be most effective. You can give recognition (and we certainly recommend it!) in a one-way communication format and still have a positive impact. However, allowing the delegate to offer input too will set up a two-way communication process that is much more meaningful and can lead to longer lasting results. When the delegate feels that his or her input is valued, you are building trust and a positive working relationship. The input you receive can help you to further improve your performance as well and make working together easier and more beneficial for the patient.

> Encouraging the delegate to be involved by offering input early in the process will help the individual experience accountability for his own performance and will set the stage for better results.

Great supervisors ask for feedback from their staff not only in terms of clinical data or reports on how the systems are working in their area but on their own performance. RNs who ask for input on their personal performance from their delegates will soon capture the respect and admiration of their teammates. Receiving feedback graciously allows the RN to hear the other person's point of view without being defensive or angry. The RN can further explore the points being made and decide whether the feedback is something that he or she can use to improve his or her performance or behavior in the job setting.

> Being clear on outcomes you wish to achieve from the conversation and use of "I messages" will go a long way toward achieving your goals. Clarity produces the confidence that engenders respect and is an antidote to the powerless "victim" mentality.

It is important to understand that some delegates might have difficulty in participating in a two-way communication process. Others may welcome the chance and overwhelm you with their opinions! To make certain the process stays on track, you might want to review what is expected (clarifying expectations again) so that you foster an environment in which you are all working together to improve your delivery of care.

On a periodic basis, it's important to ask such questions as:

- How did these assignments work for you?
- Is there anything I could have done that would have made the day/shift/case better for you?
- How am I doing, in your perception?
- What am I doing that works well?
- What should I be working on, in your opinion?
- What ideas do you have that I could use to make things work better here?
- Did the instructions I gave you help, or was there a better way for me to communicate with you?
- What could we do differently tomorrow if we have the same assignment?

Being open to such feedback allows your delegates to know you think you are human too, and fallible. They will feel less defensive themselves when you must give them negative feedback or criticism when they know you are willing to receive it yourself. Certainly everyone will feel more free to give the positive feedback needed to keep everyone's self-esteem and motivation at the highest level.

UPWARD FEEDBACK

Most of our discussion so far has been on providing information to the delegates in terms of their performance to ensure their competency in performing delegated tasks. When soliciting feedback from delegates, you are, in effect, asking them to provide "upward feedback," or evaluative information to a superior. This can be difficult for many people because the fear of reprisal might hinder their desire to be honest. Consider your own situation—are you comfortable in providing feedback to your supervisor, as was discussed in Grant and Pat's OR situation?

We have, unfortunately, worked with some organizations where the "chain of command" was strictly enforced and communication flowed only in one direction. This top-down approach has a significant negative impact on teamwork, morale, and productivity. It is sad to see such outdated management practices in any organization, but there are ways around the limitations imposed by such a command/control environment.

CHECKPOINT 10-8

Consider the following situations:

1. Why is it so important, as an RN, to ask for feedback from others on the team?

2. Think about a situation in which you've been delegating to others. What questions could you ask to determine how you are doing?

3. Arlene, a school nurse, has given many instructions to the parents who help out in the high school when she's out in another one of the schools in her area. The school secretary tells Arlene that one of the parents was assisting when a girl came in with some concerns, and then the girl left the office sobbing. The secretary overheard the assisting parent telling the girl loudly that "You should have just said no! Well, you'd better call your parents about this pregnancy or I will!" How would you give feedback and further instructions to the assisting parent?

4. Frank, a nurse working in a poison control center, has trained a new assistant. This nurse is relatively inexperienced, and Frank is quite concerned about the first few times that she'll be on alone. How can Frank receive some feedback from his new assistant about the training process and his supervision style while giving feedback to the new nurse?

See the end of the chapter for the answers.

If you find yourself in a situation where providing feedback to a superior is forbidden and you must continue to work in that setting, you can speak to these individuals using the assertive strategy of "I messages." Rather than focusing on "you are never around when I need you," consider rephrasing the message as "I need to know where I can reach you if we get another admission." If you are not getting any feedback from this supervisor and would like to find out how you are doing, don't criticize him or her for lack of performance ("You never give me any feedback—how am I supposed to know how I'm doing?"). Instead, use the I-message technique and state, "I need to have some information from you about how I am doing. I have been here at the clinic for 3 months now, and I'd like to know if I am performing okay."

CHECKPOINT 10-9

Using I messages, give upward feedback in the following situations.

1. The charge nurse frequently gives you more patients with a higher acuity than anyone else's assignment. Other members on the team have noticed this but are reluctant to say anything on your behalf.

2. The evening supervisor was yelling loudly at you in front of patients and staff. This is something he does frequently, but no one will discuss it with him.

Recall what we discussed in the chapter on communication: Before sitting down to give feedback to a superior, be clear on the outcome you would like from the conversation. In the previous example, the person giving the I message was clear that she wanted some feedback right away. That nurse might also have had additional outcomes in mind, ranging from "I'd like to meet with you every 2 months during the orientation period so I am clear on how I am doing" to "Let me know only if I make a mistake, otherwise we'll talk again in a year." The outcomes you wish will vary, and being certain of what you really want will go a long way in making your points clear and in gaining the ear, and the respect, of your boss.

Often nurses allow position and chain of command to foster a helpless "victim" mentality. As professional nurses, you are accountable for the safety of your patients, and working conditions such as those described might hamper your ability to provide that care. It is essential to be able to provide feedback to those persons who are in a position to affect your ability to provide safe care.

In situation 1 of Checkpoint 10–9, if you are feeling overloaded and you question your ability to provide adequate care to the patients in this assignment, you must give this feedback to the charge nurse. Consider using an I message such as "I am concerned about this assignment. I will need some assistance with Mr. Smith when I do his dressing, and I will need someone to watch the rest of my patients when I begin the initial chemotherapy on Mrs. Blake. Will you be available?" Without being directly confrontational or offering judgmental feedback on the charge nurse's ability to make fair assignments, you have let her know your specific concerns and that you will need assistance throughout the shift.

Situation 2 involves a scenario that makes the work setting less than pleasant when allowed to continue. Taking control of the situation, you may consider using an I message to redirect the supervisor to another location: "I appreciate your comments and would like to have further feedback, but I need to step into the medication room to get an IV." When removed from the public arena, you can continue your discussion with additional assertive techniques (see Chapter 8). As time and the situation dictate, using the entire feedback model to give upward feedback is also effective.

CONCLUSION

Giving and receiving feedback can be risky business, but the potential for building more positive working relationships outweighs these risks. Remembering the step-by-step process and preparing your message before you speak will help you to make this a more meaningful part of your role as a professional nurse. From the impact of a simple "thank you" to the detailed exchange of the evaluation of the performance of a new task, feedback closes the loop of the delegation process. As a result, you are fulfilling your legal obligation to monitor, evaluate, and follow up, and the patients are reaping the benefits. Be sure that you incorporate specific times for offering and receiving feedback into your workday. Good job!

ANSWERS TO CHECKPOINTS

10-1

1. Twelve percent, if the concern is about a nurse or other level of care provider (i.e., physician)(www.Silencekills.com)

2. Sixteen percent. If nurses are waiting for their supervisors to confront an issue with their delegates, rather than dealing

with the concerns themselves as supervising RN, they may be waiting in vain. The nurse herself/himself must learn to offer effective performance feedback. Also, the NCSBN and state regulations require a nurse to stay engaged in the delegation process by ongoing supervision and corrective action to ensure safety and quality.

10-4

1. "Were there any learning moments for the assistant or the nurse?"

2. "Was the assistant acknowledged for accomplishing the task/activities/function?" (NCSBN, 2006)

10–8.

1. The RN, as leader of the team, must set the stage for listening to others' perceptions, being open to growth, and being nondefensive. You will engender the respect of your coworkers as you teach them how to give and receive feedback. Your nurse practice act states that you must supervise your delegates, and this means giving feedback on their performance. They'll accept feedback from you much more happily if you are able to accept it yourself. You can grow and learn from constructive information sharing. Giving feedback and discussing goals can improve performance effort up to 60%.

2. Use the questions preceding this checkpoint or others that fit your situation exactly.

3. Follow the feedback model, being certain that you get input from the assisting parent first. You might have to explain the school district's policy on confidentiality.

4. Follow the feedback model. Be prepared with a few questions for your new assistant that would, when answered correctly, help you feel more comfortable with her knowledge. Be certain to listen to how well you've been orienting her.

REFERENCES

Allen, D., & Vitale-Nolen, R. (2005). Patient care delivery model improves nurse job satisfaction. *The Journal of Continuing Education in Nursing, 36*(6), 277–282.

Connors, R., & Smith, T. (1999). *Journey to the emerald city.* Paramus, NJ: Prentice-Hall Press.

Connors, R., Smith, T., & Hickman, C. (1994). *The Oz principle: Getting results through individual and organizational accountability.* Paramus, NJ: Prentice-Hall Press.

Cox, K. (2003). The effects of intrapersonal, intragroup and intergroup conflict on team performance effectiveness and work satisfaction. *Nursing Administration Quarterly, 27*(2).

Goode, C., et al. (1993). What kind of recognition do staff nurses want? *American Journal of Nursing, 93,* 64–68.

Hersey, P., & Duldt, B.W. (1989). *Situational leadership in nursing.* Norwalk, CT: Appleton & Lange.

Jenks, J.M., & Kelly, J.M. (1985). *Don't do—delegate!* New York: Franklin Watts.

Kouzes, J., & Posner, B. (1993). *Credibility.* San Francisco: Jossey-Bass. The original study cited was from A. Bandura and D. Cervone, Self-evaluation and self-efficacy mechanisms governing the motivational effects of goal systems, *Journal of Personality and Social Psychology, 45* (1983).

LaMonica, E. (1983). *Nursing leadership and management, an experiential approach.* Monterey, CA: Wadsworth Health Sciences Division, 139.

Maxfield, D., Grenny, J., McMillan, R., Patterson, K., & Switzler, A. (2005). *Silence kills: The seven crucial conversations for healthcare.* Retrieved from www.SilenceKills.com. VitalSmarts, L.C.

National Council of State Boards of Nursing. (1990). *Concept paper on delegation.* Chicago: Author.

National Council of State Boards of Nursing. (2006). *Joint statement on delegation— American Nurses Association (ANA) and the National Council of State Boards of Nursing (NCSBN).* Retrieved July 23, 2007, from https://www.ncsbn.org/Joint_statement.pdf.

O'Neil, K. K., & Gajdostik, K. L. (1989). The head nurse's managerial role. *Nursing Management, 20,* 39–42.

Powell, S. (2007, July/August). Benefits to team briefings. *Healthcare Executive, 22*(4), 54–57.

Press Ganey, Inc. (2007). *Hospital check-up report: Nurse and hospital employee perspectives on American health care.* South Bend, IN. Retrieved from www.PressGaney.com/employee_report.

Samuel, M. (2006). *Creating the accountable organization.* Katonah, NY: Xephor Press.

The Joint Commission. (2007a). *Root causes of sentinel events, 1995–2006.* Retrieved July 23, 2007, from http://www.jointcommission.org/NR/rdonlyres/FA465646-5F5F-4543-AC8F-E8AF6571E372/0/root_cause_se.jpg.

The Joint Commission. (2007b). *2008 national patient safety goals.* Retrieved July 23, 2007, from http://www.jointcommission.org/PatientSafety/NationalPatient-SafetyGoals/08_hap_npsgs.htm.

Know How to Evaluate: How Well Has the Delegation Process Produced the Outcomes I Want to Achieve?

Ruth I. Hansten and Marilynn Jackson

CHAPTER SKILLS

- Describe the relationship of continuous, problem-related, and periodic evaluation in the delegation and supervision process.
- Identify the impact of learning styles on how we communicate with assistive personnel.
- Evaluate your organization for critical thinking facilitation.
- Reflect on your personal accountability for developing critical thinking skills.
- Apply the critical thinking problem-solving process to a clinical problem.

RECOMMENDED RESOURCES

▶ Read the following books by Rosalinda Alfaro-LeFevre:
  - Alfaro-LeFevre (2009). *Critical thinking and clinical judgment: A practical approach to outcome-focused thinking* (4th ed.). Philadelphia: Saunders-Elsevier.
  - Alfaro-LeFevre (2009). *Applying nursing process: A tool for critical thinking* (7th ed.). Philadelphia: Lippincott-Williams & Wilkins.
  - Alfaro-LeFevre, R. (2007–2008). *Critical thinking indicators: 2007–2008.* Evidence-based version available from http://www.alfaroteachsmart.com/cti.htm.
▶ Use the 10-step critical thinking problem-solving process (with each step in order) to solve a pesky problem in your life or practice.

It's 6 a.m. on a medical surgical acute care nursing unit. A nursing assistant who was assigned to answer call lights reports to the charge RN, "Oh, by the way, about midnight Mr. Peterson in Room 555 complained of chest pain and was diaphoretic. I decided it was because he'd been coughing too much and asked the other RN to give him a sleeping pill. I think he's okay." The charge nurse races down to the room, finds that Mr. Peterson is, in fact, having a myocardial infarction, calls the Rapid Response Team, and rushes him, monitored, to the cardiac unit. (Hansten, 1991)

As in any situation involving people and judgment, there are several possible problems as well as several times when the error could have been caught before it was too late for the patient. In this case, one would expect the nursing assistant to have known that all complaints of chest pain must be immediately reported to the nurse in charge. She was definitely overstepping her job description by diagnosing the origin of the pain and taking her own interventions. However, was this the first time throughout the entire shift that the charge nurse and the assistant crossed paths to discuss the patients? Where was the supervision by the charge nurse? Did the charge nurse make rounds and check the patients herself? An "eyeball" assessment of a sleeping patient often yields the necessary information to avoid a tragedy; in this case, however, the patient was stable and did not reflect the minor arrhythmias and ischemia his heart was certainly experiencing. A fourth issue is present: What about the second nurse who administered a sleeping pill without assessing the reasons for it? One wonders if the patient was experiencing the chest pain as the nurse gave the medication.

CHECKPOINT 11–1

Keeping in mind what you have learned about the delegation process, what went wrong in this situation?

EVALUATION: CONTINUOUS, PROBLEM RELATED, AND PERIODIC

Evaluation is a familiar word and process to all RNs. Evaluation, as a part of the nursing process, is continuous, as we consider whether our interventions are achieving the projected outcomes for each nursing diagnosis. In this chapter, we'll discuss evaluation of the delegation process itself. How well the process is working will yield important information on the performance of the systems we have created and the people to whom we delegate. Evaluation will allow us to give useful feedback, both positive and negative, and to learn from the feedback that is given to us by our coworkers. In this chapter we'll cover some of the issues we have discovered that commonly interfere with successful completion of the process.

With the current nurse shortage, the National Council of State Boards of Nursing and the American Nurses Association seized the opportunity to create a combined statement in 2006 to clarify 21st century nurse delegation and supervision competencies. They include four main steps: 1) assess and plan the delegation; 2) communicate directions; 3) surveillance and supervision; and 4) evaluation and feedback (NCSBN, 2006, p. 4). From our experience working with nurses across the country, we discovered that some nurses have not built into their day a plan for evaluating the care. If evaluation and feedback are not planned, the chances that evaluation will occur by accident are really quite slim. Does this make a difference in results or outcomes? Absolutely. In 2001, Standing, Anthony, and Hertz evaluated the results of working with assistive personnel. When deficiencies were noted, about 61% were related to the nursing assistant not completing a task that was assigned or not following proper standard processes. However, the RN's delegation skills were often at the root of the problem. They found that 13.9% of the care deficiencies were related to RNs not providing appropriate communication, and 12.4% were due to a lack of ongoing supervision. When outcomes were determined by routine observation, more positive events occurred, but when there was no direct ongoing supervision, problems occurred (Standing, Anthony, & Hertz, 2001, p. 21). As RNs, we are accountable for the care given to the patient, and we retain a sacred trust with the public to assure that care is administered appropriately.

One of the most productive stages of the delegation process includes the portion covered in this chapter: evaluation of the results of the process, with a careful analysis of each step of the process to ensure that the cycle of delegation has been complete and effective. In the situation of Mr. Peterson, evaluation of a problem situation yielded important information for the growth of the personnel involved and for improving the quality of the care delivered. Often, when evaluating, we discover that we've missed some essential points from preceding parts of the process. There were many errors in the chest pain incident:

- Before we question the people involved and find out more, we can at least assume that the delegate did not report appropriately.
- We can also guess that the charge nurse did not make a practice of giving and receiving feedback frequently throughout the shift.
- In this case, an evaluation of a particular incident (a problem evaluation) reveals that the shorter term, ongoing evaluation throughout the shift might not have been proceeding as effectively as it could have been.
- Checkpoints between the supervising RN and the delegate were missing.
- A long-term view of the situation will certainly reveal that the nursing assistant's performance must be evaluated and feedback given in relation to her past performance.
- The communication systems used in this unit's selected care delivery system might need some changing.

Within any organizational setting, there is the need for continuous (ongoing), incident- (problem-) related, and periodic evaluation. Whether it is broken down on a shift-by-shift, daily, case, product line, program, or delegate basis, evaluation is integral. Just as the nursing process of assessment, planning, intervention, and evaluation is a circular, never-ending continuum, evaluation is a continuous part of the delegation process as the delegating nurse constantly checks reality with what was projected in terms of job descriptions, expected behaviors, and outcomes.

The feedback related to the process of evaluation is received in two forms.

1. Data reporting and the RN's personal assessment of the client situation and the actual process by which care is delivered will yield some of the information necessary to evaluate the process and the people who perform the process.
2. Performance feedback (see Chapter 10) is a two-way, reciprocal action in which the RN coaches and guides the delegates and receives feedback from them related to the RN's performance as well.

Evaluation of specific problems or situations, whether they have to do with personal performance or systems performance, will consistently be a part of the RN's job in his or her appraisal during the delegation process. Feedback must be given, and problem solving, both short term and long term, is necessary.

Periodic evaluation considers the effects of systems and people performance on the overall goal achievement of the team. What outcomes have been expected, and what outcomes have been evidenced? The RN looks for what is working well and what problems or trends need attention to improve the quality of care and takes steps to resolve recurring issues. Periodic evaluation of the performance of the team members is also a part of this type of evaluation.

The evaluation phase of the delegation process is represented graphically in **Figure 11–1**.

CONTINUOUS EVALUATION

Checkpoints, Timelines, and Parameters for Reporting

Depending on the healthcare setting where you work, you have integrated a method by which you can receive and give feedback or share information and clinical data on a regular, ongoing basis in your clinical work. The communication is two way: to and from you as the RN and to and

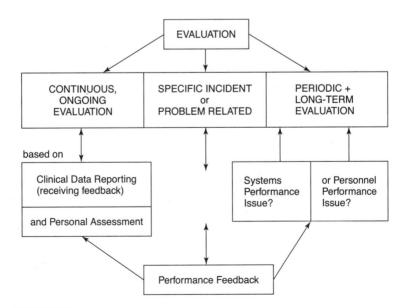

FIGURE 11–1 The Evaluation Process

from the delegates. This data sharing makes it possible for you to evaluate the clinical situation and to make decisions about further assessment and interventions that might be necessary for a specific patient or case. If you have not yet incorporated a plan for your day or case that includes communication and checkpoints and evaluation, it's time to build that into your daily work. In a psychiatric day care setting, for example, the supervising RN might receive data from assistive personnel several times throughout the day about a client who is experiencing an acute depressive episode. He or she may also spend one-on-one time with that patient to make decisions about further treatment modalities. Getting the necessary data in a timely manner from the assistive personnel depends on having checkpoints, timelines, and parameters for reporting.

As we have discussed previously in this book, it's essential for you to know what you want. Knowing what kinds of things you need to find out from assistive personnel is fundamental to your own ability to clearly express your requirements to the delegates. We again review the journalist's list of questions necessary for evaluation: who, what, when, where, how, and why.

Be clear with the delegate about:

- Who should be doing which tasks, and to whom
- What kinds of data are necessary
- When, where, and how it will be reported to you

This is basic information that is often assumed to be understood, and the expectation is not shared by all delegates and supervisors. (Is it okay to chart only essential information? What kinds of data are important?) "Why" shows delegates what kinds of things you are concerned about and helps them grow while they become another set of eyes and ears. For example, in acute care, if a delegate is assigned a group of tasks, including data collection such as vital signs, he or she needs to know when to report to you any vital signs that are abnormal and what constitutes "abnormal." Parameters for reporting are essential and are often forgotten, especially when you delegate to another RN who is floating to your area. Keep in mind that when you became a renal nurse specialist, you didn't know how much urine to expect the first 48 hours posttransplant, and the float RN or assistive personnel won't know either. Guidelines for reporting help avoid unpleasant surprises. Wherever you work, take time to think about how you implement the following and whether the communication is in a written and/or oral format.

+ Checkpoints—How often do you get together to share data? (This is a two-way street, as shown by the double arrows in Figure 11–1.) Before people go to breaks or meals, knowing what has been happening is essential. Where and how can delegates find you if needed?

+ Timelines—Are all personnel certain of when to report which data? Which are okay merely to chart and which need immediate attention? How often should the delegate expect that you'll report changes or update them on the client's situation? Are you clear about this expectation when delegating?

+ Parameters for reporting—Are you worried about the bleeding on the dressing or in the chest tube with Mrs. Smith? If so, how much bleeding should be expected in the next 2 hours? Are you wondering whether Mr. Potter's daughter has been in the home with him to discuss transport to the rehabilitation center for physical therapy (PT)? How soon do you need to know about the travel arrangements that have been made? Just as you appreciate (and need!) specific parameters for reporting patient condition changes to the physician, your delegates need specific parameters as well. Do you provide them?

If you found the answers to the preceding questions were difficult to come by or if the questions raised some concerns about whether information is being shared appropriately and in a timely manner, now is the time to determine what can be done about interruptions in the continuous flow of important information among the members of the healthcare team. As we discuss the problems that might become evident as a part of your evaluation process, you can use some of the suggestions to help you proceed with solving the communication flow issue.

Learning and Communication Styles

As you thought about how you are giving and receiving clinical information and feedback continuously with members of your healthcare team to evaluate whether outcomes have been achieved, you may have overlooked the importance of understanding how people best learn. This one issue commonly creates problems in the delegation process that become evident as you gather data and evaluate, and it is closely related to how well you assessed your delegate and acted on those assessment data.

People have preferred modes of learning that can affect their ability to retain and implement your instructions to them. Let's take a closer look at how learning and communication styles can influence the manner in which you discussed the work to be done with the delegates and the achievement of outcomes.

Global versus Linear Learning

Some of the delegates need to know the total, overall goals and the global picture before they are able to begin working most effectively; others want more detailed instructions of the steps to be accomplished, with less regard for the total view. When discussing the work at hand, it's best to give the overall outcomes to be achieved for the motivational value and for those who need that type of information to get started, while giving more detailed information to those who need it. For example, if you are discussing an assignment in a long-term care setting, you will want to tell the group about the outcomes you wish to achieve with Mrs. Ventelli: "The patient and family, along with the multidisciplinary team group, determined that we'd all work for the goal of getting her home by Christmas with a home health aide coming in several times a week for chores and personal care [overall picture for the global learners]. This means she will be gradually increasing her physical therapy (PT) and ambulation by 10 minutes three times per day. The rehabilitation aides will use this graph in the room to chart Mrs. Ventelli's responses. Let me know before afternoon break how well it's gone today" [more detail for the linear learners]. In this way, each person on the team is more clear about the work he or she needs to do and what kind of information you are expecting in return.

Visual, Auditory, and Kinesthetic Learning

Those of you who were very glad that we've included graphic representations and models to aid in your assimilation and integration of the material are probably visual learners. Very observant, these people might have difficulty understanding or remembering oral directions. (Have you ever been given directions verbally at the convenience store or gas station when what you really wanted was a map of the area?) It is very frustrating for visual learners to hear directions only. These people will be able to do their jobs more effectively if given written directions, and even better when the care map or plan is visually represented by symbols or in a graph-like format. Visual delegates might want to make up

> Considering global versus linear learning styles, as well as visual, auditory, and kinesthetic learning styles will help you communicate more effectively throughout the delegation process.

their own assignment sheets or write up personal notes (called "brains" in many settings) to make certain they are organized and will give appropriate feedback to the RN in a timely manner. It's best when written information on assignments, reporting timelines, and so on is available for clarity and legal reasons as well as to facilitate the accomplishment of the process. We'll discuss the topic of documentation more fully later on in this chapter.

Visual learners want to "see" what you're telling them in a written or graphic format; auditory learners want to hear from you; kinesthetic learners want "hands on" assistance or practice.

Many organizations have specific (written) policies for reporting times, checkpoints, and so on. Certainly all healthcare organizations across the continuum expect some kind of formal charting of patients' responses and other clinical data. Computerized patient clinical data might be available in a real-time manner; however, it is not a substitute for the RN's interpretation and discussion of the implications with the delegates.

Auditory learners need to hear from you. They won't be satisfied with a written assignment but will want to discuss it with you. This is their preferred method of communication, and despite the time it takes to talk about what needs to be done and how, it's essential to save time later by being clear in asking for and receiving feedback or clinical data reporting. We have observed negative consequences in systems where delegates were given only written instructions to be followed, without discussion, before beginning their work. Because health care in any setting is a dynamic process, what is written as an instruction one minute might be inaccurate at best, dangerous at worst, in the next minute. Relying on "routine" in any setting has created many problems. Be aware that some of the problems can be related to the necessity for auditory learners to personally hear from you. Since those who evaluate the root causes of errors, such as The Joint Commission, determined that improved handoff communication is a goal for patient safety, we recommend that a handoff template be used to standardize and simplify processes and avoid duplication or omissions of information (The Joint Commission, 2007). Research related to the report model used shows that the type of information exchanged and the method impacts care planning (Hays, 2003; Dowding, 2001; Hansten, 2003.)

CHECKPOINT 11-2

The authors recommend that shift report and other hand-off communication should be based on a template for communication. Why?

With so many delegates speaking English as a second language, it's important to understand the necessity of clarity in both written and oral communication. When determining delegates' ability to understand, get immediate feedback from them by asking them what their plan for the day/shift/case is. Although it is uncomfortable to determine these issues, it's even more uncomfortable when unclear communication causes a patient problem. Many organizations use written universal symbols to help multilingual patients, staff, and families understand each other.

Kinesthetic learners are those who need to "do" rather than hear about it. Some delegates might feel comfortable with trying to complete a task with verbal instruction, but kinesthetic learners will need to experience an active learning process of watching and helping with the task or procedure, then doing it with a supervising nurse. When giving instructions such as parameters for reporting, it might not suffice for this delegate to be told that "the dressing should not have more than 1 or 2 more centimeters of bleeding on it, and please let me know the amount of additional drainage before you go to break." For these delegates, you might need to go with them to the patient's room and describe and show them what you mean. When asking a delegate to complete the patient's clothing checklist, paying special attention to suicide prevention articles, it won't suffice for them to read the procedure and discuss it with you. They'll have to work through it in a patient situation with a supervising nurse to feel comfortable with the process.

Because all of us have a combination of preferences of learning modes, it's best to use as many of them as possible when communicating and asking for feedback in the form of data reporting. Keep in mind that just because a delegate might have a combination of styles that is different from yours doesn't mean it will detract from his or her ability to do the job. It does mean, however, that you will need to adjust your methods of communication as you learn what works best with that staff member. Before you proceed, complete Checkpoint 11–3.

CHECKPOINT 11–3

1. Thinking about your communication links in the system in your workplace, how do you make certain you respond to the preferred learning and communication styles of those with whom you work?

2. Have you ever been frustrated with those with different learning styles? For example, what would the following example lead you to believe? (Use information you have learned in all the preceding chapters.)

I have told Delegate A several times today that she needs to empty the dirty linen cart, and it hasn't been done yet. Is Delegate A

a) lazy?

b) hard of hearing?

c) new to the English language, so that she might not have understood?

d) a visual or kinesthetic learner who needs written instructions or actual demonstration?

e) of a culture that differs from yours, so that she might not interpret your instructions as a priority due to your method of communication?

f) lacking motivation and being resentful and subordinate?

g) misunderstanding what you expect?

Looking at this example, it would seem that further assessment and evaluation are necessary to determine what is really going on here. Does the RN have the extra time and energy to spend in frustration and anger, or would time be better spent finding out what the real issue is behind this? (You have learned many skills for working with these issues: the assertiveness formula, the collaborative resolution model, and the feedback process. You have also learned how to assess the delegate to determine how to delegate effectively based on your appraisal.)

Importance of Personal Assessment

Although we have mentioned this previously, whether you are evaluating achievement of outcomes on a patient-by-patient basis, doing ongoing evaluation as the shift progresses, evaluating a specific unusual occurrence, or completing a more global evaluation of the processes and systems you are using for delivery of care, nothing can substitute for your own personal assessment and evaluation. Using assistive personnel has allowed RNs to gather data with the additional eyes and ears of others, leaving more time for the RNs to perform professional nursing tasks and processes more thoroughly. However, keep in mind that the RN is the supervising authority. You are being paid to use the nursing process, solve problems, and think about maintaining and improving the quality of the care or service provided to your clients on a short-term and long-term

As a supervising (delegating) nurse, you'll often find yourself using the same skills you've used with patients (assessing their readiness and preferred learning and communication methods) with your delegates and coworkers. If it works for the RN to adapt to the patient's needs, it is certainly effective to utilize the same skills with the other members of the healthcare team.

basis. Nothing can substitute for the time you spend evaluating the situations you are faced with each day.

Besides evaluating the results achieved by your interventions according to your treatment plan as in the nursing process, you must evaluate the efficacy of the delegation process and the performance of the delegates. If you are a public health nurse who has been examining the data of the growing rate of tuberculosis and AIDS in your community and have reviewed reports of specific cases from many assistive personnel, nothing can substitute for some on-site assessment and evaluation of selected patient cases. If you work in ambulatory care and a medical assistant or LPN often gives the injections in your well-baby clinics, supervising the process and observing and evaluating his or her ability to perform the functions of the job description are essential to your ability to evaluate the systems you are using as well as the performance of the delegates. If you work in home health care and you've made a home assessment visit, you know that there is no other professional or assistant that can put together the medical, psychological, social, and practical aspects of the patient's and family's lives to determine the plan of care and how to best capitalize on the patient's strengths.

If you work in acute or long-term care and you are so busy at the desk being "in charge" that you never actually see the patients, you are missing a valuable and essential part of your job. You are able, in a moment's time, to "eyeball" a patient and observe very quickly any changes in condition. In a few seconds, you have taken in the patient's respiratory rate, depth, and comfort; skin color and moisture; body habitus and expression—all the visual and auditory cues. Asking a short question will allow you to make a preliminary assessment of cognitive functioning as well. Combining your observations with the clinical data and your experience with your scientific knowledge is a part of the art of nursing. You use this special art to evaluate, decide what additional data are needed, and come to a conclusion about what else needs to be done. The patient assessment and/or evaluation data that you complete by your clinical assessment also yield valuable information about the delegation process and how well it is going. Is care being completed by the delegates? Are changes in condition being appropriately reported? How does the environment appear? Where have the assistive personnel been concentrating their efforts? How are we proceeding as a team in achieving the planned outcomes?

Nothing can substitute for your own personal assessment and evaluation.

Evaluation is another part of the delegation process that encourages you to make decisions about what data can be gathered by others and what data must be generated by your own senses. Again, nursing judgment must be used in each specific situation to determine how much of the evaluation can be based on reports and data collected by others, just as which tasks to delegate and the amount and type of supervision needed were determined in each situation in the beginning of the delegation process. A neonatal nurse specialist at a receiving hospital is the very best person to determine which questions to ask nurses at another hospital before transport of a critical infant can take place, even if a secretary calls with a cursory report. Nothing can substitute for the "eyeball" assessment and evaluation of the situation by another nurse. Even though this book is dedicated to helping nurses make the very best use of assistive personnel, we wish to caution all nurses to maintain patient contact so that the delegation process, and assistive personnel, can best be evaluated.

Give yourselves credit for that art of nursing, the judgment based on your experience and scientific knowledge. Think about how often we use it in our daily lives: when you and a friend are at the mall and you see someone walking past, you might comment, "Boy, that person has COPD: looks like he left the oxygen at home!" or "My goodness, that pregnant woman has 4+ pitting edema up to her calf, and with that flushed face I wonder if she's had her pressure taken recently?" Or in conversation with a friend at church or the grocery store, you might say, "With the sleep and appetite disturbances, I wonder if he's tried drugs or psychotherapy for that depression. Has he ever said anything about feeling that he'd like to never wake up? Any other suicidal ideation?" It's impossible to take the nursing process or the "art" out of a nurse at any age or in any setting. Because your nursing abilities are second nature, don't assume that all humans are endowed with these special abilities, but instead, give yourselves credit for your expertise and use it for evaluating and improving the care you provide!

CHECKPOINT 11-4

Consider your own work environment. What kinds of information about the effectiveness of the delegation process and the performance of the delegates can be obtained from your own personal assessment? What kinds of information do you retrieve from your evaluation of the patient, the chart, or other written materials?

SPECIFIC INCIDENT OR PROBLEM-RELATED EVALUATION: CRITICAL THINKING

Because you are the supervising nurse, incidents or problems will definitely occur, if not daily, then at least frequently enough that these "unusual occurrences" will consume a fair amount of your time. Evaluating the situation is essential for resolving the problem or situation. In the first situation we discussed (the case of the chest pain), there were many possible errors and several times when the problem could have been resolved. For example, ongoing checkpoints and two-way feedback were missing. The other RN might not have assessed the patient before giving the sedative. The nursing assistant could have reported the problem.

The charge RN stepped in immediately when the information was shared to solve the short-term problem: finding out whether the patient had a myocardial infarction (MI) and what kind of treatment was necessary to provide immediately. After the emergency issues were resolved, there remained another concern. Why did this problem occur, and how could it be prevented from happening again? In this case, evaluation of the problem uncovered the need for more information from the other RN (to determine what steps would be necessary) and for performance feedback for the nursing assistant. (In Chapter 10 we discussed the process of performance feedback. As Figure 11–1 illustrates, performance feedback supports the entire evaluation process.) Now let's take a closer look at the RN's responsibility for evaluating incidents and resolving problems.

Many nurses have reported to us that they wish that their managers were better at resolving problems and incidents. They often share their frustration with the slow progress they've seen in improving and repairing systems and personnel performance. These RNs have clearly evaluated specific incidents or have determined trends or recurring problems. They have begun the evaluation and problem-solving process by analyzing situations and coming up with ideas of what is wrong and what should be done. Most of the work in resolving the problem is already complete! Ideas like these should be shared and used with the managers of the departments to improve the quality of care and outcomes achieved instead of being kept bottled up in individual and collective frustration! The managers cannot possibly "fix" everything (including people's performance) alone. Each RN has the accountability to be involved in the short-term and long-term improvement of care.

Defining Critical Thinking

As discussed in Question 52 of *The Nurse Manager's Answer Book* (Hansten and Washburn, 1993) and again in our *Toolbook for Health Care Redesign* (Hansten and Washburn, 1997), there is a step-by-step process to use when evaluating an incident or problem. We have used this model with countless healthcare professionals and have incorporated research related to critical thinking skill development.

Critical thinking skills are essential as professional nursing moves increasingly into cognitive work rather than task-oriented psychomotor practice, that is, brain-work: coordination, leadership of the interdisciplinary team, focusing on outcomes rather than merely tasks.

As nurse executives and managers call for improved critical thinking on the part of their staff, educational groups have responded by concentrating on these skills. The National League for Nursing (NLN) requires schools of nursing to teach, measure, and evaluate improved critical thinking of nursing students. Many studies from various perspectives have evaluated this topic, leading to improved methods of teaching critical thinking. Although varying definitions are seen in the literature, this skill set is basically creative problem solving as a continual process. A sample of definitions follows.

> Critical thinking is a certain mindset or way of thinking, rather than a method or a set of steps to follow. Critical thinking is clear thinking that is active, focused, persistent, and purposeful. It is a process of choosing, weighing alternatives, and considering what to do. Critical thinking involves looking at reasons for believing one thing rather than another in an open, flexible, attentive way. (Kyzer, 1996, p. 66)

> Critical thinking is a complex form of thinking and can be defined as the rational examination of ideas, inferences, assumptions, principles, arguments, conclusions, issues, statements, beliefs, and actions. It is reasoning in a way that generates and examines questions and problems. During this type of thinking, the individual weighs, clarifies, and evaluates evidence, conclusions and arguments (Bandman, 1988, as quoted in Stark, 1996, p. 168). The process of critical thinking may actually be part of and integrated into an individual's inner self, incorporating intuition and feelings in the problem-solving process. (Gross, 1991, as quoted in Stark, 1996, p. 168)

[Critical thinking is] purposeful, self-regulatory judgment which results in interpretation, analysis, evaluation, and inference, as well as explanation of the evidential, conceptual, methodological, criteriological, or contextual considerations upon which that judgment was based. (Facione & Facione, 1996, p. 129)

Despite some variance in definitions, it is clear that critical thinking, ongoing problem solving from an organizational and clinical perspective, and clinical nursing judgment are closely aligned. Intuition has also been discussed (see "novice to expert" portion of Chapter 5, "Know Yourself") as a part of critical thinking. One study, based on qualitative research that shows that the use of intuition in clinical judgment making is an important part of the critical thinking process, gives evidence that as the level of nursing proficiency increases from beginner to expert, and as the amount of clinical experience increases, the use of intuition to make clinical nursing judgments increases significantly, concluding that "participants working in short term care, with a high level of education, adequate work experience (5–10 years) and using both practical and theoretical (intermediate) nursing knowledge, used intuitive decision making" (Lauri, et al., 2001, p. 89). Where clinical judgment meets regulation of professional practice, the National Council of State Boards of Nursing were commended by the 2004 Institute of Medicine report, "Keeping Patients Safe: Transforming the Work Environment of Nurses" to distinguish human errors from willful negligence and intentional misconduct (IOM, 2004). The NCSBN then developed TERCAP, the "Taxonomy of Error, Root Cause Analysis, and Practice-responsibility." Using a large case database, they were able to categorize practice categories, several of which are related to attributes of critical thinking: "clinical reasoning," "attentiveness," and "interpretation and implementation of authorized provider orders" (NCSBN, 2007). We as a profession are beginning to categorize in helpful ways our ability to think and act in our chaotic and complex practice environments.

How does one recognize expert critical thinkers, besides the fact that patient problems are resolved effectively and potential errors are avoided? Instead of stating, "This is the way we've always done it," they move beyond the norm or daily routine to being open to possibilities and asking "why?" They look for patterns and trends in individual patient situations as well as patients in a category, such as a disease process. They see the big picture, use intuition, and get input from others when solving problems (Stark, 1996, p. 169). In what almost seems like an updated scout creed, educational research supports that the ideal critical thinker is

- habitually inquisitive,
- well informed,
- trustful of reason,
- open minded,
- flexible,
- fair minded in evaluation,
- honest in facing personal biases,
- prudent in making judgment,
- willing to reconsider,
- clear about issues,
- orderly in complex matters,
- diligent in seeking relevant information,
- reasonable in the selection of criteria,
- focused in inquiry, and
- persistent in seeking results that are as precise as the subject and the circumstances may permit (Facione & Facione, 1996, p. 130).

CHECKPOINT 11-5

The NCSBN developed TERCAP (The Taxonomy of Error, Root Cause Analysis, and Practice-responsibility, 2007) partially in response to the 2004 Institute of Medicine report "Keeping Patients Safe: Transforming the Work Environment of Nurses." Name some of the identified thinking practices that contributed to nursing errors in this large database.

Further research with hundreds of graduates nationwide has shown that critical thinking skills and the disposition toward critical thinking are vitally important in the exercise of workplace decision making, leadership, clinical judgment, professional success, and effective participation in a democratic society (Jones, 1994). Certainly this is not a new thought to nurses and nurse managers and the patients who reap the results of noncritical thinkers in various situations. For example: A nurse dutifully charts that there is no urine all night (as was ordered under "strict I and O") but does nothing with the information, or a nurse pages the same physician again and again with no response as the patient's pressure falls and heart rate increases, but the nurse does not problem solve beyond that same paging number until the patient arrests.

Several principles seem to emerge related to research results:

+ Certain characteristics assist the individual to gain critical thinking skills, including
    - foundations of knowledge and experience,
    - attitudes of openness and attentiveness,
    - thinking strategies (thinking from all perspectives, seeing patterns, gathering all facts and ideas),
    - skills (problem solving, prioritization, technical, time management, assertiveness, negotiation, communication) (Kyzer, 1996, p. 4).
+ Critical thinking can be learned.
+ When an individual obtains concepts, theories, and knowledge, personal experiences combine with that memory to become "productive memory" or the basis for critical thinking (Whiteside, 1997, p. 154).
+ Use of a model can assist nurses in clinical areas to improve their ability to think critically (Whiteside, 1997, pp. 159–160).
+ The organization shares some responsibility in providing barriers or supports to critical thinking.

Rosalinda Alfaro-LeFevre, a leading international author and lecturer on the subject of critical thinking in nursing, uses Critical Thinking Indicators™ as evidence-based descriptions of actual nursing behaviors or actions that demonstrate critical thinking in clinical practice. **Exhibit 11–1** presents the required knowledge, characteristics, attitudes, intellectual skills, and competencies that, according to Alfaro-LeFevre, are related to critical thinking—her view of the expert nurse is a holistic being who uses both right and left brain and emotional intelligence to create an environment for healing and actual health for her patients!

EXHIBIT 11–1   Examples of Critical Thinking Indicators™ (CTIs™)[1]

Definition: Critical Thinking Indicators™ (CTIs™) are evidence-based descriptions of behaviors that demonstrate the knowledge, characteristics, and skills that promote CT in clinical practice. CTIs™ give concrete descriptions and examples and are listed in context of what's likely to be observed

---

[1]Adapted with permission from Critical Thinking Indicators™. © 2003 R. Alfaro-LeFevre. Comprehensive list of CTIs™ available at: www.AlfaroTeachSmart.com. Critical Thinking Indicators™ and CTIs™ are registered trademarks of Rosalinda Alfaro-LeFevre.

when a nurse is thinking critically in the clinical setting.[2] The complete list of CTIs™ and support material is available at www.AlfaroTeachSmart.com.

CTIs™ Demonstrating Required Knowledge

Clarifies nursing vs. medical responsibilities; manifestations of commonly encountered problems and complications; related anatomy, physiology, and pathophysiology; reasons behind interventions, medications, and diagnostic studies; policies and procedures and reasons behind them; nursing process and research principles; ethical and legal principles; spiritual and cultural concepts.

CTIs™ Demonstrating Charcteristics/Attitudes of Critical Thinkers

- Self-confident: expresses ability to think through problems and find solutions

- Inquisitive: seeks reasons, explanations, and new information

- Honest and upright: speaks and seeks the truth, even if the truth sheds unwanted light

- Alert to context: looks for changes in circumstances that may warrant a need to modify thinking or approaches

- Open and fair-minded: shows tolerance for different viewpoints; questions how own viewpoints are influencing thinking

- Analytical and insightful: identifies relationships; shows deep understanding

- Logical and intuitive: draws reasonable conclusions (if this is so, then if follows that . . . because . . .); uses intuition as a guide to search for evidence

- Reflective and self-corrective: carefully considers meaning of data and interpersonal interactions; corrects own thinking; observant for mistakes; identifies way to prevent mistakes

- Sensitive to diversity: Expresses appreciation of human differences related to values, culture, personality, or learning style preferences; adapts to preferences when feasible

---

[2]Alfaro-LeFevre, R. (2009). *Critical thinking and clinical judgments: A practical approach to outcome-focused thinking,* 4th Ed. Philadelphia: WB Saunders.

CTIs™ Demonstrating Intellectual Skills/Competencies

Nursing Process and Decision-Making Skills: assesses systematically and comprehensively; recognizes assumptions and inconsistencies; checks accuracy and reliability; identifies missing information; distinguishes relevant from irrelevant; supports conclusions with facts (evidence); sets priorities/makes decisions in a timely way; determines outcomes specific to each client; reassesses to monitor responses and outcomes

---

Organizational Barriers and Supports for Critical Thinking

The barriers and supports of an organization for problem solving and critical thinking deserve additional commentary. The organization that has characteristics similar to those of individuals who are effective critical thinkers will help improve those skills in the nurses it employs. For example, if the qualities listed in Exhibit 11-2 are true of your organization, your road to expertise in this pivotal skill will be swift! Use **Exhibit 11– 2** evaluate your organization for support of the process.

Strategies for improving critical thinking in an organization stem from improving the organizational climate by practicing critical thinking in all areas and rectifying those areas in the list in Exhibit 11–2 that need improvement. Loosening up to develop new ideas and risk-taking behaviors could mean using games, exercises, role playing, puzzles, or any number of strategies that open up the creative right side of the brain. The use of case studies or other simulated experiences will help produce the episodic memory that is necessary for building up experience and the potential for using that invaluable intuition. Most effective is the on-site mentoring of a clinically astute manager, supervisor, or clinical nurse specialist who is able to ask the right questions and help staff in real-time coaching as incidents occur. (See our discussions of managerial rounds in *Toolbook for Health Care Redesign*, Hansten & Washburn, 1997, pp. 20–22, 236.)

Potential benefits from focusing on critical thinking skill development for all healthcare workers in an organization are numerous. Although it is difficult to draw a direct cause–effect relationship with the improvement of thinking and the improvement of patient care, nursing leaders across the country tell us they expect to see the following improvements related to enhanced critical thinking:

EXHIBIT 11-2   Organizational Evaluation for Critical Thinking Facilitation

❑ Organizational culture or rules that would cause an individual employee to avoid creative problem solving and risk taking have been changed, and the new culture encourages empowerment and rapid action on problems.

❑ Critical thinking is modeled by managerial levels, with on-site mentoring focused on coaching rather than blaming.

❑ Education focuses on improving these abilities with use of case studies, experiential learning, and guided problem solving with expert mentors and preceptors.

❑ Education evaluates its effectiveness and does not attempt to do too much in too little time.

❑ Preceptors and mentors are also used for orientation, cross-training, or focused development activities.

❑ Multidisciplinary teams share their experiences and work together with open communication so that learning can take place across disciplines.

❑ Participative management is present, with supportive employee–managerial relationships.

❑ Mistakes are seen as a chance to learn and grow, and the punitive aspects are deemphasized.

❑ Questions, new ideas, and risk taking are supported (adapted from Kyzer, 1996).

Outcomes related to critical thinking

- improved patient care as measured by fewer incidents (falls, medication errors, omissions), decreased length of stay, fewer return visits to the hospital, emergency department, or intensive care unit
- better patient satisfaction related to appropriate discharge instructions, attention to patient priorities while under care of an RN, smooth transitions from one point of care to another
- increased resolution of problems, care issues, system glitches
- less blaming, more "How can I fix this problem?"
- improved staff morale and less turnover in all disciplines as interdisciplinary teamwork improves and as all workers feel more empowered to effect change both within the patient care realm and with organizational systems

Personal Accountability for Developing Critical Thinking Skills

Your job as a critical thinker is exciting and rewarding: developing these skills will assist you in your goal of delivering excellent patient care and will allow you to actually solve some of the problems that have frustrated you and have been an impediment to your practice! (See **Exhibit 11–3**.)

EXHIBIT 11–3   Personal Accountability for Developing Critical Thinking Skills

❑ As you identify your current point in the journey from novice to expert, consider how you can continue to grow through additional education, consultation with those more experienced when questions occur, and working enough to immerse yourself in your specialties. Consider obtaining certification in your current specialty.

❑ Reflect on the way you think, and review those steps you miss most often.

❑ Learn from your mistakes and the mistakes of others. "What steps in the process did I (or my unfortunate colleague) miss this time?"

❑ Recognize your personal indicators that alert you to when you aren't able to think as well, such as illness, short staffing, or stress at home that reduces focus on work issues. Redouble efforts at that time to resist jumping to conclusions, not challenging your assumptions, or being close-minded due to time constraints. This might include stress-reduction techniques or asking a coworker to hear your thinking out loud.

❑ Participate in or lead discussions of clinical scenarios.

❑ Participate in a mentorship or preceptor program, either as a participant or as a mentor. You will learn as you teach others.

❑ Trust your intuition, your gut feelings. If something (a lab value, a physical assessment parameter, an organizational problem) seems odd or out of the ordinary, ask why.

❑ Use the four types of questions and/or the positive problem-solving process (Falkof and Moss) as a model for intermittent measurements of your critical thinking processes (adapted from Kyzer, 1996, pp. 74–75).

We have developed the checkpoints and case studies in this book to assist in development of critical thinking skills. Although we cannot provide actual mentorship or experiences in this written format, we have attempted to begin the process that can be used by clinical instructors to develop preceptorships, real-time case studies, and peer consultation. Based on our work with thousands of nurses across the nation, we recognize that the use of a model or a guide will provide an essential link for those who are learning creative problem solving and are developing their critical thinking skills.

Falkof and Moss's classification scheme (Girvan, 1989) uses four levels of questioning for improving critical thinking. When a charge nurse finds that he has been given two fewer people than he expected for staffing this shift, the following questions will help him critically think through this situation:

1. Factual questions—test knowledge and comprehension—develop the thinking skills of cognition and memory. "What is the way we have staffed this unit in the past? Who is present and what are their abilities? Who are our patients this shift? What skill levels are needed to care for these patients today?"

2. Interpretive questions—test application and analysis—develop convergent thinking. "What principles were used in staffing based on acuity, and how were they applied today? How can we apply past knowledge to the current patient population?"

3. Creative questions—test ability to synthesize information—develop divergent thinking. "What possible reasons would cause the short staffing, and can the situation be altered? What other ways can I think of to do safe patient care, given the people we have today, if no help is possible? What care tasks can be done differently, or what can be left for later or done by someone else? What other methods can we use to obtain help?"

4. Evaluative questions—test ability to evaluate—develop affective thinking skills (Girvan, 1989). "How will I evaluate the outcomes we achieve by trying to solve this staffing problem from a short- and long-term perspective? What is good about this problem? How will I know if we have been successful at the end of this shift?"

Positive Problem-Solving Process

Think back to the clinical problem we discussed at the beginning of the chapter. We will use this example to discuss the process of positive problem solving and then use the additional examples of the case studies for practice. If you become frustrated during this process, consult with a peer or a mentor to assist you. Remember that the critical thinking process is continuous and doesn't stop after one or two potential solutions have been tried and found wanting. Results are measured, and if the right solutions haven't been found, the process returns to the beginning.

1. What signs cause you to think there is a problem? Here you must think about the frame of reference, reasons that this problem might exist, attitude, and assumptions. This step gives the problem solver a chance to reflect on the characteristics within himself that will affect his ability to solve the problem effectively. The emotional intelligence issues of intrapersonal intelligence (being aware of how moods, presuppositions, or past experiences might affect thoughts and behaviors) and interpersonal or social intelligence (understanding how the internal environment of others involved in the problem might affect their thoughts and behaviors) must be consulted in the very first step of the process (Merlevede, Bridoux, & Vandamme, 2003, p. 7). If reflection on attitudes, assumptions, and the effects of frame of reference does not occur at the inception of problem solving, the planned solutions might not achieve the desired results. Be very specific about the exact nature of the problem, incident, or error. (Patients who have an MI need to go to the critical care unit [CCU]. A patient didn't get appropriate care because the RN didn't know about his symptoms. The symptoms weren't reported.) Use the following questions to further define the problem.

    +   How is my frame of reference affecting my interpretation of this situation? (Because I work night shift, do I expect that others should see their patients less frequently or that nursing assistants should not need to report to the RNs?)
    +   What are the reasons that this problem might exist? (Is this a performance problem? Is there shared accountability with the RN and the assistive person who did not report the symptoms? Is this an educational need, i.e., does the nursing assistant misunderstand what to report? Why was the RN unavailable, and why did the other RN give a sleeping pill without verifying her assessment?)
    +   How does my attitude affect this problem-solving process? (Do I dislike that nursing assistant and hope she gets fired because she hasn't helped me with my care for ages?)

✦ What are my assumptions? (I need to verify what happened. It is possible the second RN did assess the patient, but the patient didn't give any indication of pain to her. It's also possible that the charge RN did assess the patient as well. I need to talk to all involved to find out each person's perceptions of the truth.)

2. What is good about this situation? To challenge your brain, identify three aspects of the situation that are positive. (Remember collaborative resolution?) This step allows the creative juices to flow. When we ask this question, we begin to change our mindset. Instead of "Oh no, not another problem!" we can open up the creative right brain to begin to see other possible solutions. Try it in your personal life; it really works! We encourage all readers to apply this question to all situations that they encounter when the same old problems keep reappearing. The statement "Oh, no! We are out of linen again for the 30th time this month!" should be a trigger to use the full positive problem-solving process and, especially, to ask what is good about the problem. (The good things about the patient situation in the chest pain example are numerous: the patient didn't die; this incident allows us to teach the assistant and the other nurses; we can look more closely at our methods of communicating clinical data; we can examine how nursing assistants have been taught what things to report; and we can evaluate whether that program is working effectively.)

3. What should have been happening instead of what did happen? Here, discuss specific and measurable criteria. These will be your criteria for knowing when the problem has been effectively resolved. (The nursing assistant would have reported the pain; the patient would have been transferred to CCU; the other RN would have assessed him further or at least asked if the charge nurse had time to assess him before the sedative was given; and, in the long term, this type of miscommunication of relevant and critical patient data will not occur.) From an organizational perspective, one of the most glaring problems in this example is that an assistive person did not report serious data in a timely manner. She made a decision about the implications of the patient's complaint and decided to make an intervention on her own. We would be able to tell that the problem was resolved if this staff member reported appropriately at all times. Another problem is the lack of checkpoints and

sharing of information throughout the shift. If a system were set up by which that could occur, then information would be shared on an ongoing basis each shift. The outcomes for the patients would ultimately be avoidance of complications and, potentially, discharge as planned. In this situation, absence of lawsuits based on poor quality of care could be another outcome.)

4. Have I identified the real problem or do I need more information? Step four is an opportunity to consider whether or not enough information has been gleaned or if there might be other routes to explore. For example, have we actually talked to all the people that were involved in this situation? What does the nurse that gave the medication say about her role? Is there something inherently missing in the way that our shift is set up? Are all our routines effective? Many problems will not be solved for the long term without further exploration.

5. Do I need to do something about this? Ask yourself this question to determine accountability and ownership. The following questions will help make a determination about when you should get involved. Some of us like to be involved in everything, but we become overly taxed and ineffective from spreading ourselves too thin and assuming others' responsibilities. Other individuals seem to take accountability more lightly and would not consider this to be their problem to solve. To determine that, ask these questions:

   + **Does it affect me, my patients, or our team goals?** (YES!) Also ask yourself this related question: Is this a real problem or is it something I can let go? (No, patients' lives could be threatened if I let this go.)
   + **What will happen if I don't do anything about this?** (Another patient could die. This is a good reason to deal with the incident. It's also true that someone else might do something about it, but I am not willing to allow this kind of incident to continue. The next time it could happen to me!)
   + **What will happen if I try to resolve this problem?** (Be aware and prepared for the fact that addressing a problem can cause conflict, but don't let concerns about conflict get in your way. You know how to deal with that. Keep your mind on what can happen that will be better: If this communication problem is solved, perhaps lives will be saved. Also be aware of organizational politics. If this nursing assistant is the director of nursing's best friend, you'll have to weigh that into the equation.

However, we hope that you will respond ethically and put the client or those you serve in the priority position.)

+ **Am I the person who can solve this problem (or prevent this type of incident from occurring in the future), or should this problem be dealt with by another person or department?** Remember to consider who else might be affected. (In the chest pain incident, the short-term situation definitely required the action of the charge nurse. The long-term solution for this problem will rest with the charge nurse as well as the manager. The errors are too serious to leave for quick, undocumented verbal feedback.) Consideration of who else might be affected due to your action or inaction will help you determine other stakeholders. For example, quick transfers to the CCU without warning at change of shift are unpleasant, although necessary, for all involved, including the lab workers who drew the stat blood, the CCU staff, the staffing clerks, and the transporters.

6. What can we do about these problems? Consider three possible solutions in terms of the following:

+ immediate corrections of the short-term problem
+ long-term resolution so the situation does not occur again
+ people/departments/resources that need to be involved
+ the solutions' potential side effects to other individuals and departments
+ a timeline for evaluation

Without judging the feasibility of each idea, list some possible plans for resolving the problem. Here, the charge nurse might list a variety of ideas: 1) fire the nursing assistant, a solution that would require the manager's help; 2) educate the nursing assistant about what to report; 3) plan for checkpoints and evaluation at intervals throughout the shift; 4) ask other charge nurses for ideas; 5) research the situation more fully and get some feedback from all the people involved; 6) talk to the manager about this and give him or her a list of possible alternatives.

Consider what should be done first. (In this case, the charge nurse decides to get more information from the others and then talk to the nurse manager. The manager will need to know about this very soon because of the risks inherent in the situation, and he or she will want to be involved. The charge nurse will also think of how to better supervise in an ongoing manner and report the plan to the manager at the same time.)

Be certain you have considered the solutions' potential side effects to other departments or individuals. (Will this affect other departments to which this individual floats if she is fired? What could happen if she improves?)

Plan the steps for implementation of the solutions or follow-up, keeping in mind the positive results you will enjoy because of your efforts. Remember the need to involve all individuals who will be affected when changes are made. (Depending on the amount of responsibility given to charge nurses in the job description, the charge nurse will be working with the manager to give performance feedback to the assistant and the other nurse. The charge nurse will be implementing the plan for better supervision. The manager, or perhaps the charge nurse if he or she has a "hiring/firing" supervisory role, will probably be engaged in the progressive discipline process for the assistive person. Don't forget to implement this excellent plan!)

Evaluate your results by the objective criteria you designed. Is the situation/problem vanishing? (Is the nursing assistant reporting all information? How is your system of checkpoints working? Are you getting the information you need from the assistive personnel? When will you judge that the nursing assistant is competent?)

If related incidents continue to occur, the solutions aren't working and a new plan needs to be developed. (Perhaps this nursing assistant will never report appropriately and it's time for her to progress to a different job.) It's possible that the real problem hasn't been defined or that the symptoms you saw were caused by something else. Perhaps the facts weren't fully disclosed, or you did not fully research the incident. Maybe communication with all those who needed to be involved hasn't occurred or the solutions haven't been given enough time to do their magic! Again, remember that the process is ongoing—continuous, just as is the nursing process—and includes evaluation to be certain that the applied solutions are still working.

We encourage each professional nurse to complete as much of the problem-solving process as is authorized in his or her work setting. As we have noted, managers must be notified of problems and should be involved in developing and carrying out the solutions. However, as reforms in our national system continue and health care adopts the business trend of flattened hierarchies, increased accountability and responsibility will be granted to each employee. Each RN will become more empowered to act in the best interests of the patients for whom he or she cares and will be more involved in activities that once were considered the province of managers.

The five-step process of evaluation and follow-up for specific incidents or problem situations can be applied to any clinical setting. To review the steps just outlined, see **Exhibit 11–4.**

EXHIBIT 11–4   A Positive Approach to Problem Solving

The following worksheet can be used as a teaching tool for positive problem solving.

1. What signs tell you that something is wrong here? What is the exact nature of the problem, incident, or error? Be specific. Consider your
    *   frame of reference (shift, position, etc.)
    *   reasons that this problem might exist
    *   attitude (do you have a personal investment or bias?)
    *   assumptions (have you verified the evidence?)
2. What is good about this situation? Identify three aspects of this situation that are positive.
3. What should be happening instead of what did happen? These are your criteria for success. Be specific and measurable so that you know when you have solved the problem.
4. Define the problem. Do we have enough information to determine the root causes?
5. To determine accountability and ownership, ask yourself: Do I need to do something about it?
    *   Does it affect me, my patients, or our team goals?
    *   What will happen if I don't do something about this?
    *   What could happen if I do?
    *   Should I be solving this problem, or do I need someone else (who is affected)?
6. What can be done about it? Consider three possible solutions in terms of:
    *   immediate corrections of the short-term problem
    *   long-term remedies so the situation does not occur again
    *   people/departments/systems/resources that need to be involved
    *   the solutions' potential side effects to others
    *   a timeline for evaluation

Source: Adapted from *Toolbook for Health Care Redesign* (Hansten & Washburn, © 1997, p. 193), Aspen Publishers.

The process of evaluation of a specific situation or incident includes many of the principles of the conflict management process as well as the nursing process. Evaluation must focus on the short-term situation as well as on how the problem could be avoided in the future.

CHECKPOINT 11–6

Think of a problem incident or situation that has occurred in your facility or work setting in the last month. Was it related to the delegation process? Was it related to problems within the system or with the performance of personnel or both? How did you go about helping to solve it, immediately and long term?

PERIODIC EVALUATION

Whether you are a charge nurse or staff nurse working with assistive personnel or are involved in upper management, you will need to take some time for periodic evaluation of the work and how the delegation process has been proceeding. Depending on the site in which you work, this might be on a shift-by-shift basis as each case is finished or every several months.

We worked with one subacute care facility that had recently changed shift times for the professional nurses and the assistive personnel. When their shift was completed, assistants went home without reporting what had happened during those 8 hours. It's obvious that this created some difficult situations as the RNs attempted to find out what had been done, how the patients responded, and what was left to be completed. The RNs spent a lot of time looking for charted information and asking the patients or family members. Although their observations within the patients' rooms and their rounding afforded them valuable information about the performance of their delegates, some of the information could have been handled much more efficiently by verbal communication. It's obvious that evaluation needed to be done on a shift-by-shift basis at a minimum in addition to checkpoints throughout the shift.

Again, as an RN you'll need to use your nursing judgment, in addition to consulting the policies, to decide when your periodic evaluation needs to occur.

One community care agency developed a policy that required RNs to meet with the home health aides and rehabilitation aides twice per month to discuss progress on the long-term cases. Nurses who at first complained about the amount of time this would take discovered that it actually saved them time when they reflected on whether the plan of care was working, gave and received feedback from their delegates, and decided whether the system and the personnel were performing as required. The team members were able to celebrate the outcomes they achieved with their patients as well!

An ambulatory respiratory rehabilitation clinic employed respiratory therapists, physical therapy/occupational therapy aides, a secretary/receptionist, and an LPN (LVN), all supervised by an RN. In this situation, the team met at the beginning and end of each case to plan the care and evaluate outcomes and also to evaluate their process of delegation. Often personnel performance issues were discussed and feedback was given. Each time, the RN asked for feedback about how the system worked for the delegates and, ultimately, for the patients and their families. When the clinic expanded its services to include general respiratory patients who were receiving ongoing outpatient care from the pulmonologists, some of whom were being referred to the rehabilitation clinic, the periodic evaluation of the system and personnel performance changed. Personnel were evaluated on a quarterly basis by the managing RN, and systems functioning was discussed in the staff meetings every month. The case-by-case evaluation of outcomes for the rehabilitation clinic patients continued. The staff handled personnel performance issues as they came up by using the feedback process, as we discussed in the previous chapter.

Overall evaluation includes asking some questions related to the delegation process. At the end of a shift, for example, an RN can ask the questions listed in **Exhibit 11–5**. When you have reviewed these questions, proceed to Checkpoint 11–7.

EXHIBIT 11–5   Questions for Overall Evaluation

1. Did we accomplish our goals? What patient outcomes have been achieved?
2. If so, did the outcomes have anything to do with the manner in which work was delegated and assigned? If so, what worked well so that I can use it again the next time?
3. What didn't work? Why?
4. If there was a problem, did it have anything to do with how I delegated?
   a. Did I know my own job description, roles, and responsibilities?
   b. Did I allow any personal barriers to get in the way?
   c. Did I know the roles, job descriptions, and characteristics of my delegates?

    d. Did I match the jobs to the delegates appropriately? Were jobs prioritized?

    e. Did I communicate clearly and assertively?

    f. Was conflict handled?

    g. Did I use checkpoints, timelines, and parameters for reporting?

    h. Have I given feedback as needed, both negative and positive?

CHECKPOINT 11–7

All but two of the personnel in an acute care surgical unit were on over-time this shift. Although the number of staff assigned matched what had been designated by the department's acuity system, all the RNs were behind and didn't have breaks. Joe and Marty, unit aides, completed their work early and were ready to go home on time. What possibly could have gone wrong with the delegation process in this case?

See the end of the chapter for the answers.

CASE STUDY ANALYSIS OF EVALUATION

In this case study, we will review the three types of evaluation (continuous, periodic, and specific incident related) and setting up timelines, check-points, and parameters for reporting in a community health setting.

Continuous Evaluation: Bob, a visiting nurse in a large metropolitan area, is supervising a challenging child abuse case. The mother has had two previous children who were mentally disabled from what has been surmised to have been head trauma. Because the charges were unproved previously, the judge awarded custody of her new twins to this natural mother, despite the concerns of the social worker, child welfare worker, mental health professional, and mental health worker. Until the case can be appealed, Bob is attempting to coordinate the team's activities as well as supervise the work of a chore worker who has been placed in the home to help do the food purchasing and preparation and provide some assistance with feeding the babies. How will Bob best evaluate and give necessary instructions to Evelyn, the chore worker?

_____

_____

_____

_____

Discussion: Bob will discuss the overall case with the chore worker and plan to visit at least twice weekly himself. The chore worker, Evelyn, will understand the global picture in terms of the desired outcomes (the twins to be healthy and safe and the mother to be able to handle the situation) and will be given details, both written and oral, about what to look for: signs that would indicate Mom is not coping well, problems with the infants, and how to recognize if Mom has been using drugs again. Evelyn and Bob will make the first visit together to be certain the step-by-step process of care and reporting is followed. In this way, the mother will know what to expect from both Evelyn and Bob in the ensuing weeks. Evelyn will be able to tell Bob how quickly he or the caseworker (or the emergency network) should be notified if problems occur and will report to Bob after each visit for at least the first month. On each visit, Bob will evaluate the babies, the mother, and the care that Evelyn is giving.

In this case we've reviewed some of the basic principles of evaluation on a continuous basis—discussing the parameters, timelines, and check-points for reporting. Bob will have given and received feedback (clinical data reporting) from a clinical situation based on Evelyn's data gathering and his own personal assessment.

Periodic Evaluation: Beginning on a daily basis, then moving to a weekly, biweekly, and monthly basis, Bob completed a more long-term, periodic evaluation of the plan of care and outcomes and how the team's process was proceeding. At the end of 1 month, which proceeded rather smoothly, Bob and the rest of the interdisciplinary team discussed the case. Bob evaluated the plan against the goals and projected outcomes: Is the mother able to cope with the twins with the support she has been given? This is being measured by whether or not the twins are gaining weight and thriving, a lack of evidence of abuse or neglect, and the mother's self-report of being in control. The assessment of all the support professionals agrees with the mother's statement that she has been able to care for the babies and herself without incident. Despite all the concerns of the staff, periodic evaluation yields positive results. Based on our evaluation model, what two questions does Bob need to ask himself at this point?

_____

_____

_____

_____

Discussion

1. How is the system working? (So far, so good. We'll need to keep up the continuous evaluation and communication, however. We seem to have matched the right person with the right work, and our communication in the delegation process has been effective.)

2. How is the personnel performance affecting the results of this case? (The people involved have been doing an excellent job! It's time for positive feedback for all the professionals who have been so deeply concerned and involved in this case!)

Specific Incident Evaluation: The twins seemed to be consuming formula at a faster rate, and this means Evelyn has had to pick up groceries more often. One day, on returning home from the market, she noted that their mother was fast asleep on the couch, a cigarette burning in the ashtray, while the twins were howling from hunger. It was difficult to arouse Mom, so Evelyn fed and changed the twins. The mother stated she had been up late the night before trying to get them settled and was exhausted. Evelyn, having been an exhausted new mother herself, decided not to report this incident as a possible problem unless it occurred again. Several days later, the twins were again screaming as Evelyn arrived, but this time Mom had left the used syringe out on the kitchen table. How would you, as a supervising RN, evaluate this incident? Use the questions in the table in Checkpoint 11–8 to guide your evaluation.

CHECKPOINT 11–8

Answer each question in the space provided.

1. What signs tell you something is wrong here?	The potential problem could have been reported earlier.
2. What's good about this incident?	The twins are okay. The drug abuse evidence will help get the children ultimately to a safe foster home. This is a great teaching example to use for the future.
3. What should be happening? What is the exact nature of the problem, issue, or error? By what objective criteria will I know if the problem is solved?	

4. Have I defined the problem? Do I need more information?	
5. Do I need to do something about it?	
6. What can be done?	
7. Weigh potential positive and negative impact for each solution.	
8. Plan steps and implement the proposed short- and long-term solutions.	
9. Evaluate the short-term results by objective criteria.	
10. Evaluate the long term results. Was the problem solved?	
(Are new/additional strategies needed?)	

See the end of the chapter for the answers.

DOCUMENTATION AND THE DELEGATION PROCESS

As we travel the country talking to nurses during and after seminars and consulting projects, we are often asked, "How do I document the delegation process?" We have several recommendations based on the particular situation and the degree of seriousness of the problem. Many nurses voice concerns about creating visible "proof," in the form of documentation, to demonstrate that they have indeed completed their responsibility as a supervisor of a delegated act.

To record the process of evaluation and feedback, many facilities have developed policies, procedures, or forms to be completed. For example, if a specific problem or error has occurred, you might be asked to fill out an "Unusual Occurrence Report" or "Incident Report," or participate in a Root Cause Analysis process. In these cases, follow the guidelines you've been given at your workplace. Generally, the actual observable problem is recorded in the chart objectively, but any interpersonal performance feedback is not documented on the patient record. (For example, if a medication was omitted, record that it was omitted and what you did to care for the patient. The facility incident report is generally a form that is used for communication to the healthcare agency's insurance company and often asks who was responsible for the incident and what form of follow-up was done.) If the problem is significant, a Root Cause Analysis might be performed, as recommended by The Joint Commission. Personnel feedback and evaluation is documented on such forms as interim performance progress notes, performance appraisal forms, or other anecdotal notes that are often kept by managers. As a delegating nurse, you might be asked to give written information to your manager about what you've discussed with your delegate when performance has been exceptional in either direction.

Documentation of the matching of the jobs to the delegate is often completed through assignment sheets or daily task lists. We recommend that you check to find out whether these are saved, and for what time period, in your department. We also recommend that you keep notes on your daily activities. Whatever method you currently use to keep track of your work for the case or the shift is an acceptable way to make a notation that you talked to Pam about the difficulty she was having in performing a task, but if the problem continues or becomes more serious, you will want to use a more formal method of documentation and alert the appropriate management person.

CHECKPOINT 11-9

1. Think of all the people that help you when you are in an emergency (or other challenging) situation in your healthcare setting. List them and what they do.

Example: A code in an acute care facility:

a) secretary: called the needed physician, called for stat labs

b) unit runner: ran specimens to lab

c) lab technician: took the stairs to get to the patient more quickly to draw blood

d) nursing assistant: reported the bloody stools, blood pressure drop, and stayed to get supplies

e) student nurse: answered other call bells

f) pastoral care: got coffee and gave support to family

g) LPN: gave medications to other patients while code progressed

h) a new nurse: recorded during code

    i)   code team: all did their jobs

    j)   housekeeping: cleaned room for quick transfer

    k)   admitting clerk: found room for patient

    l)   supervisor: called in staff for ICU to help save patient

2. Discuss with your coworkers the successes you have enjoyed in the last week.

3. How can you and your team plan to celebrate your successes more often?

When you've done the delegation process well and followed all the steps, and a delegate makes an error, how can you support your decision to delegate that task? Your decision is endorsed by delegating according to state statutes, your facility job description, and validated competencies or skills checklists. You will save your notes from the day that record that you did instruct and verify competency. (This information is not charted in the patient record, however.) Many organizations have established guidelines and policies about delegating that could support your decision. Your follow-up and feedback given to the delegate will be documented in some way by your manager, and an "Unusual Occurrence Report" will be completed according to specific agency rules.

An excellent example of documentation of delegation by RNs to unlicensed care providers in specific settings (such as residential programs for the developmentally disabled, licensed adult family homes, and licensed boarding homes for assistive living) has been used by the State of Washington's Department of Social and Health Services. As Harris points out,

> Specific policy and procedures must be written by a facility to delineate the scope of responsibilities to be delegated. . . . The successful completion of training and/or competency evaluation as required under [Medicare regulations of 1989] would be the minimum requirement for delegation of additional responsibilities to a home healthcare aide. Additional criteria include demonstration of ability to perform instructions from professional nurse; demonstrated successful interaction with home care team; interest and initiative for this responsibility; and additional training and supervision for a delegated responsibility. (Harris, 1993, p. 55)

The following forms have been developed by the State of Washington in collaboration with Aging and Adult Services to provide a backup to the nurse delegation provisions in the nurse practice regulations. The first form (**Exhibit 11–6**) is a checklist to assist the nurse in determining whether the delegation is appropriate and the assistant has had adequate training. This first checklist form is no longer used, and the information is incorporated into the subsequent forms used in 2007. However, because the checklist is a good review of the steps of problem solving for delegation and can be used by novices to reflect on their critical thinking about the process, it is retained for your perusal. The forms used in Washington state are included in the Appendix. The first form in Appendix 11-A, Nurse Delegation: Credentials and Training Verification, identifies the competencies and the training of the home health aide, ascertains which task(s) is to be delegated and that the nursing assistant has been taught and instructed and takes on accountability for performance of the task.. The next form in Appendix 11-A, Nurse Delegation: Consent for Delegation Process, clarifies patient/client consent and partnership in the healing process. The subsequent forms follow the delegation process: Nursing Visit Instructions for Nursing Task, and Assumption of Delegation, when a new RN takes over a case. Other contingencies and more detailed instructions are included in the following forms: PRN Medication, Rescinding Delegation, and Changes in Medical/Treatment Orders. These forms show the nurse's participation with the assistant in making certain that the instructions for the delegate are related to the patient's preferred outcomes and that the assistant is competent. If the nurse determines that the delegation must be rescinded due to the assistant's performance, the form titled Rescinding Delegation will also support tracking of the supervision process. When another nurse assumes the responsibility for delegating, the documentation will support the rationale as well as the resident's choice. Initial instructions for a nursing task carefully describes the procedures, predictable outcomes, potential risks, and what to report. What an excellent example of checkpoints, timelines, and parameters for reporting! PRN medication delegation (if it is delegated) is carefully recorded on the form Nurse Delegation: PRN Medication. If a change of physician orders for delegated medications occurs, the RN must verify the change with the physician and make a decision about whether a site visit is necessary, whether delegation must be rescinded, or whether the new task can be added to the instruction list. These decisions are guided by the documentation in the final form in Appendix 11–A Nurse Delegation: Change in Medical/Treatment Orders.

EXHIBIT 11-6   Checklist for the Delegation of Specific Nursing Tasks

Delegated Task	Client/Patient

YES NO

❑ ❑ Does the nurse hold a current license to practice as a registered nurse in Washington?

❑ ❑ Is the setting in a certified community residential program for the developmentally disabled, a licensed adult family home, or a licensed boarding home contracted to provide assisted living services?

❑ ❑ Is the task within the nurse's areas of responsibility (scope of practice)?

❑ ❑ Has the specific care task been approved for delegation?

❑ ❑ Has the nurse assessed the patient's clinical and behavioral status and determined the patient to be in a stable and predictable condition that does not require the nurse's frequent presence and evaluation?

❑ ❑ Has the nurse considered the potential risk of harm for the individual patient and determined that the task can be properly and safely performed by the nursing assistant?

❑ ❑ Has the nurse analyzed the complexity of the nursing task and determined the knowledge, psychomotor skills, and training needed by the nursing assistant to competently perform the task?

❑ ❑ Has the nurse assessed the level of interaction required, considering language or cultural diversity that may affect communication or the ability to accomplish the task to be delegated, as well as methods to facilitate the interaction? Has the nurse verified that the nursing assistant:

❑ ❑ is currently registered or certified as a nursing assistant in Washington State in good standing without restriction?

❑ ❑ has a certificate of completion issued by the Department of Social and Health Services (DSHS) indicating completion of Core Delegation Training for Nursing Assistants?

❑ ❑ is willing to perform the task in the absence of direct or immediate nurse supervision and accept responsibility for his or her actions?

YES NO

❑ ❑ Has the nurse assessed the ability of the nursing assistant to competently perform the delegated nursing task in the absence of direct or immediate supervision?

❑ ❑ Has the nurse informed the patient, or authorized representative, of the delegation and the nursing assistant's training and obtained written, informed consent from the patient, or authorized representative?

❑ ❑ Has the nurse taught the nursing assistant how to perform the task, including return demonstration under observation to verify competency to perform the task safely and accurately, and documented the training? Has the nurse provided specific and written delegation instructions to the nursing assistant that the nursing assistant understands including the following:

❑ ❑ the rationale for delegating the nursing task

❑ ❑ that task is patient specific and not transferable

❑ ❑ that task is not transferable to another nursing assistant

❑ ❑ the nature of the condition and purpose of the delegated nursing task

❑ ❑ the procedure to follow to perform the task

❑ ❑ the predictable outcomes and how to deal effectively with them

❑ ❑ the risks of the treatment

❑ ❑ the interactions of prescribed medications

❑ ❑ how to observe and report side effects, complications, or unexpected outcomes and appropriate actions to deal with them, including specific parameters for notifying the registered nurse, the physician, or emergency services

❑ ❑ the action to take in situations where medications are altered by physician orders

❑ ❑ how to document the task in the patient's record

❑ ❑ how task was taught, including content and that a return demonstration was correctly done

❑ ❑ If delegating administration of PRN medications, has the nurse provided written parameters specific to an individual patient that provide guidelines for the nursing assistant to follow when deciding to administer the PRN medication and the procedure to follow for administration?

YES   NO

❑   ❑   Is there a plan of nursing supervision describing how frequently the nurse will supervise and evaluate the performance of the delegated nursing task by the nursing assistant and reevaluate the patient to ensure continued appropriateness of delegation, which must occur at least every 60 days?

❑   ❑   Has the nurse completed any records required by the Secretary of Health for evaluation?

Nursing Assistant's Name	Nurse's Signature

Source: Used with permission of State of Washington Department of Social & Health Services.

As delegation to unlicensed healthcare personnel becomes even more widespread in the future, documentation such as this will be adopted across the healthcare continuum. If you are concerned about the absence of adequate job descriptions or competency checklists, or if you feel you need a form such as those in the appendix, begin now to identify how you can be involved in planning documents that can be initiated to record your professional practice.

CHECKPOINT 11–10

In our work across the nation, nurses and other healthcare providers state they do not make it a habit to stop and evaluate, make course corrections, or celebrate success. Name one way that you could commit to increase your celebration of success in your job/role/practice.

CONCLUSION

Evaluation is an integral part of our daily nursing practice, yet unfortunately we rarely take enough time to carefully appraise our ability to use this part of the nursing (and delegation) process. In this chapter, you've found this topic explored in its various facets, emphasizing the need for continuous evaluation throughout the shift, visit, or case so that clinical and performance feedback can be offered effectively to shift course and correct any problems that might be occurring. The use of checkpoints, timelines, and parameters will assist you in that process. Nothing can substitute for your own personal assessment and evaluation of a situation because you are uniquely prepared by your scientific education, your experience, and your intuition. When a specific incident occurs, you use critical thinking skills then move forward using the positive problem-solving process to creatively challenge assumptions and implement logical, planned solutions, continuously measuring for success along the way. When you function in a leadership or supervisory role (and nearly 100% of nurses do!), you implement periodic evaluations of how the delegation process is working and how assistive personnel are functioning so that planned client outcomes can be most effectively achieved. Evaluation allows us to make the system work better and to applaud what's working well in our team efforts.

CELEBRATE THE SUCCESS OF THE TEAM!

Whether you work in an intensive care unit (ICU), a public health department, or any other healthcare arena, health care is a serious business. Supervising other people and delegating work to them is a complex and often anxiety-laden proposition. But when you learn to delegate properly, using the skills we have presented in this handbook, you'll gain the confidence needed to grow professionally, and safe, effective, high-quality patient care can be delivered.

Due to the stressful nature of working with others, nurses might focus only on the potential for error and the actual problems that occur. It sometimes seems they have little time to do anything else. However, as an RN and as a leader of your healthcare team, you are in the very best position to help your coworkers also focus on the most wondrous work you are doing! The outcomes of your efforts are evidence of the existence of all that is good and full of light in this harried, violent, and often frightening world.

You have helped create a new family, a haven for love and nurturing, because you and your team provided family planning information or infertility therapy and prenatal care; you taught the mother about nutrition and sexually transmitted diseases and made sure she received financial assistance. Or you might have been the nursing care team who helped birth the baby

Think of what you have accomplished, not alone but together with the members of your team, you and your delegates.

and gave him his first bath, or supervised and supported the new family as they attempted a sleepy adjustment at home.

Perhaps you were a part of the nursing care team who helped keep another disabled child in school, teaching the teachers to suction, providing therapy in the rehabilitation setting, or nudging the child once again out of a crisis in the pediatric intensive care unit. Maybe you are one of the group of healthcare professionals who are intent on finding the answer to preventing this child's disability through research or public health measures.

Victories are continual, each day, in all settings of the healthcare continuum, whether you've saved a life during a code or whether you gently cared and provided support as a peaceful, sheltered death ensued. Nurses are there in the most challenging, difficult, joyful, or tragic episodes of human life. And you are not alone.

Maybe it was your team that helped someone's grandmother come to terms with Grandfather's inability to recognize her or his past. Or you might have been the ones who treated Grandfather when his suicide attempt followed the first diagnosis of his disease. From the emergency department to the psychiatric long-term care unit, you have been there for them, working together as a team.

So recognize your unique contribution to this world, and recognize all the people that help make it happen. And celebrate the success of the team!

ANSWERS TO CHECKPOINTS

11-2 Research would indicate that the type of information exchanged and the report method impacts care planning and would therefore impact patient outcomes. Patient safety organizations and the Joint Commission recommend standardization of communication so that omissions are avoided, processes are simplified, and duplication is avoided. A template also acts as a "thinking model" for novices and helps develop their ability to think beyond the list provided as they no longer have to spend vital intellectual energy on remembering which information to include.

11-5 The database showed deficiencies in the following critical thinking categories as the origin for nursing errors:

1. Clinical reasoning

2. Attentiveness

3.   Interpretation and implementation of authorized provider orders. (NCSNB, 2007)

11–7.   Using the questions in Exhibit 11–5, consider possible alternatives. Evaluation of this shift might show that the following could have occurred. Personal barriers of the nurses could have been in the way; perhaps they did not assign all the work they could have to the aides, consistent with their job descriptions. Perhaps the RNs did not know the extent of responsibilities that could be assigned or did not trust Marty and Joe. Checkpoints did not reveal that RNs were behind and that the others were getting work completed so that tasks could be reassigned. Marty and Joe might not have been asked to do things they could have done, or perhaps their job descriptions are too limited and need to be reevaluated. Did all RNs communicate their needs assertively and clearly and ask for help? It doesn't seem that feedback of a clinical nature flowed freely in all directions. Other issues could be part of the problem: disorganization, people unfamiliar with the department, emergencies, inaccurate acuity system, performance of the RNs and/or the delegates.

11–8.   (Refer to steps as given in Exhibit 11–4.) 1. What signs tell you something is wrong? Evelyn could have reported the first problem so that Bob could have visited to determine whether drug abuse was a problem. 2. What is good? Evelyn reported it now and was very observant. The twins are still intact. 3. If all had gone well, she might have reported this earlier, or one of the other professionals could have seen other signs. The objective criteria we'd use to determine whether the problem was solved are that any and all possible symptoms of drug abuse or child abuse or neglect in the home would be reported for further follow-up. 4. Do we need more information to determine the real issues here? Yes, we do need to fully investigate this problem, but right now we should act. (In other words, we can't freeze and avoid our responsibility to identify what needs to be done immediately. See step 6 for some of the actions we could take.) 5. Should we do something? Yes, this might be a good chance to give more instruction to Evelyn. It will help other patients in the future. 6. What should Bob do? Bob should talk with the manager about his plan but will probably give feedback to Evelyn and determine if this is a learning need, or if Bob should have communicated his expectations more clearly, or if there is a system glitch. Is it to be expected that a new mother would be difficult to rouse? This is certainly difficult to tell, and Bob should be careful to be positive about all that Evelyn did well in this situation. Also, he should determine whether she left him a message about this that was not given to him. First, Bob must secure emergency care for the mother and the twins; then he must look at how the incident occurred and how to avoid it in the future, using his feedback model to let Evelyn know about his concerns.

11-10   Although the answer will be variable based on each individual's situation, here are a few options:

1.   Be clear about my own goals and the patient/family goals at the beginning of each day/shift/case.

2.   Keep track of the patient/family goals on a dry erase board, computerized record, or other jotted note.

3.   Be ready to recognize progress toward goals and openly discuss with team members.

4.   Create a ritual of "celebrating success" toward the end of the work day or case. Review goals and celebrate progress or attainment.

5.   Ask other team members to help remember "success rounds" or "success checkpoints."

6.   In addition to verbal praise and recognition of goal attainment, consider adding rewards in addition to operational benefits such as "getting off on time." "Latte gift cards" or other awards can be offered for improvements in teamwork or reaching longer term goals.

7.   A personal commitment to stop and recognize successes may be the most important step to enjoying the impact each person makes on the health of our communities.

REFERENCES

Alfaro-LeFevre, R. (2007–2008). *Critical thinking indicators.* Retrieved July 30, 2007, from www.Alfaroteachsmart.com; http://www.alfaroteachsmart.com/cti.htm. Reprinted with permission.

Bandman, E. (1988). *Critical thinking in nursing.* Norwalk, CT: Appleton & Lange, 5–6.

Dowding, D. (2001). Examining the effects that manipulating information given in change of shift report has on nurses' care planning ability. *Journal of Advanced Nursing, 33*(6), 836.

Facione, N.C., & Facione, P. (1996, May/June). The disposition toward critical thinking. *Journal of General Education, 44*, 129–136.

Girvan, J. (1989). Enhancing student decision-making through use of critical thinking/questioning techniques. *Health Education, 20*(7), 48–50.

Gross, R. (1991). *Peak learning.* New York: Putnam and Sons, 141–167.

Hansten, R. (1991, April). Delegation: Learning when and how to let go. *Nursing, 91*, 126.

Hansten, R. (2003). Streamline change of shift report. *Nursing Management, 34*(8), 58.

Hansten, R., & Washburn, M. (1993). *The nurse manager's answer book.* Gaithersburg, MD: Aspen Publishers.

Hansten, R., & Washburn, M. (1997). *Toolbook for health care redesign.* Gaithersburg, MD: Aspen Publishers.

Harris, M.D. (1993). Competent, supervised, unlicensed personnel will contribute to high-quality, in-home health care. *Home Healthcare Nurse, 11*(6), 55.

Hays, M. (2003). The phenomenal shift report. *Journal for Nurses in Staff Development, 19*(1), 25–33.

Institute of Medicine. (2004). *Keeping patients safe: Transforming the work environment of nurses* (Recommendation 7.2, p. 15).

Jones, E.A. (1994). *Defining important CT skills for college graduates to achieve.* Paper presented at the Sixth International Conference on Thinking. Boston, MA.

Kyzer, S. P. (1996). Sharpening your critical thinking skills. *Orthopaedic Nursing, 15*(6), 66–76.

Lauri, S., et al. (2001). An exploratory study of clinical decision making in five countries. *Journal of Nursing Scholarship, 33*(1), 83–90.

Merlevede, P., Bridoux, D., & Vandamme, R. (2003). *Seven steps to emotional intelligence.* Williston, VT: Crown House Publishing.

National Council of State Boards of Nursing. (2006). *Joint statement on delegation: American Nurses Association and the National Council State Boards of Nursing.* Retrieved July 23, 2007, from https://www.ncsbn.org/Joint_statement.pdf.

National Council of State Boards of Nursing. (2007). TERCAP (Taxonomy of error, root cause analysis and practice-responsibility). Retrieved August 3, 2007, from www.ncsbn.org/441.htm.

Standing, T., Anthony, M., & Hertz, J. (2001). Nurses' narratives of outcomes after delegation to unlicensed assistive personnel. *Outcomes Management for Nursing Practice, 5*(1), 18–23.

Stark, J. (1996). Critical thinking for outcomes-based practice. *Seminars for Nurse Managers, 4*(3), 161–171.

The Joint Commission. (2007). 2008 national patient safety goals. Retrieved July 23, 2007, from http://www.jointcommission.org/PatientSafety/NationalPatientSafetyGoals/08_hap_npsgs.htm.

Washington State Department of Social and Health Services. Retrieved August 1, 2007, from http://www1.dshs.wa.gov/search.shtml. All forms are present by number; example for form 1381 "Nurse Delegation: Changes in Medical/Treatment Orders," access http:/www1.dshs.wa.gov/word/ms/forms/13_681.doc.

Whiteside, C. (1997). A model for teaching critical thinking in the clinical setting. *Dimensions of Critical Care Nursing, 16*(3), 152–162.

Appendix 11–A

NURSE DELEGATION FORMS

- NURSE DELEGATION: Credentials and Training Verification
- NURSE DELEGATION: Consent for Delegation Process
- NURSE DELEGATION: Nursing Visit
- NURSE DELEGATION: Instructions for Nursing Task
- NURSE DELEGATION: Assumption of Delegation
- NURSE DELEGATION: PRN Medication
- NURSE DELEGATION: Rescinding Delegation
- NURSE DELEGATION: Change in Medical/Treatment Orders

NURSE DELEGATION:
NURSING ASSISTANT CREDENTIALS AND TRAINING

RESIDENT'S NAME (LAST, FIRST, MIDDLE INITIAL)	DATE OF BIRTH (MM/DD/YYYY)	CLIENT ID NUMBER

NURSING ASSISTANT'S NAME

☐ The RN Delegator has viewed certificates documenting this individual's credentials:

     ☐ NA-R or NA-C
     ☐ WA State Certificate/Registration Number   _____
     ☐ Renewal Date   _____
     ☐ Basic Caregiver's Course (Date)   _____
     ☐ ND for Nursing Assistants (Date)   _____

The RN Delegator has verified that the nursing assistant's registration or certificate is in good standing without restriction (Date)

RN DELEGATOR SIGNATURE	DATE

Delegated Task(s): (Check One or More Below)

☐ MEDICATION ADMINISTRATION:

     ☐ ORAL   ☐ RECTAL SUPPOSITORY
     ☐ GASTROSTOMY TUBE   ☐ ENEMA
     ☐ TOPICAL (SKIN/NOSE/EAR/EYE)   ☐ INHALATION
     ☐ VAGINAL SUPPOSITORY   ☐ OTHER: _____

☐ OSTOMY CARE   ☐ DRESSING CHANGE (CLEAN TECHNIQUE)
☐ URINARY CATHETERIZATION (CLEAN TECHNIQUE)   ☐ NEBULIZER/OXYGEN
☐ GASTROSTOMY FEEDING   ☐ BLOOD GLUCOSE MONITORING
☐ OTHER: _____   ☐ OTHER: _____

My signature below verifies that I have been informed, taught and instructed to perform the delegated task(s) and I accept responsibility for performing them as delegated. I have been given information on how to contact the RND if I am no longer able or willing to do these tasks, or the resident's health care orders change.

NURSING ASSISTANT SIGNATURE:	DATE

NURSING ASSISTANT'S NAME

☐ The RN Delegator has viewed certificates documenting this individual's credentials:

     ☐ NA-R or NA-C
     ☐ WA State Certificate/Registration Number   _____
     ☐ Renewal Date   _____
     ☐ Basic Caregiver's Course (Date)   _____
     ☐ ND for Nursing Assistants (Date)   _____

The RN Delegator has verified that the nursing assistant's registration or certificate is in good standing without restriction (Date)

RN DELEGATOR SIGNATURE	DATE

Delegated Task(s): (Check One or More Below)

☐ MEDICATION ADMINISTRATION:

     ☐ ORAL   ☐ RECTAL SUPPOSITORY
     ☐ GASTROSTOMY TUBE   ☐ ENEMA
     ☐ TOPICAL (SKIN/NOSE/EAR/EYE)   ☐ INHALATION
     ☐ VAGINAL SUPPOSITORY   ☐ OTHER: _____

☐ OSTOMY CARE   ☐ DRESSING CHANGE (CLEAN TECHNIQUE)
☐ URINARY CATHETERIZATION (CLEAN TECHNIQUE)   ☐ NEBULIZER/OXYGEN
☐ GASTROSTOMY FEEDING   ☐ BLOOD GLUCOSE MONITORING
☐ OTHER: _____   ☐ OTHER: _____

My signature below verifies that I have been informed, taught and instructed to perform the delegated task(s) and I accept responsibility for performing them as delegated. I have been given information on how to contact the RND if I am no longer able or willing to do these tasks, or the resident's health care orders change.

NURSING ASSISTANT SIGNATURE:	DATE

DSHS 10-217 (REV. 12/2002) (AC 01/2003)

To register concerns or complaints about Nurse Delegation, please call 1-800-562-6078 Toll Free.

COPIES: Original - Record   Copy - RN Delegator   Copy - Other

NURSE DELEGATION:
CONSENT FOR DELEGATION PROCESS

1. CLIENT NAME				2. DATE OF BIRTH	3. ID. SETTING *(Optional)*

4. CLIENT ADDRESS	CITY	STATE	ZIP CODE	5. TELEPHONE NUMBER

6. FACILITY OR PROGRAM CONTACT	7. TELEPHONE NUMBER

8. FAX NUMBER	9. E-MAIL ADDRESS

10. SETTING	11. CLIENT DIAGNOSIS	12. ALLERGIES
Certified Community Residential Program for Developmentally Disabled		
Licensed Adult Family Home		
Licensed Boarding Home		
Private Home		

13. HEALTH CARE PROVIDER	13. TELEPHONE NUMBER

CONSENT FOR THE DELEGATION PROCESS

I have been informed that the Registered Nurse Delegator will only delegate to caregivers who are capable and willing to properly perform the task(s). Nurse Delegation will only occur after the caregiver has completed state required training (WAC 246-841-405(2)(a)) and individualized training from the Registered Nurse Delegator. I further understand that the following task(s) may never be delegated:

- Administration of medication by injections (IM, Sub W, IV)
- Sterile procedures
- Central line maintenance
- Acts that require nursing judgment

If verbal consent is obtained, written consent is required within 30 days of verbal consent.

16. CLIENT OR AUTHORIZED REPRESENTATIVE SIGNATURE	16. TELEPHONE NUMBER	17. DATE

18. VERBAL CONSENT OBTAINED FROM	19. RELATIONSHIP TO CLIENT	20. DATE

My signature below indicates that I have assessed this client and found his/her condition to be stable and predictable. I agree to provide nurse delegation per RCW 18.79 and WAC 246-840-910 through 970.

21. RDN NAME (PRINT)	22. TELEPHONE NUMBER

23. RDN SIGNATURE	24. DATE

To register concerns or complaints about Nurse Delegation, please call 1-800-562-6078
Copy in client chart and in RND file

INSTRUCTIONS
NURSE DELEGATION:
CONSENT FOR DELEGATION PROCESS

All fields are required unless indicated *"OPTIONAL"*

1. Client Name	Enter ND client's name *(last name, first name)*.
2. Date of Birth	Enter ND client's date of birth *(month, date, year)*.
3. ID. Setting	*OPTIONAL* Enter client's ID number as assigned by your business OR enter setting "AFH," "BH," "DDD Program," "In-home."
4. Client Address	Enter the address where the client currently resides, including street address, city, state and zip code.
5. Telephone Number	Enter the telephone including area code where the client can be reached.
6. Facility or Program Contact	Enter the name of facility or name of individual to contact at the facility. Enter N/A if client resides in own home.
7. Telephone Number	Enter the telephone including area code if different from 5 above.
8. Fax Number	Enter the fax number at the facility if available.
9. E-mail Address	Enter e-mail address of client or facility if available.
10. Setting	Check the appropriate box.
11. Client Diagnosis	Enter client's diagnoses that affect the delegated task.
12. Allergies	List known allergies or "N/A" if none.
13. Health Care Provider	Enter name of client's health care provider.
14. Telephone Number	Enter telephone number including area code of provider named in 13.
15. Client or Authorized Representative Signature	Read the statement to the client/authorized representative and explain the nurse delegation process to them before obtaining verbal consent. Print the name. Written consent must be obtained within 30 days of verbal consent.
16. Telephone Number	Ask them to enter their telephone number if different from 5 above.
17. Verbal Consent Obtained From	Date the signature.
19. Relationship to Client	Enter the relationship of the person to the client named in 18 above.
20. Date	Date when you obtained verbal consent.
21. RND Name	Print your name.
22. Telephone Number	Enter your telephone number including area code.
23 & 24. RND Signature and Date	Sign and date your signature.

NURSE DELEGATION:
NURSING VISIT

1. CLIENT NAME	2. DATE OF BIRTH	3. ID. SETTING *(Optional)*

4. CHECK ALL THAT APPLY

- [ ] Initial Client Assessment *(See attached)*
- [ ] Initial Caregiver Delegations
- [ ] Supervisory Visit
- [ ] Condition Change
- [ ] Other

5. CLIENT REQUIRES NURSE DELEGATION FOR THESE TASK(S):

DUE TO:

6. REVIEW OF SYSTEMS: *Only check changes in condition from last assessment*

- [ ] Cardiovascular
- [ ] Respiratory
- [ ] Integumentary
- [ ] Diet/Weight/Nutrition
- [ ] Endocrine
- [ ] Psych/Social
- [ ] Neurological
- [ ] ADL
- [ ] Musculoskeletal
- [ ] GU/Reproductive
- [ ] Sensory
- [ ] Cognition
- [ ] GI
- [ ] Pain
- [ ] *No Change*

7. NOTES

8. Caregiver (CG) Training/Competency (Check or date all that apply)

A. CG Evaluated	B. Observation or Demonstration	C. Verbal Description	D. Record Review	E. Training Needed	E. Training Completed	F. Other *(specify)*
1.)	[ ]	[ ]	[ ]	[ ]	[ ]	[ ]
2.)	[ ]	[ ]	[ ]	[ ]	[ ]	[ ]
3.)	[ ]	[ ]	[ ]	[ ]	[ ]	[ ]
4.)	[ ]	[ ]	[ ]	[ ]	[ ]	[ ]
5.)	[ ]	[ ]	[ ]	[ ]	[ ]	[ ]

9. [ ] Check here if additional notes/caregiver name on page 2.

10. [ ] Client stable and predictable   [ ] Continue delegation   [ ] See rescind form

I have verified, informed, taught and instructed the caregiver(s) to perform the delegated task(s). The caregiver(s) has indicated that he/she accepts responsibility for performing the task as delegated. The caregiver(s) has been given the information on how to contact the RND if he/she is no longer able or willing to do these task(s) or resident healthcare orders change.

11. RND SIGNATURE	12. DATE	13. RETURN VISIT ON OR BEFORE

To register concerns or complaints about Nurse Delegation, please call 1-800-562-6078
DISTRIBUTION: Copy in client chart and in RND file

NURSE DELEGATION:
NURSING VISIT

1. CLIENT NAME	2. DATE OF BIRTH	3. ID. SETTING *(Optional)*

17. NOTES

8. Caregiver (CG) Training/Competency (Check or date all that apply)

A. CG Evaluated	B. Observation or Demonstration	C. Verbal Description	D. Record Review	E. Training Needed	E. Training Completed	F. Other *(specify)*
6.)	☐	☐	☐	☐	☐	☐
7.)	☐	☐	☐	☐	☐	☐
8.)	☐	☐	☐	☐	☐	☐
9.)	☐	☐	☐	☐	☐	☐
10.)	☐	☐	☐	☐	☐	☐
11.)	☐	☐	☐	☐	☐	☐
12.)	☐	☐	☐	☐	☐	☐
13.)	☐	☐	☐	☐	☐	☐
14.)	☐	☐	☐	☐	☐	☐
15.)	☐	☐	☐	☐	☐	☐
16.)	☐	☐	☐	☐	☐	☐
17.)	☐	☐	☐	☐	☐	☐
18.)	☐	☐	☐	☐	☐	☐
19.)	☐	☐	☐	☐	☐	☐
20.)	☐	☐	☐	☐	☐	☐

I have verified, informed, taught and instructed the caregiver(s) to perform the delegated task(s). The caregiver(s) has indicated that he/she accepts responsibility for performing the task as delegated. The caregiver(s) has been given the information on how to contact the RND if he/she is no longer able or willing to do these task(s) or resident healthcare orders change.

19. RND SIGNATURE	20. DATE	21. RETURN VISIT ON OR BEFORE

To register concerns or complaints about Nurse Delegation, please call 1-800-562-6078
DISTRIBUTION: Copy in client chart and in RND file

INSTRUCTIONS
NURSE DELEGATION: NURSING VISIT

All fields are required unless marketed "*OPTIONAL*"

1. Client Name — Enter ND client's name *(last name, first name)*.

2. Date of Birth — Enter ND client's date of birth *(month, date, year)*.

3. ID. Setting — *OPTIONAL* Enter client's ID number as assigned by your business OR enter setting "AFH," "BH," "DDD Program," "In-home."

4. — Check the box or boxes that apply to how you are using this form.

5. Client Requires Nurse Delegation For These Delegated Task(s) — List the task(s) you are delegating and the reason why the client needs to have the task(s) delegated.

6. Review of Systems — Check the box for "No change" if client's condition is unchanged from your last client assessment. If client's condition is changed from your last assessment, check the appropriate category box. If a category box is checked, complete a note in Box 7 below.

7. Notes — Describe change in client's condition in this box if a category box (other than "No change) is checked above.

8. Caregiver Training Competency — A. List the name of each caregiver evaluated at this visit.
B.-D. Check the box.
E. Check box or insert the date for training needed or completed.
F. OPTIONAL In this column, enter any other method of determining competency not already listed.

9. OPTIONAL — Check this box if a second page is used for additional note/caregiver names.

10. — Check all boxes that apply. If "Rescinding delegation" box is checked, you must complete "Rescinding Delegation" form, DSHS 13-680.

11 & 12. RND Signature and Date — Sign and date your signature.

13. Return Visit On Or Before — Enter a date or the number of days within the 90 day time frame that you will return for the next supervisory visit.

14. — See number 1, above

15. — See number 2, above

16. — See number 3, above

17. — See number 7, above

18. — See number 8, above

19 & 20. — See number 11 & 12, above

21. — See number 13, above

Be sure to sign and date both pages if a second page is used.

NURSE DELEGATION:
INSTRUCTIONS FOR NURSING TASK

1. CLIENT NAME	2. DATE OF BIRTH	3. ID. SETTING *(Optional)*

4. DATE TASK DELEGATED

5. DELEGATED TASK AND EXPECTED OUTCOME

Complete 6 & 7 only if medication(s) delegated:

6. LIST SPECIFIC MEDICATION(S) DELEGATED ON THIS DATE

7. DATE AND WHO VERIFIED DELEGATED MEDICATIONS

8. STEPS TO PERFORM THE TASK: Check here if additional teaching aide(s) attached

Report Side Effects or Unexpected Outcomes To:

9. RND NAME (PRINT)	10. TELEPHONE NUMBER

11. WHAT TO REPORT TO RND

12. HEALTHCARE PROVIDER NAME	13. TELEPHONE NUMBER

14. WHAT TO REPORT TO HEALTHCARE PROVIDER

EMERGENCY SERVICES, 911

15. WHAT TO REPORT TO 911:

16. RND SIGNATURE	17. DATE

CALL RN WHEN:

- Medications change
- New orders received
- Client dies
- Client is admitted to ER, hospital, or SNF

- Client moves
- Client condition changes
- Problem/unable to perform nursing task

To register concerns or complaints about Nurse Delegation, please call 1-800-562-6078
Copy in client chart and in RND file

INSTRUCTIONS
NURSE DELEGATION:
INSTRUCTIONS FOR NURSING TASK

All fields are required unless indicated *"OPTIONAL"*

1. Client Name   Enter ND client's name *(last name, first name)*.

2. Date of Birth   Enter ND client's date of birth *(month, date, year)*.

3. ID. Setting   *OPTIONAL* Enter client's ID number as assigned by your business OR enter setting "AFH," "BH," "DDD Program," "In-home."

4. Date Task Delegated   Enter the date task is first delegated.

5. Delegated Task and Expected Outcome   Enter the name of the task and what outcome is anticipated. Separate task sheet is required for each task.

6. List Specific Medication(s) Delegated on This Date   *OPTIONAL* **Only complete if medications are delegated.** Enter the name, dose, frequency and route of each medication delegated.

7. Date and Who Verified Delegated Medications   Enter the date verified and with whom.

8. Steps to Perform the Task   Steps to perform the task should be written in detail here. Check box and describe if additional material(s) are attached. For example: medication information sheet, task procedure sheet, etc.

9 & 10. RND Name and Telephone Number   Print RND name and telephone number with area code.

11. What to Report to RND   List side effects or unexpected outcome to report to RND.

12 & 13. Healthcare Provider and Telephone Number   Enter the name of the healthcare provider and telephone number with area code.

14. What to Report to Healthcare Provider   List side effects and unexpected outcome to report to the healthcare provider.

15. What to Report to 911   List signs and symptoms to report to 911.

16 & 17. RND Signature and Date   Sign and date your signature.

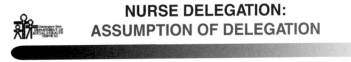

NURSE DELEGATION:
ASSUMPTION OF DELEGATION

1. CLIENT NAME	2. DATE OF BIRTH	3. ID. SETTING *(Optional)*
4. FACILITY OR PROGRAM NAME *(OPTIONAL)*		5. TELEPHONE NUMBER
6. REASON/DATES FOR ASSUMING DELEGATION		

I agree that I know the client through my assessment, the plan of care, the skills of the nursing assistant, and the delegated task(s). I agree to assume responsibility and accountability for the delegated task(s) and to perform the nursing supervision. I have informed the client and/or authorized representative of this change. I have informed the nursing assistant, case manager and client of this change.

7. ASSUMING RND SIGNATURE	24. DATE

To register concerns or complaints about Nurse Delegation, please call 1-800-562-6078
Copy in client chart and in RND file

INSTRUCTIONS
ASSUMPTION OF DELEGATION

All fields are required unless indicated *"OPTIONAL"*

1. Client Name	Enter ND client's name *(last name, first name).*
2. Date of Birth	Enter ND client's date of birth *(month, date, year).*
3. ID. Setting	*OPTIONAL* Enter client's ID number as assigned by your business OR enter setting "AFH," "BH," "DDD Program," "In-home."
4. Facility or Program Name	*OPTIONAL* Enter name of facility/program contact.
5. Telephone Number	*OPTIONAL* Enter telephone number of facility/program contact including area code.
6. Reason /Dates for Another RND to Assume Delegation	Enter reason other RND rescinded and the date you assume responsibility for delegation.
7 & 8. Assuming RND Signature and Date	Sign and date your signature.

NURSE DELEGATION:
PRN MEDICATION

TO BE COMPLETED ONLY IF PRN MEDICATIONS ARE DELEGATED

1. CLIENT NAME	2. DATE OF BIRTH	3. ID. SETTING *(Optional)*

4. DATE ORDERED	5. NAME OF MEDICATION	
6. DOSE/FREQUENCY/ROUTE		
7. NOT TO EXCEED	8. REASON FOR MEDICATION	
9. SYMPTOMS FOR ADMINISTRATION AND AMOUNT TO BE GIVEN		
10. NOTES		
11. RND SIGNATURE		12. DATE

4. DATE ORDERED	5. NAME OF MEDICATION	
6. DOSE/FREQUENCY/ROUTE		
7. NOT TO EXCEED	8. REASON FOR MEDICATION	
9. SYMPTOMS FOR ADMINISTRATION AND AMOUNT TO BE GIVEN		
10. NOTES		
11. RND SIGNATURE		12. DATE

4. DATE ORDERED	5. NAME OF MEDICATION	
6. DOSE/FREQUENCY/ROUTE		
7. NOT TO EXCEED	8. REASON FOR MEDICATION	
9. SYMPTOMS FOR ADMINISTRATION AND AMOUNT TO BE GIVEN		
10. NOTES		
11. RND SIGNATURE		12. DATE

To register concerns or complaints about Nurse Delegation, please call 1-800-562-6078
Copy in client chart and in RND file

INSTRUCTIONS
PRN MEDICATION

All fields are required unless indicated *"OPTIONAL"*

1. Client Name	Enter ND client's name *(last name, first name)*.
2. Date of Birth	Enter ND client's date of birth *(month, date, year)*.
3. ID. Setting	*OPTIONAL* Enter client's ID number as assigned by your business OR enter setting "AFH," "BH," "DDD Program," "In-home."
4. Date Ordered	Enter the date PRN medication ordered.
5. Name of Medication	Enter the name of the medication ordered.
6. Dose/Frequency/Route	Enter dose, frequency of medication to be given and enter route of medication. Examples: PO, Supp, Topical, Drops, etc.
7. Not to Exceed	Enter maximum number of doses in a specified time period, if applicable.
8. Reason for Medication	Enter action or reason medication is given.
9. Symptoms for Administration and Amount to Be Given	Enter behavior/symptom client will display when this medication is needed. Enter the dose that should be given when this behavior/symptom is observed.
10. Notes	Enter any additional information regarding this administration of this medication.
11 & 12. RND Signature and Date	Sign and date your signature.

Repeat boxes 4 through 12 for each additional PRN medication ordered at this time.

NURSE DELEGATION:
RESCINDING DELEGATION

1. CLIENT NAME	2. DATE OF BIRTH	3. ID. SETTING *(Optional)*

4. FACILITY OR PROGRAM NAME *(Optional)*	5. TELEPHONE NUMBER

6. Reason for Rescinding: (Check all that apply)

A. Client died	F. NA not competent	K. Rescinding facility includ-
B. Client's condition changed	G. NA not willing	ing clients and nurse
C. Frequent staff turnover	H. NA credential expired	assistant
D. Client/authorized repre-	I. NA No longer working	L. Other (specify)
sentative requested	with client	
E. Task not performed correctly	J. Client safety compromised	

7. TASK RESCINDED

8. NAMES OF CAREGIVERS	9. ALL TASKS	10. MEDICATIONS			11. BLOOD SUGAR	12. OTHER/SPECIFY
		ORAL	TOPICAL	DROPS		
1.)						
2.)						
3.)						
4.)						
5.)						
6.)						
7.)						
8.)						
9.)						
10.)						

13. Case Manager Notified (when appropriate)

14. NAME OF CASE MANAGER NOTIFIED	15. DATE

16. ALTERNATIVE PLAN FOR CONTINUING THE TASK

17. RND SIGNATURE	18. DATE

To register concerns or complaints about Nurse Delegation, please call 1-800-562-6078
Copy in client chart and in RND file

INSTRUCTIONS
RESCINDING DELEGATION

All fields are required unless indicated *"OPTIONAL"*

1. Client Name Enter ND client's name *(last name, first name)*.

2. Date of Birth Enter ND client's date of birth *(month, date, year)*.

3. ID. Setting *OPTIONAL* Enter client's ID number as assigned by your business OR enter setting "AFH," "BH," "DDD Program," "In-home."

4. Facility or Program Name *OPTIONAL* Enter name of facility/program contact.

5. Telephone Number *OPTIONAL* Enter telephone number of facility/program contact including area code.

6. Reason for Rescinding Mark the boxes next to the reason for rescinding. Mark all that apply.

7. Task Rescinded Enter name of task rescinded. If medication, list name. This applies to all caregivers delegated for this task.

8. Names of Caregivers Enter name of individual caregiver rescinded. If all, enter "ALL."

9. All Tasks Enter "X" under all tasks next to name of appropriate caregiver(s)

10. Medications Enter name of individual medication if appropriate. If all, enter "ALL."

11 . Blood Sugar Enter "X" if blood sugar rescinded.

12. Other/Specify *OPTIONAL* List other tasks rescinded or list date if appropriate.

13. OPTIONAL Check the box if appropriate. Case Manager must be notified if ALL tasks (client condition has changed) are rescinded or ALL caregivers (client unable to receive needed services).

14. Name of Case Manager Notified Enter case manager name, if notified.

15. Date Enter date the case manager was notified.

16. Alternative Plan for Continuing the Task Describe how client's needs will continue to be met.

17 & 18. RND Signature and Date Sign and date your signature. The date the form is signed is the date of rescinding, unless otherwise noted in #7.

Repeat boxes 4 through 12 for each additional PRN medication ordered at this time.

NURSE DELEGATION:
CHANGE IN MEDICAL/TREATMENT ORDERS

1. CLIENT NAME		2. DATE OF BIRTH	3. ID. SETTING *(Optional)*

4. DATE RND WAS NOTIFIED	5. BY WHOM	6. CHANGES IN ORDER(S)
		☐ New Med. ☐ Change in a delegated med
		☐ Change in a nursing tank ☐ New nursing tank

7. HOW WAS THE CHANGE RECEIVED? ☐ Written ☐ Faxed ☐ Verbal	8. EFFECTIVE DATE OF CHANGE

9. Only complete if number 7 was a verbal order.

NAME OF PERSON PROVIDING VERIFICATION	TITLE OF PERSON PROVIDING VERIFICATION

DATE OF VERIFICATION

10. NURSING TASK(S)   ☐ New task(s) sheet required   ☐ Current task(s) sheet(s) updated
☐ No change to task(s) sheet(s)

NURSING TASK/ORDER

11. This medication(s) was: ☐ New   ☐ Changed

12. DATE ORDERED	13. NAME OF MEDICATION(S)	14. START DATE	15. STOP DATE

16. STRENGTH/DOSE	17. MEDICATION FREQUENCY	18. ROUTE	19. NOT TO EXCEED

20. REASON FOR MEDICATION(S)

Optional Task Sheet: (21-29)

21. STEPS TO PERFORM THE NEW TASK(S)

22. EXPECTED OUTCOME OF DELEGATED TASK(S)

Report side effects or unexpected outcomes to:

23. RND NAME (PRINT)	24. TELEPHONE NUMBER

25. WHAT TO REPORT TO RND

26. HEALTHCARE PROVIDER	27. TELEPHONE NUMBER

28. WHAT TO REPORT TO HEALTHCARE PROVIDER

29. WHAT TO REPORT TO EMERGENCY SERVICES, 911

Select Only One of the Following

30. ☐	Delegate immediately. No site visit required. The above order and instructions have been communicated to the delegated caregiver(s) and this form should be added to the client's chart. **OR**
31. ☐	A site visit required for training or assessment prior to delegation. The caregiver may not perform the task until the site visit is completed.

32. RND SIGNATURE	33. DATE

To register concerns or complaints about Nurse Delegation, please call 1-800-562-6078
Copy in client chart and in RND file

INSTRUCTIONS
NURSE DELEGATION:
CHANGE IN MEDICAL/TREATMENT ORDERS

All fields are required unless indicated *"OPTIONAL"*

1. Client Name Enter ND client's name *(last name, first name)*.

2. Date of Birth Enter ND client's date of birth *(month, date, year)*.

3. ID. Setting *OPTIONAL* Enter client's ID number as assigned by your business OR enter setting "AFH," "BH," "DDD Program," "In-home."

4. Date RND was Notified Enter date you were notified of change.

5. By Whom List name and title of individual who notified delegating nurse of change/new task or medication.

6. Change in Orders Check appropriate box to indicate a change or a new task/medication.

7. How Was the Change Received Select the method used by the healthcare provider to communicate the change.

8. Effective Date of Change Enter date the change was ordered by healthcare provider.

9. If Verbal Was Selected in #7 above Insert the name, title (MD, ARNP, PA) and date the order was verified.

10. Nursing Task/Orders What was the order, and does it require a new task sheet or a change to the current instructions.

11. This Medication Was *OPTIONAL* Complete 11-20 **only** if a medication was involved. Indicate whether the medication was changed or new. Complete all boxes (11-20) for **each** medication changed or ordered new.

12. Date Ordered Enter the date this change was ordered.

13. Name of Medication(s) Enter name of medication(s) ordered.

14. Start Date Enter the date the new/changed medication was first administered.

15. Stop Date Enter, if applicable, last date to administer this medication.

16. Strength/Dose Enter strength of medication and dose to be administered.

17. Medication Frequency Enter how often medication is to be administered.

18. Route Enter route for medication to be administered. *Ex: PO, Supp, Topical, Drops, etc.*

19. Not to Exceed Enter maximum number of doses in a specified time period, if applicable.

20. Reason for Medication Enter the reason the client takes this medication. Repeat #11-20 for each new or changed medication.

INSTRUCTIONS
NURSE DELEGATION:
CHANGE IN MEDICAL/TREATMENT ORDERS

Continued . . .

21 - 22. Steps to Perform New Task/Medication	OPTIONAL Complete 21 & 22 **only** if using this form for a task sheet. Enter results expected by providing this task/medication.
23 - 24. RND Name and Telephone Number	Print your name and telephone number including area code.
25. What to Report to RND	Enter symptoms or side effects for all tasks, medications on this sheet to be reported to you.
26 - 27. Healthcare Provider Name and Telephone Number	Enter healthcare provider name and telephone number including area code.
28. What to Report to Healthcare Provider	Enter symptoms or side effects for all tasks, medication on this sheet to report to healthcare provider.
29. What to Report to Emergency Services, 911	Enter symptoms or side effects for all tasks, medications on this sheet to report to emergency services (911).
30 - 31. Delegate Immediately OR Site Visit Required	Choose **only one** (#30 **OR** #31) to indicate whether caregiver(s) may provide the new task/medication immediately or whether a training visit (on site) is necessary prior to delegation. IN EITHER CASE, THE DOCUMENTATION IN THE CLIENT FILE MUST REFLECT WHEN DELEGATION FOR THE NEW TASK/MEDICATION BEGAN.
32 - 33. RND Signature and Date	Sign and date your signature.

Index

Page numbers followed by ex or f denote exhibits or figures respectively.